D1217564

MEDICAL DEPARTMENT, UNITED STATES ARMY

SURGERY IN WORLD WAR II

THE PHYSIOLOGIC EFFECTS OF WOUNDS

By

THE BOARD FOR THE STUDY OF THE SEVERELY WOUNDED
North African-Mediterranean Theater of Operations

OFFICE OF THE SURGEON GENERAL

DEPARTMENT OF THE ARMY

WASHINGTON, D. C., 1952

The volumes comprising the history of the Medical Department of the U. S. Army in World War II are divided into two series: (1) The Administrative and Operational series which constitutes a part of the general series of the history of the *U. S. Army in World War II,* published under the direction of the Office of the Chief of Military History, and (2) the Professional, or clinical and technical series, published as *The Medical Department of the United States Army* under the direction of the Office of The Surgeon General. Both series are being prepared by the Historical Unit, Army Medical Service. This volume is one of a number of surgical volumes to be published in the latter series.

For sale by the Superintendent of Documents, U. S. Government Printing Office
Washington 25, D. C. - Price $3.50 (Buckram)

THE MEDICAL DEPARTMENT OF THE UNITED STATES ARMY

The Physiologic Effects of Wounds

By

The Board for the Study of the Severely Wounded
North African-Mediterranean Theater of Operations

Members

Henry K. Beecher, M. D.
Formerly Lt. Colonel, MC, A. U. S.

Charles H. Burnett, M. D.
Formerly Major, MC, A. U. S.

Seymour L. Shapiro
Formerly Captain, SnC, A. U. S.

Fiorindo A. Simeone, M. D.
Formerly Colonel, MC, A. U. S.

Louis D. Smith, Ph. D.
Formerly Captain, SnC, A. U. S.

Eugene R. Sullivan, M. D.
Formerly Lt. Colonel, MC, A. U. S.

Tracy B. Mallory, M. D.*
Formerly Lt. Colonel, MC, A. U. S.
Chairman
*Deceased

Report of the Board edited by Henry K. Beecher.

This volume was prepared by the Historical Division, Army Medical Library, under the direction of Colonel Joseph H. McNinch, MC, U. S. A., Editor in Chief; Associate Editor, Sylvia Gottwerth.

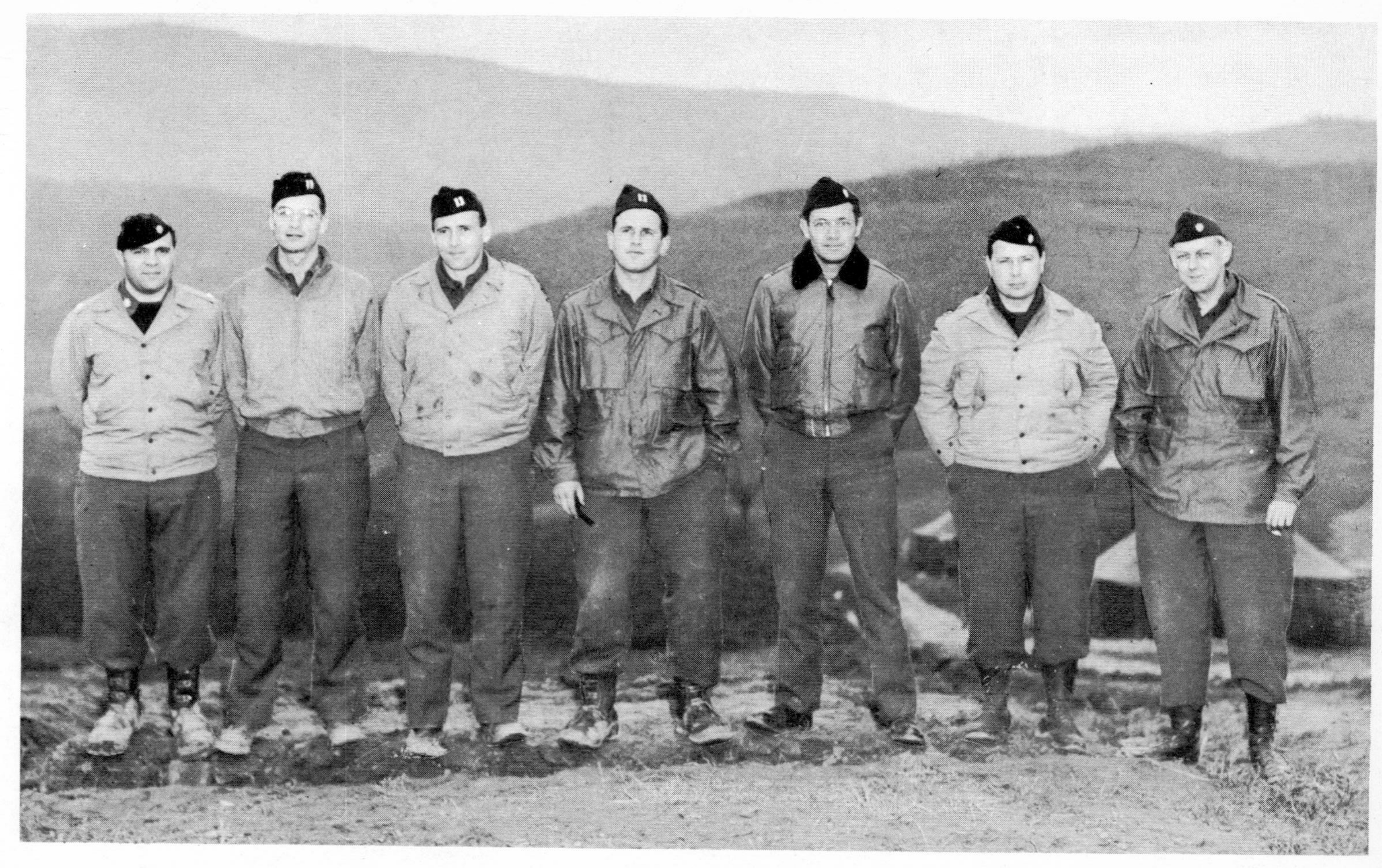

THE BOARD FOR THE STUDY OF THE SEVERELY WOUNDED. *Left to right:* Lt. Col. (later Colonel) Fiorindo A. Simeone, Capt. (later Major) Charles H. Burnett, Capt. Louis D. Smith, Capt. Seymour L. Shapiro, Lt. Col. Henry K. Beecher, Maj. (later Lt. Colonel) Eugene R. Sullivan, Lt. Col. Tracy B. Mallory. Monghidora, Italy, 1944.

Foreword

Severe surgical shock following trauma is not commonly encountered in the medical practice of any group during peacetime. When it occurs it is the result of unexpected accident, and adequate provision for careful study has seldom been available. Consequently, although considerable noteworthy experimental work had been done on shock in animals since World War I, little opportunity has existed to study this serious condition in man. When the United States entered World War II, much information required for handling battle casualties with serious injuries was not available. The need for whole-blood replacement for resuscitation was incompletely understood. The significance of blood volumes, infection, continuing hemorrhage, the anatomic location of the injury, and the limitations of analgesic and anesthetic agents was not fully appreciated although all these subjects had been understood in a seemingly adequate manner.

The brunt of this lack of information and training in U. S. Forces was carried by the Medical Service of the North African and later the Mediterranean Theater. Until June 1944, when their forward medical service was organized to study the severely wounded, they were the only theaters with sizable numbers of ground troops steadily in contact with the enemy. For nearly 2 years they experienced battle casualties at rates almost continuously above 50 per 1,000 per annum, and for nearly 10 months of this period their battle casualties were above 100 per 1,000 per annum. The ingenuity, resourcefulness, and thoroughness with which Medical Department personnel performed under these trying circumstances are exemplified by the work of the individuals of the MTO Board for the Study of the Severely Wounded and the progressive steps taken by them to initiate their studies without special provision or support.

The Board's studies on human casualties under battle conditions contributed much information of immediate practical value for the handling of wounded as well as pointed the way for many basic studies required for the future. The data were accumulated under the rigors of field conditions, at times under fire, and the work was often begun in the shock tents a few minutes after a wounded subject fell. This research was unique for American Forces during World War II and provided information on the resuscitation and treatment of the severely wounded that cannot be procured from any other source. Aside from its significance as a contribution to medical knowledge, this report must stand as a tribute to the men who showed that it could be done.

GEORGE E. ARMSTRONG
Major General, U. S. Army
The Surgeon General

Preface

On 3 September 1944, the Commanding General, North African Theater of Operations, appointed a Medical Board to Study the Treatment of the Severely Wounded, his action following by only two days a recommendation by the Surgeon of that theater that such a board be appointed. Appendix A includes the Surgeon's communication and the order appointing the Board, together with data concerning its organization and operation.

Each of the authors of this volume was a member of the Board as formally established. Before that time several of us had been interested individually in various aspects of the physiologic and pathologic changes in the severely wounded, and the chapters of this volume include our observations both as members of the Board and as individual investigators. The background against which the study was undertaken is described fully in the Introduction.

At the time this study began, our attention was focused in considerable part on anuria in the wounded. This interest continued, but it early became apparent that to limit ourselves to the study of anuria was undesirable and actually impossible. Thus at the end of the work we have found, almost inevitably, that what we have is a kind of physiologic atlas of the severely wounded. In producing it we have followed the trend that medicine as a whole has taken: Probably there are few new things to be learned in studies of gross morphology, but certainly much remains to be found in the domain of function. So too it may be with the wounds of battle. They have already been accurately described in terms of structural loss, but there are great deficiencies in our knowledge of the effects of wounds on the function of organs. If this study has contributed in a useful way toward filling these gaps, our effort will have been justified.

The several chapters of this volume have been written by the member or members of the Board responsible for those particular phases of the investigation. The aim has been to present factual observations, with a minimum of essential supplementary remarks to orient the reader. We have, therefore, in most instances deliberately avoided detailed discussion of the data. Many of the findings were provocative to us, and we hope they will be to others; in any event the mass of data accumulated in this battlefront study provides a basis for contemplation and further work. From these data the reader who may differ with our views can construct his own and perhaps more accurate interpretations and conclusions.

For those who have not had a similar experience, it may be difficult to judge which things caused trouble during the course of the work and which were not important. Of real importance were the winds that blew some tents down, split others, upset stoves, knocked bottles off shelves, and stirred up endless clouds of dust that swirled around our hilltop at Monghidoro and invaded the laboratory. The rain and mud were unpleasant but not of real consequence until the dampness began to interfere with the spectrophotometer. When we were up in the Apennines, water froze and the cold at night caused solutions to alter and saturated solutions to crystallize out. Troublesome as these things were, they were overcome either by waiting until the environmental conditions had improved, or by the ingenuity of our technicians.

Supplies and equipment needed for our studies were for the most part delivered promptly and in adequate quantity but occasionally delays in arrival of items influenced the progress of our observations. In only two instances was absence of supplies of material consequence. We never succeeded in obtaining equipment to make desired oxygen determinations, and materials for renal clearance studies arrived so late that only a few cases could be studied.

Although the spectacular "artificial moonlight" produced by great floodlights reflected from clouds lighted up the out-of-doors at night and was much used in the months of the Northern Apennines Campaign, we never escaped from the necessity of working in blacked-out tents, and in poorly lighted tents it was easy to overlook cyanosis or icterus.

The major consideration at all times was that our studies must not delay or otherwise interfere with the treatment of the wounded soldier. The necessity of not interfering with the therapy due the wounded man was important. The patient's good came first; it was trying but necessary sometimes to let observations go, knowing that an unfortunate shortcoming would be present in the case under study. During periods of heavy action, when the cases best suited for study were coming in, the man covering the shock tent needed all the maneuvering skill of a combat pilot to keep out of the way of those responsible for the care of the wounded man. At times he failed, all of us failed, to get the observations needed for completeness.

Sometimes a patient would be accessible to us for only a few hours and then would be evacuated to the rear, never to be seen again. Most of the patients were followed into the postoperative period, but some were evacuated at, for our purposes, their most enlightening stage, or sometimes, because of the tactical situation, we were obliged to move forward or back and leave them.

We realize that those accustomed to working in the atmosphere of leisure and with the laboratory facilities of peacetime can find much to criticize here. We had to get what we could when we could, and record it "on the go." Our observations are published as recorded at the time and without later attempt to identify and compare individual cases in all the various aspects of the study. It will be readily appreciated that identical data could not be obtained on all cases. We present the results without apology. Moreover, we believe that what we were able to do indicates the soundness of our attempt to study the wounded in the line of combat where they fell.

Finally, we are bound to acknowledge the extraordinary spirit of the newly wounded, those with whom we dealt. They did all they could to help us in this work.

HENRY K. BEECHER, M.D.
(Formerly Consultant in Resuscitation and Anesthesia, North African-Mediterranean Theater of Operations)

Boston, Massachusetts
23 February 1952

Contents

The Physiologic Effects of Wounds

Introduction

A report is spread that there is, in some country or other, a giant as big as a mountain; and men presently fall to hot disputing concerning the precise length of his nose, the breadth of his thumb, and other particulars, and anathematize each other for heterodoxy of belief concerning them. In the midst of all, if some bold sceptic ventures to hint a doubt as to the existence of this giant, all are ready to join against him, and tear him to pieces.—*Attributed to Voltaire*

Shock—the Background

Although warriors have died of their wounds from the beginning of time, the first scientific approach to an analysis of how and why they die was made during World War I. In that war the wound surgeon lifted his eyes from the shattered limb to inquire with some degree of precision about the nature of the processes that a wound may initiate in the body as a whole. Because, even if the limb were amputated and every organ of the body was sound, death was likely to occur as the terminal event of a profound disturbance known as wound shock.

World War I revealed wound shock as a complex problem. Its nature was not solved nor were sufficient observational data accumulated to permit clear identification and subsequent analysis. Certain pre-existing hypotheses (vasomotor exhaustion, acapnia, adrenal exhaustion) were discredited, but other concepts inadequately supported by facts (traumatic toxemia, the distinction between shock and hemorrhage) were substituted. These concepts centered on wound shock as an entity not accounted for by hemorrhage, infection, brain injury, blast, asphyxia of cardiorespiratory origin, fat embolism, or any other clearly demonstrable lethal effect of trauma. World War I thus recognized a problem of shock but left it wrapped in mystery.

At the end of World War I the so-called shock problem was transferred to the experimental laboratories of medical science. Attempts were made to resolve it by physiologic and chemical techniques under a wide variety of experimentally induced circumstances. As the methods of initiating experimental shock were multiplied, the term itself became broadened, so that it included a number of processes that appeared to have one feature in common —a reduced effective volume flow of blood with inadequacy of the peripheral circulation and resulting tissue asphyxia. In the clinic as well as the laboratory, shock became separated from wounds, and "medical shock," "obstetrical shock," "burn shock," "shock due to infection," and other types were described as entities. So-called shock became synonymous with the process of dying from almost any cause unless death was practically instantaneous or, as Henderson[1] stated, "unless one is burned alive." The phrase, "the problems of shocks," was used by Mann[2] to describe this confusion of definition.

In the welter of animal experimentation during and after World War I there were certain findings pertinent to the original problem. Bayliss and Cannon[3] had imitated wound shock by crushing and lacerating the thigh muscles of anesthetized animals. This was supposed to produce a destruction of tissue but not a very great extravasation of blood. Failure to measure the factor of blood and fluid loss in the local area of trauma (and, as shown later, failure to recognize the superimposed clostridial infection) enabled Cannon[4] and other experimenters to propose that toxic products of tissue disintegration were absorbed into the general circulation, causing what was termed traumatic toxemia. Parsons,[5] Parsons and Phemister,[6] and Blalock[7] measured the local blood and fluid loss in traumatized legs by precise methods and showed that it was far greater than had been suspected and quite sufficient to account for the reduction in blood volume observed.

It was thus made clear that estimation of the amount of hemorrhage in an injured man must include the blood extravasated into the tissues as well as that poured on the ground or caught by the dressings. It was also found necessary to consider the blood volume that remained in circulation

[1] HENDERSON, Y.: Fundamentals of asphyxia. J.A.M.A. **101**: 261–266, July 22, 1933.

[2] MANN, F. C.: *In* Bulletin on Shock, minutes of third meeting of Subcommittee on Shock, Division of Medical Sciences, National Research Council, 18 May 1942, p. 117.

[3] BAYLISS, W. M., and CANNON, W. B.: Sections IV, V, and VI in Report VIII, Traumatic Toxaemia as a Factor in Shock, Special Report Series, No. 26, Medical Research Committee. London, H. M. Stationery Office, 1919.

[4] CANNON, W. B.: Traumatic Shock. New York, D. Appleton and Co., 1923.

[5] PARSONS, E.: Experimental shock and hemorrhage. Tr. A. Resid. & ex-Resid. Physicians, Mayo Clin. (1929) **10**: 106–108, 1930.

[6] PARSONS, E., and PHEMISTER, D. B.: Haemorrhage and "shock" in traumatized limbs; experimental study. Surg., Gynec. & Obst. **51**: 196–207, Aug. 1930.

[7] BLALOCK, A.: Experimental shock; the cause of the low blood pressure produced by muscle injury. Arch. Surg. **20**: 959–996, June 1930.

in terms of plasma and red cells, for the proportionate loss of these elements varied under different circumstances. The phenomena of hemoconcentration and hemodilution were thus made understandable. Nevertheless certain investigators insisted on using the physical state of the blood to define shock as an entity, and confusion was introduced by proponents of the thesis that shock could not exist unless hemoconcentration was present.

In a critical review of the shock problem in 1942, Wiggers[8] commented that contributions to the literature on shock appeared to be directed toward the support of one or another favored theory. Experimental conditions, he stated, had not been carefully evaluated and conclusions, rather than facts, were emphasized. "Beneficial effects," Wiggers said, "are claimed for various forms of therapy in instances in which it was never shown that the subjects were in a state of shock which would have proved fatal without treatment."

Obvious loss of blood (hemorrhage), or plasma (burns), or water and electrolytes (dehydration), or all elements (trauma) were generally accepted as clearly recognized initiating factors in shock. Beyond these, however, experimenters continued to search for other mechanisms by which the volume of blood returned to the heart might be reduced. Belief in a generalized increase in capillary permeability, a concept introduced with "traumatic toxemia," held sway for years, and many investigators insisted that this, and only this, accounted for the "true" shock that had been witnessed in World War I.

Analysis of the course of events in progressive circulatory failure was pressed in the attempt to identify and define a phase-line that ushered in what was called an "irreversible" state. It had been claimed in World War I that the seriously wounded could be resuscitated by appropriate measures if their condition was attributable to hemorrhage alone, but that if profound shock had been superimposed on hemorrhage or had appeared independently of hemorrhage, all measures, including blood transfusion, were futile. The term "irreversible" was used by some with specific reference to the function of tissues or the closely linked processes of intermediary metabolism. It was used in this sense by the Subcommittee on Shock[9] of the National Research

[8] WIGGERS, C. J.: The present status of the shock problem. Physiol. Rev. **22**: 74–123, Jan. 1942.

[9] SUBCOMMITTEE ON SHOCK, Committee on Surgery, Division of Medical Sciences, National Research Council: Shock, p. xxi (Preface). *In* NATIONAL RESEARCH COUNCIL, DIVISION OF MEDICAL SCIENCES. Burns, Shock, Wound Healing and Vascular Injuries. Military Surgical Manuals, vol. V. Philadelphia, W. B. Saunders, 1943.

956507 O—52——2

Council: " . . . the process of shock brings about certain changes in the function of the tissues which, after a time, become irreversible."

By others the term "irreversible" was applied to the dynamics of the circulatory system itself. It was held that at some point in the deterioration of the organism in shock the circulatory failure became irreversible and the subject displayed this change by becoming nonreactive to transfusion. "Apparently," as Wiggers[10] wrote, "at a certain stage an adequate circulation cannot be restored by merely filling the system as one does an automobile radiator." The same writer expressed his surprise at "how well tissues or organs withstand a very low rate of blood flow before they cease to function or are unable to revive."

Thus the assumption was made that at one moment restoration of blood volume could stay the progress of death, but in the next moment it would be unable to do so. It seemed reasonable to believe that if this phase-line could be identified by experiment and an analysis be made of the physiologic processes then in motion, corrective measures might suggest themselves. But even under precisely controlled laboratory experimentation, minor variations in conditions may determine whether the animal lives or dies. Subtle differences in environmental temperature, anesthetic agents, age, and previous nutritional state of the subject, as well as other conditioning factors make it difficult to halt the cinema of life at a particular frame where one may say: Up to this point continuing life is possible—beyond this, death is inevitable. If difficult in precise experimentation, identification of the onset of irreversible shock becomes impossible when one is confronted by the results of the random trauma sustained by soldiers under combat conditions. Although the diagnosis of "irreversible shock" appeared with some frequency on the clinical records in World War II, it was merely a pretentious way of indicating that the man had died of a lethal wound.

This, then, was the background of our knowledge of wound shock when World War II began. It was entered with the concept that (1) plasma to restore the bulk of the blood in the intravascular space and (2) sodium chloride solution for dehydration and electrolyte depletion of the interstitial space were therapeutic measures adequate to the purpose of adjusting homeostasis in a wounded man. As the war progressed, this concept changed. It soon became clear that much precise information about the physiologic state of a wounded

[10] See footnote 8.

man was wanting, and efforts toward this end culminated in establishment of the Board for the Study of the Severely Wounded in the Mediterranean Theater of Operations. The chronology of events leading to a better understanding of the disturbed physiology of the severely wounded and their management in World War II may be traced through several phases, beginning with the preliminary one of planning for the treatment of shock.

Management of Severely Wounded in World War II

Preliminary Planning for Treatment of Shock

The first problem encountered in the combat area was the need for whole blood transfusion, for while plasma was in plentiful supply, it proved inadequate for the purposes envisioned. An extract from a "Report on the Activities of the Surgical Section of the 77th Evacuation Hospital," dated 10 December 1942, provides a baseline for a review of the planning for the treatment of shock in World War II. This unit shipped from England with Torch Forces and entered on the landing at Oran.

> The W.I.A. [wounded in action] had for the most part either succumbed to or recovered from any existing shock before we saw them. However, later traumatic cases came to us in shock and some of the early cases were found to be in need of whole blood transfusions. There was plenty of reconstituted blood plasma available. However, some cases, particularly those with large blood loss, were in dire need of whole blood. We had no transfusion sets, although such are readily available in the United States, no sodium citrate, no sterile distilled water, and no blood donors. Transfusion bottles were borrowed from the British, sodium citrate was purchased from a French pharmacy, a water still appeared from some unexplained source, our enlisted men who had been working long hours volunteered as donors, and whole blood transfusions were given. It would seem that there is grave need of provision for whole blood at the locality and time of definitive treatment.

The initial decision to rely on plasma rather than blood transfusion for the resuscitation of the wounded appears to have been based in part on the view held in the Office of The Surgeon General of the Army, and in part on the opinion of the eminent civilian investigators summoned by the National Research Council to act as advisers to the Armed Forces. The Committee on Transfusions first met on 31 May 1940. The Army representative made the following statement: "If the theaters of operations are mostly outside the United States . . . the Army would likely discourage the use of blood banks. If war should come closer they might want to use blood that could be transported by airplane or specially devised refrigeration. In more distant places where blood could not be collected locally, plasma, either plain or dried, would have to be used." The representative of the Navy also favored "dried blood" (plasma).

The following is quoted from a report of the meeting submitted to the Chairman of the Committee on Surgery, National Research Council, under date of 24 July 1940:

> The greater part of the day was devoted to a consideration of whole blood and blood plasma and blood serum transfusions. The consensus of opinion was that the greatest emphasis should be placed on the use of blood plasma for the following reasons: (1) Most instances of shock are associated with hemoconcentration and a given quantity of plasma is more effective than an equal quantity of whole blood in treatment; (2) blood plasma is approximately as effective in the treatment of hemorrhage as is whole blood; (3) the difficulties of preservability and transportability of plasma are considerably less than those of whole blood; and (4) matching and typing are not necessary when pooled plasma (suppression of iso-agglutinins) is used.

The last two reasons given may have been concessions to the position taken by the representatives of the Army and Navy; the first two, however, appear to reflect the prevailing concept of wound shock held by experts at that time. The efficacy of blood in the treatment of hemorrhage had been established in World War I. In small quantities it had been preserved and transported considerable distances, even up to regimental aid posts. It had been recorded that "in cases of profound shock accompanied by loss of blood, excellent results are obtained from direct blood transfusion."[11] Robertson[12] had cast doubt on the efficacy of various fluids used as "substitutes" for blood in World War I (gum acacia, gelatin) and called attention to the fact that their beneficial effects were often slight. "The only means available of increasing the oxygen-carrying power of the blood is the addition of new red blood cells," he had said. "This constitutes the unique value of blood transfusion." Whole blood transfusion also had become universally employed in surgery in civil life.

It is of real interest, therefore, to inquire into the process of reasoning

[11] Fraser, J., and Cowell, E. M.: A clinical study of the blood pressure in wound conditions. Report II, sec. 1, Special Report Series, No. 25, Medical Research Committee. London, H. M. Stationery Office, 1919, p. 49–71.

[12] Robertson, O. H.: Memorandum on blood transfusion. Report IV, Special Report Series, No. 25, Medical Research Committee. London, H. M. Stationery Office, 1919, p. 143–180.

that led the Committee on Transfusions of the National Research Council to take the position that "most instances of shock are associated with hemoconcentration and a given quantity of plasma is more effective than an equal quantity of whole blood in treatment." This concept can be traced back to observations on the wounded made in World War I by Cannon, Fraser, and Hooper[13] who reported that counts of red cells in blood taken from the capillary bed were high, particularly when compared with those of venous blood. This also was a keystone in the establishment of shock as an entity distinct from hemorrhage and led to the widely accepted hypothesis of a generalized increase in capillary permeability. "Hemoconcentration was found to furnish a practical means for differentiating shock from hemorrhage, but the enormous potential value of this sign was not comprehended by the members of the Special Committee on Wound Shock nor has it been sensed by physicians during the 20 years since that time," wrote Moon[14] in 1938. The manual on shock[15] (1943), prepared under the auspices of the Committee on Surgery of the Division of Medical Sciences of the National Research Council, also set forth this erroneous concept.

The other statement of the Committee on Transfusions, namely, that "blood plasma is approximately as effective in the treatment of hemorrhage as is whole blood," appears to have found origin in conclusions drawn from laboratory experiments that were purposely designed so that the number of variables could be rigidly limited. Transference of these conclusions to a situation that introduced a number of additional variables was an error of human reasoning. An example may be found in the widely quoted experiments of Rous and Wilson[16] (1918). These authors made a precise determination of the limits within which plasma may replace the loss of whole blood in acute hemorrhage induced in rabbits. In summarizing the results of their experiments these authors stated that "however desirable transfusion may be, it is not essential to recovery from even the severest *acute* hemorrhage, if

[13] CANNON, W. B.; FRASER, J., and HOOPER, A. N.: Some alterations in the distribution and character of the blood. Report II, sec. 2, Special Report Series, No. 25, Medical Research Committee. London, H. M. Stationery Office, 1919, p. 72–84.

[14] MOON, V. H.: Shock and Related Capillary Phenomena. New York, Oxford University Press, 1938.

[15] NATIONAL RESEARCH COUNCIL, DIVISION OF MEDICAL SCIENCES. Burns, Shock, Wound Healing and Vascular Injuries, prepared under the auspices of the Committee on Surgery of the Division of Medical Sciences of the National Research Council. Military Surgical Manuals, vol. V. Philadelphia, W. B. Saunders Co., 1943.

[16] ROUS, P., and WILSON, G. W.: Fluid substitutes for transfusion after hemorrhage. J.A.M.A. 70: 219–222, Jan. 26, 1918.

only the blood bulk can be restored in other ways." The conclusion drawn from this and subsequent observations by others[17] led to formulation of the statement by the Committee on Transfusions. The brief description of a rabbit in which up to three-fourths of the blood volume, as measured by the hemoglobin depletion, had been withdrawn and replaced by plasma contains one phrase that is significant: "The least exertion would cause the animal to pant heavily."

Presumably the rabbit had no semblance of a wound other than the needle puncture. Substitute for the rabbit housed quietly in its cage a wounded soldier picked up by litter bearers and transported by ambulance, who has in addition an extensive and painful wound with continuing extravasation of blood and plasma into adjacent tissues. Then add sedation, roentgenographic examination, anesthesia, and surgical operation with a further loss of blood. It is obvious that the introduction of these and other variables, purposely and of necessity excluded from the original experiments, may completely negate the conclusion. Both errors, the association of wound shock with hemoconcentration and the estimation regarding the effectiveness of blood plasma, are understandable in view of the paucity of observations made in World War I concerning the disturbed physiology of wounded men.

Restoration of the blood bulk in the intravascular space by infusion of a colloid solution that might be expected to stay within the confines of the semipermeable membrane of the capillary walls was envisioned during World War I. This was a projection of the Starling[18] concept elaborated by Scott[19] in 1916. Tests were made of the properties of soluble starch, dextrin, gelatin, and gum arabic, and preparations of the latter were given extensive field tests, particularly by the British, guided by the basic experiments of Bayliss.[20]

The advent of human plasma, as a result of the development of methods that enabled it to be preserved and packaged in desiccated form, appeared to provide a final answer to the problem of the restoration of blood bulk by infusion. The treatment of shock and hemorrhage was thus reduced to the simple terms of the exchange of fluid between the intravascular space and

[17] BAYLISS, (see footnote 20) for example, had shown that "more than one-half of the blood in the cat can be replaced by gum solutions with satisfactory results."

[18] STARLING, E. H.: On the absorption of fluids from the connective tissue spaces. J. Physiol. 19: 312–326, May 1896.

[19] SCOTT, F. H.: The mechanism of fluid absorption from tissue spaces. J. Physiol. 50: 157–167, Feb. 1916.

[20] BAYLISS, W. M.: Intravenous injections to replace blood. Report I, Special Report Series, No. 25, Medical Research Committee. London, H. M. Stationery Office, 1919, p. 11–41.

the interstitial space under clearly defined physicochemical laws. Extension of this same reasoning led to the proposal that because the serum albumin fraction of the blood as prepared by Cohn[21] packaged a high proportion of the total colloid osmotic activity of the serum in small liquid volume, it was peculiarly appropriate to military needs. It was postulated that the interstitial fluid compartment would provide the necessary diluent unless the patient were badly dehydrated.

This oversimplified physicochemical approach, which was an extension of the World War I quest of Bayliss aided by the availability of refined and human-derived preparations, not only failed to take into account the variables described, but also placed undue emphasis on a single physicochemical property of the blood; namely, the osmotic activity of the plasma proteins. Not only was the important function of the red cells as oxygen carriers ignored, but also their contribution to the total blood mass under abnormal circumstances. Both the magnitude of the initial loss of whole blood occasioned by wounding and the significance of a continuing seepage of blood and its fluid components into the tissue spaces were underestimated. And finally, an effort to restore and maintain blood bulk based on colloid preparations, either derived from human proteins or otherwise, presupposes a space bounded by a semipermeable membrane—not one in which large areas of the membrane may have been rendered freely permeable by the direct effects of trauma.

Evolution of Knowledge During World War II

The evolution of the management of the seriously wounded during World War II may be divided into three phases for purposes of description, although it is apparent that as phases they are not pencilled with the clarity observed in phase-lines on a tactical map. A first phase may be recognized in which efforts to identify the gross nature of the problems and devise immediate solutions predominate. Cobwebs of theory and hypothesis were swept away by simple observations and precise definitions. This was followed by a phase during which all efforts centered on the development and perfection of the practical art of resuscitation. In the final phase systematic and precise meas-

[21] Cohn, Edwin J.: Memorandum on the preparation of normal human serum albumin. Report No. 1, Subcommittee on Blood Substitutes, Division of Medical Sciences, National Research Council (acting for Committee on Medical Research, Office of Scientific Research and Development), 11 February 1942.

urements were made that for the first time described the actual physiologic state of the wounded man as it was observed on the field of battle.

A search among the records of World War II for novel and challenging hypotheses regarding the nature of shock is likely to prove disappointing. The very abundance of facts and experience discouraged "hot disputing" and debate. And yet from this experience emerged certain concepts that, when fully grasped, will be found no less significant because they appear simple and direct.

First Phase: Identification of the Problem

Although in retrospect the North African Campaign was but a brief curtain raiser for the sustained action that was to come later, it stands historically as a period in which the major problems of the management of the wounded were clearly identified. The campaign was over before many needs of the military organization could be met, but the foundation for future action was secured.

The Surgical Consultant, North African Theater of Operations (U. S. A.), reported for duty in Algiers on 7 March 1943. His first official report, submitted under date of 24 March 1943, following a period of temporary duty in II Corps on the southern Tunisian front, was a Memorandum on whole blood transfusion. Further data were collected and a formal report on whole blood transfusion was made to the Theater Surgeon, NATOUSA, on 16 April 1943. The following conclusions and recommendations were made.

Conclusions

a. There is a need for whole blood transfusion in the treatment of a significant proportion of the wounded. Plasma is not an adequate substitute in these cases.

b. Adequate and conventional safeguards that govern blood transfusion are difficult or impossible to attain in forward echelons.

c. The British Base Transfusion Unit has demonstrated the feasibility of supplying large amounts of whole blood to the combat area.

Recommendation

That a central laboratory be established in NATOUSA to provide whole blood, intravenous solutions, distilled water, and plasma.

The Italian Campaign had progressed to the establishment of the Anzio Beachhead before the distribution of preserved blood from a central laboratory was realized. In the meantime, however, the evacuation hospitals and later the field hospitals employed for forward emergency surgery were encouraged to establish their own blood banks with supplies requisitioned for that purpose.

Following this decision on therapy, the next important question that faced the Surgical Consultant in southern Tunisia in March and April 1943 was whether casualties were dying of irreversible shock—in fact, whether wound shock, unassociated with hemorrhage and other clear results of trauma, existed as an important problem in World War II. It was obvious that a precise definition was necessary if this question was to be answered, for, as was noted in the Report of the Surgical Consultant dated 2 July 1943:

In Field Medical Records, Case Reports, and Death Reports, as well as in verbal discussions among Medical Officers, the term "shock" is used with vague definition or quite commonly with no definition whatsoever. In the case reports of battle casualties dying in the forward area, "shock" or "irreversible shock" is almost invariably recorded as a secondary cause of death. This is true whether the wounded man had a lethal craniocerebral wound, an overwhelming peritonitis, fulminating gas gangrene infection, or simply died of uncontrollable hemorrhage.

Circulatory failures from peritonitis, bacterial infection, intrathoracic injury, burns, and injury to the central nervous system were placed in separate categories. All other forms of circulatory failure which arise within a few hours as a result of wounding were considered as "wound shock."[22] A study was undertaken that covered the course of the evacuation of some 1,263 casualties from the battalion areas through the evacuation hospitals. No record could be found of a death from wound shock under terms of the restricted definition, in which hemorrhage could be excluded as the important factor. The conclusions drawn from this study as well as from direct observation of large numbers of wounded were expressed as follows:[23]

Under conditions that prevailed in the management of battle casualties between 20 and 25 March in the sampling area of II Corps, wound shock was not a cause of death.

This does not imply that wound shock did not occur among the survivors, but if so it appears that remedial treatment was adequate.

[22] The Battle of El Alamein (October and November 1942) was one of the first occasions on which blood and blood substitutes were used on a large scale for the resuscitation of battle casualties in forward medical units. Report No. 1, Medical Research Section, GHQ, MEF, by Lt. Col. W. C. Wilson, RAMC, described the condition of the wounded with special reference to wound shock and its treatment. The necessity for the restricted definition of wound shock was presented with great clarity.

[23] Report of Surgical Consultant, Office of the Surgeon, Headquarters, North African Theater of Operations, U.S.A., 2 July 1943. (Appendix B, 1; Par. B, 2.)

"Irreversible" wound shock does not appear to be a problem of pressing significance.

The problem of shock as observed in the Tunisian Campaign centered in the application of accepted means of treatment, rather than in the need for additional methods of management.

Second Phase: Development of Resuscitation

The second phase in the advancement of understanding of the management of the seriously wounded was development and perfection of the practical art of resuscitation. The many experienced surgeons of the Theater contributed to and shared the responsibilities of a Theater-wide educational program. Special acknowledgment is made of the contributions of Colonel Howard Snyder, Surgical Consultant to II Corps and subsequently to Fifth Army, and of Lt. Colonel Henry K. Beecher, assigned to AFHQ as Consultant in Resuscitation and Anesthesia and working on temporary duty in the forward installations. Simple and direct observations made while actually caring for battle casualties confirmed the conclusions of the Tunisian Campaign and led to the complete discard of the confused theories of traumatic shock that had been elaborated from the experience of World War I.

A highly significant product of the development of the art of resuscitation was merging of consideration of shock with consideration of the implications of the wound. Historically, wound surgery has been linked with the prevention and treatment of infection, and, as a matter of fact, in the less seriously wounded this function of surgery still is predominant. In World War II this concept was modified, as it was not applicable to the many desperately wounded casualties that came under surgical management. It was no longer valid to hold that a seriously wounded man could be resuscitated solely by measures directed toward restoring blood volume, and that when this was accomplished wound surgery could be undertaken, depending only on the time necessary for prevention of infection. Wound surgery under these circumstances assumed the new position of being in itself the climax of resuscitation. General recognition of the principle that procedures commonly grouped as "resuscitative" are but integral steps in the management of a situation that must be viewed as a whole, and that *wound surgery may in itself be the most potent act of resuscitation,* stands as a basic achievement of military surgery in World War II.

This concept was glimpsed in the Tunisian Campaign and led to the following comment in the official report of the Surgical Consultant dated 2 July 1943:

Resuscitation comes to be regarded as a sub-specialty of military surgery and as such becomes a goal in itself. One central fact must be kept in mind and, although it appears obvious, it is often overlooked both in theory and practice. *A wounded man is resuscitated not only to save life but to prepare him for necessary surgery.*

This divorce of surgeon from shock is a disquieting outgrowth of the war that cannot be too strongly condemned. Resuscitation in every case being prepared for operation is an integral part of the surgical management of trauma and must remain so if optimal results are to be achieved.

The concept was more fully developed during the Italian Campaign by Lt. Colonel Henry K. Beecher[24] who presented the following broad definition of resuscitation that includes operation as an essential component:

The enemy has produced the worst wound he could, and its consequences are cumulative—dehydration increased by unusual fluid loss in sweat and vomitus, continuing hemorrhage or plasma loss, pain making rest impossible, increasing emotional exhaustion, developing infection—these and other factors are set in operation by the initial wound. Their progress in the seriously wounded is to be checked in most cases only by surgery or by death. Resuscitative measures give a temporary stay and make successful surgery possible in the severely wounded; but in most cases true release from the consequences of the wound is effected only by surgery. Surgery is not only the goal but is itself a part of resuscitation in the broad sense. Any other view is likely to lead to unfortunate separation between the activities of the "shock team" and those of the surgical team. Care of the wounded man must be continuous and supervision uninterrupted.

This concept now appears obvious, and in fact is a principle soon grasped by the practical worker in the field. It is likely to be overlooked when conclusions are drawn from laboratory experiments purposely designed to isolate and test the efficacy of single therapeutic measures.

The establishment of wound surgery as inseparable from the management of wound shock had many practical applications. It was a strong consideration in the placement of the surgical hospital for treatment of the severely wounded alongside the divisional clearing station, as was determined in Sicily. A short litter carry placed the casualty in the hands of a competent surgical team equipped not only for resuscitation in the conventional sense but for the major procedures of surgery. It led to the close observation of a wounded man's response to blood replacement therapy. If the response was transient

[24] Beecher, H. K.: Preparation of battle casualties for surgery. Ann. Surg. **121**: 769–797, June 1945.

or unsatisfactory, it was not judged that his shock was "irreversible" or that he displayed a "negative reaction" because of widespread capillary damage, or that it was futile to try "to repair the damage done by prolonged oxygen want." It was assumed that either continuing hemorrhage or spreading infection was present, or that a dead limb required amputation or dead tissue called for excision; operation was immediately undertaken with continuing transfusions to support the patient's condition.

Another practical result was that resuscitative measures carried out in the field, forward of a surgical hospital, came to be regarded as temporary and designed only to preserve life during transportation. They thus became both qualitatively and quantitatively different from those combined with surgery. It was necessary to rely on plasma as the chief measure to support the patient during transport, but plasma was used in minimal amounts without intent to restore the blood volume flow to a normal level. The dangers of the overuse of plasma became apparent. Resuscitation within the hospital included use of additional plasma, whole blood, ancillary measures, such as bronchoscopy, oxygen therapy, and nerve block to relieve pain or to restore respiratory effectiveness if crippled by the wound, *and* initial wound surgery.

Third Phase: Documentation by Scientific Evidence

By the summer of 1944 it was evident that although nearly two years of experience had enabled the Theater to develop the procedures of resuscitation to a high peak of effectiveness, this was largely an accomplishment of the practical art and remained to a considerable extent undocumented by scientific evidence. If left in this status at the end of World War II, it would tend to be forgotten, as are many other practical lessons that emerge from the experience of war. Even the validity of the experience would be open to question. Bayliss,[25] toward the end of World War I, had written: "On the whole it is remarkable that so little positive evidence is forthcoming as to the superiority of blood transfusions. Statements are made on the basis of general impressions, rather than on convincing proof. In the nature of the case, such proof would be difficult to provide." The question was often asked whether the experience in Italy was really accepted at face value and whether the precepts that had been formulated would be transferred to the conflict in the Pacific and to civilian needs.

[25] See footnote 20.

EARLY STUDIES

Some data of a precise nature had been obtained, but they were of a fragmentary nature. Lt. Colonel John D. Stewart, a member of the Consulting Surgical Staff of the Surgeon, NATOUSA, while on temporary duty with the Fifth Army in December 1943, made arrangements with the Commanding Officer of the 2d Medical Laboratory, with the concurrence and support of the Surgeon, Fifth Army, to conduct a clinical study of the freshly wounded. A small mobile laboratory was set up at the 3d Platoon of the 11th Field Hospital on 20 January 1944. This platoon was situated near the 36th Divisional Clearing Station, northeast of Mignano, about seven miles behind the front. The objective was to study by formal biochemic methods certain aspects of shock, hemorrhage, and dehydration.

A preliminary report was submitted under date of 17 March 1944. Observations had been made on some 35 badly wounded patients immediately after admission, usually within 12 hours after wounding. A final report of this study, extended to include 100 desperately wounded observed during the first 6 months of 1944, was submitted on 2 January 1945.[26] The data indicated (1) absence of hemoconcentration in shock, (2) reduction of blood volume in shock, (3) greater reduction of red-cell concentration than of plasma protein concentration early after wounding, (4) lowering of both red-cell and plasma protein concentration later, and (5) frequency of later dehydration.

During approximately the same period (11 February through 4 June 1944) the Consultant in Anesthesia and Resuscitation, NATOUSA, and Captain Charles H. Burnett carried out an extensive study[27] on the wounded at the 94th Evacuation Hospital, observing 557 cases on the Cassino Front (Mignano) and 2,296 cases on the Anzio Beachhead. In the latter site the position of the evacuation hospital bore the same relation to the front as a field hospital. While the greatest significance of this contribution lay in formulating procedure for the clinical management of resuscitation in the seriously wounded, in 37 of the most severely wounded fairly extensive laboratory observations were made. These confirmed the absence of hemoconcentration.

Starting in March 1944 in a field hospital platoon, Captain Joseph J. Lalich,

[26] Stewart, J. D.: Observations on the severely wounded in forward field hospitals of the Fifth Army, with special reference to wound shock. Report to the Surgeon, Mediterranean Theater of Operations, U.S.A., 2 Jan. 1945. Also, J.A.M.A. **133**: 216–219, Jan. 25, 1947.

[27] Beecher, H. K., and Burnett, C. H.: Field experience in use of blood and blood substitutes (plasma, albumin) in seriously wounded men. M. Bull. North African Theat. Op. (no. 1) **2**: 2–7, July 1944.

2d Auxiliary Surgical Group, carried out a series of hematocrit and plasma protein determinations by the copper sulfate method. His findings, like those of the other workers, were quickly made available to forward surgeons and were submitted as a formal report on 12 November 1944. Attention was called to the low hematocrit readings obtained from 3 to 5 days after initial surgery despite the very liberal use of blood transfusions in resuscitation. This was a phenomenon that was exciting interest in the general hospitals in Peninsular Base Section. For the success of the vigorous program of reparative wound surgery that was being formulated, it was found necessary to provide for the liberal use of whole blood transfusion at the base.

There was need, however, for a far more comprehensive study. In the opinion of the Medical Research Committee of the Theater there was little doubt that the impetus of the tremendous program undertaken to provide so-called "substitutes" for blood in World War II would be projected into the postwar period. It might be revived with any threat of a future war. It was essential, therefore, that the so-called impressions derived from experience be documented by hard, cold facts about the condition of a freshly wounded man. To this end, everything about a seriously wounded soldier that could be observed and recorded by precise measurement should be ascertained and recorded. The collection of data needed to be extended to a sufficient number of casualties to make the findings conclusive.

ESTABLISHMENT OF BOARD FOR THE STUDY OF THE SEVERELY WOUNDED

The summer of 1944 in Italy was a period of readjustment to meet the over-all strategy of the war in Europe. Between mid-June and the end of July more than a division a week was withdrawn from the forces to train and stage for Operation Anvil, the attack in southern France executed on 15 August. Pursuit of the enemy to the north had brought the Allied armies up against the "Gothic Line," an elaborate defense system in the northern Apennines. Then on 10 September a general offensive was launched to break through into the Po Valley. As it became apparent that the Medical Service was to face a renewed heavy flow of casualties, the Medical Research Committee sponsored certain fact-finding tasks that required concentrated and carefully organized effort for accomplishment. One of these was further analysis of the state of the seriously wounded.

More information was urgently needed regarding the problem of anuria.

Kidney damage associated with crushing injuries sustained in air raids had been described as a component of the "crush syndrome" by Bywaters et al.[28] early in the war. Identification of damaged kidney function as a component of injury in the soldier seriously wounded by flying missiles on the battlefield came slowly, but experience had already suggested that it either was being overlooked or was subject to misinterpretation. Identification was slow because first of all it requires the coordinated effort of a wide variety of expert skills in the forward area to rescue desperately wounded soldiers and keep them alive until such time as suppression of kidney function manifests itself. This involves the activity of the entire medical department from the company aid-man in the field to the surgical team and nursing staff in a mobile hospital. When a gravely wounded man dies within 48 hours of being hit, the chances are that any suppression of kidney function will pass unrecognized.

In the N. R. C. Conference on Shock held on 1 December 1943, Dr. Donald D. Van Slyke had presented a communication on the "Effect of Shock on the Kidney." The concept was developed that the peripheral vascular constriction that compensated for a deficit in the volume of circulating blood in shock may practically stop the blood flow through the kidneys. Urinary excretion stops, and prolonged ischemia may be followed by permanent suppression of renal function. Although presented as a hypothesis, this concept brought a fresh point of view to a clinical problem that was beginning to be identified in the field. Under date of 16 February 1944, a letter, from which the following extract is quoted, was addressed to Dr. Van Slyke by the Surgical Consultant.

> By excellent forward surgery and the liberal use of whole blood transfusion as well as plasma, we are saving lives but also keeping certain men alive temporarily only to display the type of kidney damage you describe. This has been either complete anuria with death, or in one case a fall of urinary output to 200 cc. with ultimate recovery of kidney function. As you suggest, this phenomenon is not unique to the "crush" syndrome but may occur in any wounded man who experiences a long period of greatly reduced volume flow.

Delay in the identification of the problem of anuria in battle casualties was not solely a matter of organization or preoccupation with more pressing problems. Recognition of anuria depended on a close check of fluid intake and output, items that are difficult to secure even in well-run civilian hospitals.

[28] Bywaters, E. G. L.; Delory, G. E.; Rimington, C., and Smiles, J.: Myohaemoglobin in urine of air raid casualties with crushing injury. Biochem. J. 35: 1164–1168, 1941.

Chemical tests for azotemia were not available in the mobile hospitals. The terminal event of pulmonary edema from forcing fluids in order to correct supposed dehydration was subject to misinterpretation as a manifestation of blast injury or other result of direct trauma to the lungs.

Even when suppression of urinary excretion was recognized, other causes than the specific effects of the injury required exclusion. In the earlier phases of the war medical officers were alerted to the effects of sulfonamide administration on the kidney. Early in 1944 the widespread usage of sulfonamides was still making it difficult to clarify the problem of posttraumatic anuria. This was referred to in the Annual Report of the Surgical Consultant (1943) as follows: "Kidney damage is probably the most frequent and easily overlooked sequel of shock and is manifested by anuria or reduced urinary output. Information relative to renal damage produced by decreased volume flow of blood is particularly desired because of a close linkage with policies on sulfonamide therapy."

Even more important, however, was the use of blood transfusion in resuscitation. The question arose again and again how often blood transfusion itself might be responsible for kidney damage. To interpret posttraumatic anuria, blood given in transfusion must meet rigid specifications. It must be compatible both in type and iso-agglutinin titer. It must be collected and stored in a closed system to avoid contamination. When supplied in bulk in military operation, frequent checks must be made for free hemoglobin content both at the bank, in the forward hospital, and by examination of the recipients' plasma after transfusion.

With the increased use of transfusion in the forward area and the distribution of preserved whole blood from the central laboratory in Naples, the identification of posttraumatic anuria became tangled with that of "transfusion kidney." Informal requests came from Anzio Beachhead for distribution of Type A blood for massive transfusions in this type of recipient. The policy of issuing only Type O blood in which the iso-agglutinins had been titered was adhered to. Blood with titer 1:64 or above was labeled "for O-Type recipients only"; that with weaker iso-agglutinin titer was considered suitable for universal use. The problems of poorly preserved or contaminated blood encountered elsewhere in the field during World War II were not encountered in the U. S. Army, Mediterranean Theater.

The basic conditions outlined above had been established in Italy by late summer in 1944. The medical department personnel were expert from long experience; penicillin had replaced sulfonamides in the treatment of the seriously wounded; the Theater blood bank was issuing a liberal supply of whole blood that met the required specifications. The total situation, both military and medical, was thus favorable for an intensive study of the seriously wounded soldier. To this end, the Theater Surgeon recommended on 1 September 1944 that a Board to Study the Treatment of the Severely Wounded be appointed by the Commanding General, NATOUSA. Such a board was established on 3 September 1944 and it is the report of this Board which is presented in this volume. In retrospect, it is doubtful that this particular effort would have been feasible at an earlier date; even if undertaken it probably would not have been as productive, for reasons that have been presented.

Selection of the personnel of this Board was a matter of vital importance, and the recommendations of his Medical Research Committee were generously accepted by the Theater Surgeon. It was essential that medical officers be selected who were skilled in the techniques of clinical investigation that can be utilized without harm or discomfort to seriously injured patients. Different phases of the study required precise and critical observations in the laboratory, in the ward tents, and in the operating tent. It was essential that the members of the Board be familiar with the subjects to be studied—seriously wounded soldiers. Those finally selected had long experience in identification of the complex sequelae of wounds, and those in charge of the clinical aspects were experts in the practical art of resuscitation. Further, and most important, all had become expert in the art of overcoming, rather than being frustrated by, the retarding element of "friction" ever present in a huge military undertaking.

It is of more than passing interest to note that the minutes of the first meeting of the Committee on Transfusions of the National Research Council, already referred to, contain the suggestion "that a group of men be allowed to work in the Army, freed from any of the obligations of Army officers, who would study cases of shock as investigators. This would give opportunity to observe shock on a big scale, an opportunity to get an insight into the nature of shock." This was on 31 May 1940. In May 1945, as the Germans in northern Italy capitulated and brought the task of the Board to a conclusion, this objective had been accomplished—not precisely as visualized, but effectively. The

956507 O—52——3

members of the Board were in no way "freed from any of the obligations of Army officers," but were, on the contrary, selected because they were competent to assume the highest privilege accorded officers—the freedom of individual judgment and action. They were not a group that merely worked " in the Army"; they were of the Army.

EDWARD D. CHURCHILL, M.D.
(Formerly Colonel, MC, A.U.S., Surgical Consultant, North African-Mediterranean Theater of Operations)

CHAPTER I

Internal State of Severely Wounded Men on Entry to the Most Forward Hospital

The effects on the human body of the destructive forces of warfare have been described many times in terms of organic damage and tissue loss. Our concern was rather with the internal state of the severely wounded man. Gross tissue damage is obvious, or becomes obvious on surgical exploration, but our purpose during the first phase of this investigation was to describe the latent consequences of the wound as revealed in impairment of organic function and in abnormalities of the blood and the urine. These initial studies were made shortly after the patient entered the most forward field or evacuation hospital, before either vigorous resuscitative measures or operation had yet been undertaken. The physiologic studies were continued, whenever possible, throughout the patient's course. Other aspects of the investigation as a whole relate to diagnosis, treatment, and pathology of the severely wounded.

The very severely wounded ("nontransportable patients") were those selected for study. They were the most critically wounded or injured battle casualties to reach a forward hospital alive. With few exceptions, chiefly cases of injury,[1] the casualties[2] studied were from the "wounded in action"[3] group. The cases are listed in Appendix D.

[1] AR 40–1025, Sec V, par 79*a*, 12 Dec 44, sub: Definition [of injury]. "The term 'injury' is used here in its broad sense to include such conditions as fractures, wounds, sprains, strains, dislocations, concussions, and compressions, commonly thought of as 'accidents' . . ."

[2] ASF Manual M 807, 25 Oct 44, Glossary. "Casualty (Personnel). A soldier who is rendered unavailable for service as a result of disease, injury, or enemy action . . ."

[3] AR 40–1025, Sec II, par 26, 12 Dec 44, sub: [Definition of] WIA (wounded in action) cases. "The term will include wounds or injuries incurred as a direct result of a hostile act of a military enemy. It will not include injuries accidentally incurred while in combat, or those incurred on purely training flights or missions."

TABLE I.—TIME FROM WOUNDING TO SURGERY, MEDITERRANEAN THEATER OF OPERATIONS

Source and Period of Collection	Number of Wounded	Average Time in Hours		
		Wounding to Battalion Aid Station	Battalion Aid Station to Collecting Company	Collecting Company to Clearing Station
North of Florence, Italy (September 1944 to March 1945)	100	2.68	2.95	1.98
Loiano, Italy (April 1945) . .	47	4.65	1.43	0.93
Via Reggio, Italy (March and April 1945)	44	4.59	0.84	0.99

In all, 186 casualties were examined in the most forward hospitals by members of the Board. From previous studies made in the Theater, it was estimated that of 10,073 battle casualties in the area to reach forward hospitals alive during the period of the study, between 201 and 252 were seriously wounded. Hence the 186 studied here may be considered an adequate sample of the severely wounded in the Theater. One hundred and eight of these 186 casualties were seen at the time of admission and were studied rather completely (including blood chemistry and urine analyses) at that time. Account was taken of the nature and type of the wound, and also of the evacuation time, including the distance to be covered and the character of the terrain, since delay along the evacuation trail, the reaction of the patient to his wound, and his response to subsequent management all influence the factors under study and increase the significance of the laboratory data.

In addition to the data obtained as background material, the initial studies included determination of blood loss, of plasma protein and hemoglobin levels, analysis of other biochemic changes encountered, initial kidney function studies, and a study of liver function in the newly wounded man.

It will be observed in the tables and charts of this and following chapters that different groups and varying numbers of patients have been drawn from the total for consideration in given instances. This has been done because it was often found in comparing two or more factors that records were incomplete for the specific comparison in question and had to be omitted. As a re-

TABLE 1.—TIME FROM WOUNDING TO SURGERY, MEDITERRANEAN THEATER OF OPERATIONS—*Continued*

Source and Period of Collection	Number of Wounded	Average Time in Hours		
		Clearing Station to Forward Hospital	Forward Hospital Entry to Operation	Total Time from Wounding to Surgery
North of Florence, Italy (September 1944 to March 1945)	100	1.41	5.38	14.40
Loiano, Italy (April 1945) . .	47	0.56	8.28	15.85
Via Reggio, Italy (March and April 1945)	44	0.60	5.13	12.15

sult comparatively small numbers of cases are presented in some instances. No attempt has been made to keep the number of cases uniform in any of the various phases of the study; rather we have presented all the data that were complete for any one phase. This method was considered desirable because of the nature of the study and the exigencies under which it was carried out. In the tables throughout the study the standard error of the mean is shown whenever the data were sufficient to warrant this method of statistical treatment.

Initial Studies

Time from Wounding to Hospital Entry and Surgery

Although some of the casualties were wounded near the forward hospitals, the majority had to be transported some distance, often over mountainous terrain, by litter carry or motor transport. Since the time required to transport a patient from the place of wounding to the most forward hospital may greatly influence his condition on arrival, some indication of the length of this period in the Mediterranean Theater of Operations is given in Table 1, which shows the average progress of three groups of casualties along the evacuation route. The first group consists of 100 men selected at random from those in our study

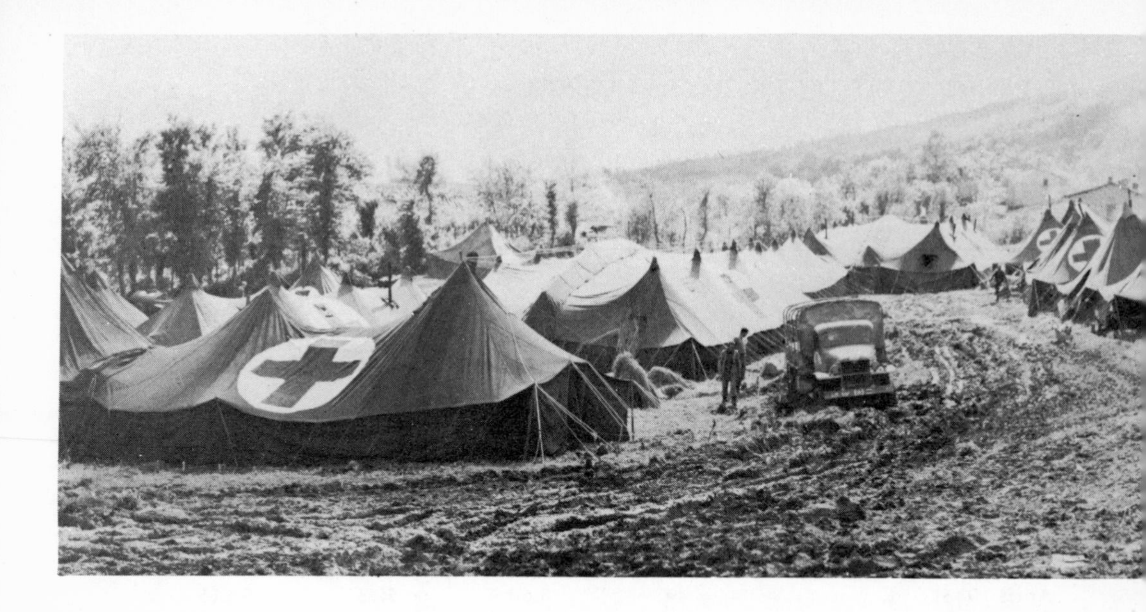

FORWARD HOSPITAL in Italy after a rain (*above*). In evacuation by jeep, as shown below, plasma could be administered during the trip, even over rough roads, but the terrain in Italy often made all types of evacuation difficult and affected the condition of the patient on his arrival at a forward hospital.

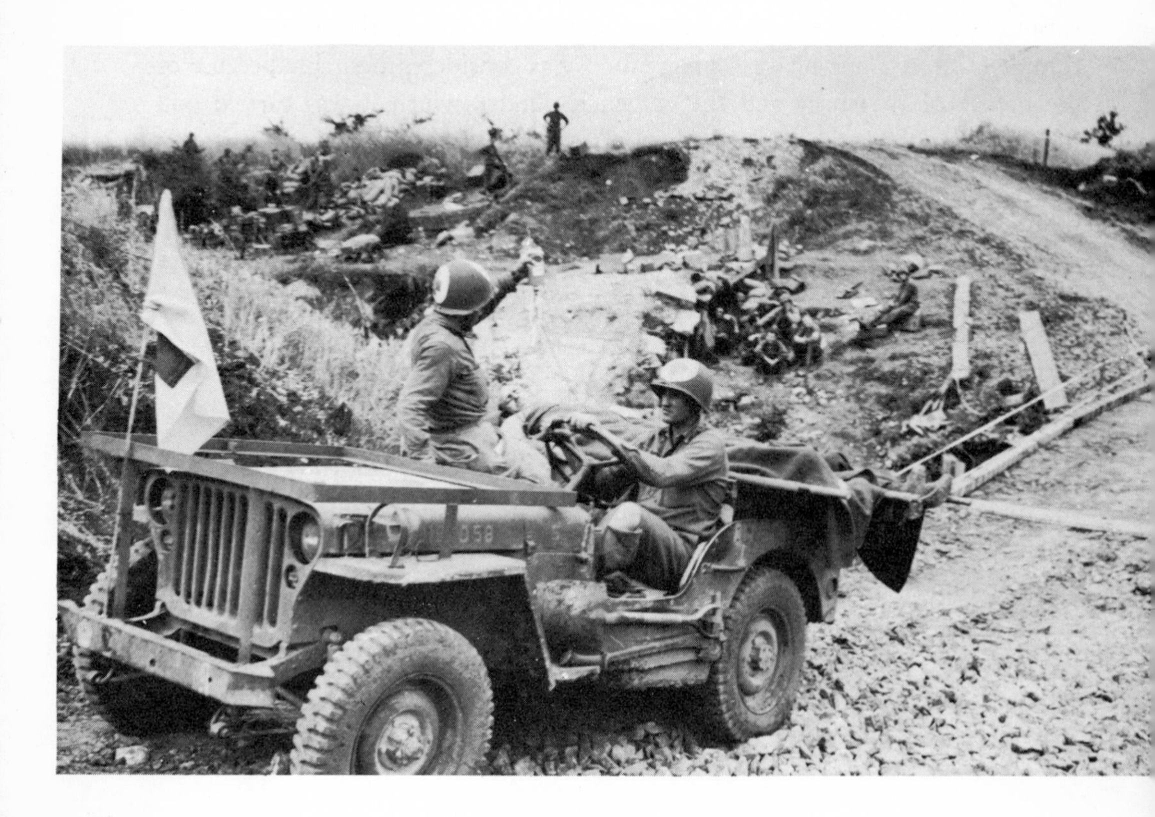

who were wounded during a relatively quiet period in the fall, winter, and spring of 1944-45. The other two groups represent men who were severely wounded during offensives in the spring of 1945. In the third locale cited, it was contended by those concerned that, considering the circumstances, evacuation had been effected rapidly. The table also shows the average time from hospital admission to surgery and the total time from wounding to surgery in the three groups.

Type and Location of Wounds

For various correlations throughout the study wounds are grouped according to their type, or location, or both. Many patients incurred multiple wounds, some multiple major wounds. For certain purposes two broad classifications of type were utilized: peripheral and nonperipheral, and this terminology will be used whenever pertinent. Nonperipheral wounds were defined as those involving the major body cavities (the abdomen, the thorax, and the interior of the skull); all others were considered as peripheral. Crush cases are excluded in some of the correlations because they were studied separately.

In the following classification the severe wounds only are considered, since they were pertinent to the study. Thus in the patients with multiple severe wounds some wounds were listed as the principal major ones; no attempt was made to record minor wounds, such as fracture of a phalanx, for example. In general, the types of wounds found in our patients were as follows:

> Severe peripheral wounds were present in 116 patients, constituting a major injury in 81 instances. Nearly all were wounds of the extremities. Thirty-three patients had peripheral wounds without fracture, 16 of which were the patient's major wound. Fifty-three of 70 patients had major peripheral wounds with fracture, and 13 had traumatic amputation of an extremity. In 10 of these 66, a major wound was also listed in another category. Three patients among those with peripheral wounds had injury to the spinal cord.
>
> Of the severe nonperipheral wounds, 34 patients had thoracic wounds (a major wound in 30 instances) and 56 patients had intra-abdominal wounds, a major wound in 50 instances. An additional 21 patients had combined thoraco-abdominal wounds and 2 patients had separate wounds of the chest and abdomen. Of the total abdominal wounds, there were 25 wounds of the liver, 20 wounds of the kidney

TABLE 2.—RELATIONSHIP OF PAIN TO MAJOR WOUND IN 215 PATIENTS

(Data Taken from Study on *Pain in Men Wounded in Battle*[1])

Type of Wound	Number of Patients	Average Age *yrs.*	Time from Wounding *hrs., average*	Total Dose of Morphine *mg., average* [2]	Latest Dose of Morphine *mg., average*	Time since latest Morphine *hrs., average*	Pain (degree and number of patients in each group)	Further Pain Relief Therapy Wanted (number of patients)
Compound Fractures of Long Bones	50	24.8±0.9	12.5±1.3	27.0±1.5 (1 pt. none)	22.6	7.0±0.8	19 none 12 slight 7 moderate 12 severe	11 yes 39 no
Extensive Soft-tissue Wounds	50	24.5±1.1	11.3±1.4	27.0±2.7 (11 pts. none)	19.5	7.2±0.6	19 none 15 slight 8 moderate 8 severe	9 yes 41 no
Penetrating Wounds of Thorax	50	24.5±0.8	9.8±1.0	25.0±1.8 (11 pts. none)	21.2	6.5±0.6	15 none 18 slight 11 moderate 6 severe	10 yes 40 no
Penetrating Wounds of Abdomen	50	22.7±0.6	7.2±0.7	29.0±2.2 (5 pts. none)	25.0	4.8±0.7	7 none 5 slight 14 moderate 24 severe	27 yes 23 no
Penetrating Wounds of Cerebrum	15	25.1±1.4	7.9±1.4	19.8±4.2 (8 pts. none)	19.8	6.2±1.5	9 none 5 slight 0 moderate 1 severe	1 yes 14 no

[1] See footnote 4, text.
[2] Patients who did not receive morphine are not included in the averages.

(treated by nephrectomy in 11 instances), and in 1 case it was not known whether a kidney or liver wound had been present. Wounds of the urinary tract involving the bladder or structures above it occurred in 9 patients. Ten patients with nonperipheral wounds had multiple major wounds.

Crush injuries were found in nine patients, and there was only one case of head injury.

Clinical Condition of Patients on Arrival at the Most Forward Hospital

Pain

The frequency and severity of pain in different types of wounds had been extensively studied under similar conditions and on the same types of patients shortly before the Board was organized and the study was therefore not repeated on these 186 patients. Part of the data obtained in the early study[4] is shown in Table 2. The incidence of severe pain was surprisingly low. The data showed that severe pain was not to be accounted for on the basis of the patients' having received less morphine or having received it earlier than patients who reported little or no pain. It was also pointed out that three factors are chiefly important in the distress of the wounded: pain, mental distress, and thirst. In the severely wounded patient in good general condition, the first two factors are important. In the man in shock, thirst is the main and often the only cause of evident distress, but it may be extreme.

Shock

Grading of Shock.—The view sometimes has been taken that shock is either present or absent in a given case and that to try to distinguish between degrees of shock is futile. In this study, however, it was found instructive to separate the patients arbitrarily into four categories; namely, those with "no shock," "slight shock," "moderate shock," and "severe shock." This was done on the basis of the criteria listed in Table 3 which in turn were based on preliminary observation of large numbers of battle casualties by members of the Board. A patient was assigned to a particular category if he exhibited the ma-

[4] BEECHER, H. K.: Pain in men wounded in battle. Ann. Surg. **123**: 96–105, January 1946; also Bull. U. S. Army M. Dept. 5: 445–454, April 1946.

TABLE 3.—GRADING OF SHOCK*

Degree of Shock	Blood Pressure (approx.)	Pulse Quality	Skin			Thirst	Mental State
			Temperature	Color	Circulation (response to pressure, blanching)		
None	Normal	Normal	Normal	Normal	Normal	Normal	Clear and distressed.
Slight	Decreased 20% or less	Normal	Cool	Pale	Definite slowing	Normal	Clear and distressed.
Moderate	Decreased 20 to 40%	Definite decrease in volume	Cool	Pale	Definite slowing	Definite	Clear and some apathy unless stimulated.
Severe	Decreased 40% to non-recordable	Weak to imperceptible	Cold	Ashen to cyanotic (mottling)	Very sluggish	Severe	Apathetic to comatose; little distress except thirst.

* It will be observed that sweating, nausea, and vomiting are not included, although these criteria were frequently referred to in World War I reports. In the Board's experience they were found to be uncommon and of no value in estimating the extent of shock. They are probably more closely related to psychologic factors, to the nature of the wound, or to reaction to morphine than they are to shock. The pulse rate can be influenced by too many unimportant factors to have value in estimating degree of shock; pulse quality, however, is important. The last three columns of the table include items not ordinarily considered in evaluating a patient's condition; since we found them useful, they are included.

jority of criteria for that category as opposed to another. These signs were inadequate, of course, for management of a case, for a comprehensive appraisal of the patient's condition must include not only an accurate concept of his present state but also a shrewd estimate of his probable course in the immediate future.

On the basis of this arbitrary classification the 186 patients under study were evaluated as to the degree of shock they had at the time of their admission to the hospital. In three of them the degree of shock could not be ascertained. Those 78 patients who were not seen on admission by any member of the Board were classified by the Board on the basis of the available clinical data and on discussion with medical officers who had seen them on admission. In the 108 patients who had been observed on admission by some member of the Board the degree of shock was probably more uniformly classified. Table 4 shows the clinical evaluation of shock and its distribution in these 108 patients as well as in the entire series. It is apparent that the distribution remained about the same when the 108 were separated from the entire group. Since the percentages were essentially unchanged when the magnitude of the cases was roughly doubled, it was assumed that the size of the sample 108 cases was adequate.

TABLE 4.—CLASSIFICATION AND DISTRIBUTION OF SHOCK

Degree of Shock	All Patients		Patients Seen on Admission by Members of Board	
	Number	Percent of Total	Number	Percent of Total
None	34	18.3	20	18.5
Slight	37	20.0	27	25.0
Moderate	55	29.5	34	31.5
Severe	57	30.6	26	24.1
Unclassified	3	1.6	1	0.9
Total	186	100.0	108	100.0

Relationship to Time from Wounding.—Examination of the records of 167 of the entire group of severely wounded men under study on whom these data

Table 6.—Wound Composition in Each Shock Category—121 Patients

Degree of Shock	Number of Patients	Major Wound Composition						Cases of Concomitant Injuries
		Penetrated Abdomen	Penetrated Chest	Lacerated Soft Tissue	Traumatic Amputation of Extremity [1]	Compound Fracture of Long Bones [2]	Miscellaneous Wounds and Injuries	
None	24	7	1	5	2	1	7 Crush	Abdominal wound and compound, comminuted fracture of humerus—1 case.
Percentage	....	29%	4%	21%	8%	4% *(8%)	29%	
Slight	24	7	3	5	2	3	1 Crush 1 Penetrated face 1 Compound, comminuted fracture of sacrum 1 Fractured vertebra	Abdominal wound and penetrating chest wound—1 case.
Percentage	....	29%	13%	21%	8%	13%	17%	
Moderate	36	13	8	5	6	4	....	Abdominal wound and penetrating chest wound—3 cases. Abdominal wound and compound, comminuted fracture of both bones of leg—1 case. Abdominal wound and compound, comminuted fracture of humerus—1 case. Chest wound and compound, comminuted fracture of arm bones—1 case. Soft-tissue wound and fractured skull—1 case. Traumatic amputation and compound, comminuted fracture of bones of other leg—1 case.
Percentage	....	36%	22%	14%	17%	11% *(19%)		
Severe	37	10	5	3	9	8	1 Crush 1 Fractured pelvis	Abdominal wound and penetrating chest wound—2 cases. Chest wound and compound, comminuted fracture of humerous—1 case. Chest wound and compound, comminuted fracture of ilium—1 case.
Percentage	....	27%	14%	8%	24%	22% *(24%)	5%	

[1] Includes some cases in which surgical amputation was undertaken early.
[2] Percentages marked with asterisk include the compound fractures listed under concomitant injuries.

were complete failed to show any correlation between the time from wounding until examination (clinical appraisal and blood analysis) and the presence or severity of shock (Table 5). The time elapsed in each of the four groups was approximately the same. There was, however, a striking correlation between severity of shock and blood loss, as will be shown later.

TABLE 5.—RELATIONSHIP OF DEGREE OF SHOCK ON HOSPITAL ENTRY TO TIME FROM WOUNDING—167 CASES

Degree of Shock	Number of Cases	Average Time from Wounding to Hospital Entry *Hours*
None	29	6.7±0.9
Slight	36	7.6±0.8
Moderate	52	6.4±0.5
Severe	50	6.9±0.7

Relationship to Wound.—Table 6 indicates the wound composition of 121 patients in each shock category. It merits some comment. If the two types of serious extremity wounds—traumatic amputation of extremities and compound fractures of long bones—are combined (the two are often very similar as to blood loss), it can readily be seen from Table 7 that the incidence of such wounds rose progressively in each category of increasing severity of shock. In the section on Blood Loss it will be shown that the greatest loss of hemoglobin occurred when the wound involved compound fracture of the long bones or

TABLE 7.—INCIDENCE OF COMBINED CASES OF SERIOUS EXTREMITY WOUNDS (MAJOR OR CONCOMITANT INJURY) IN EACH SHOCK CATEGORY

Degree of Shock	Number of Cases	Incidence of Traumatic Amputation or Compound Fracture of Long Bones *Percent of all such cases in each shock group, Table 6*
None	4	16.6
Slight	5	20.8
Moderate	14	38.9
Severe	18	48.6

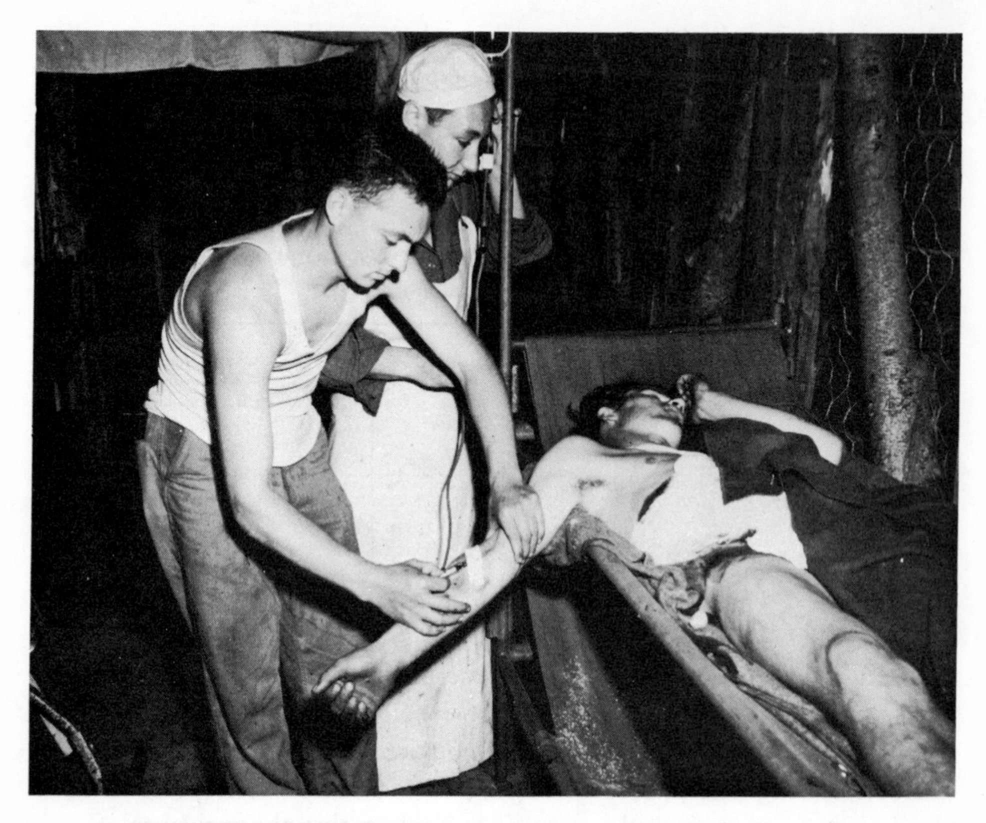

A SEVERELY WOUNDED MAN receives treatment in the forward area.

traumatic amputation of an extremity. Since most patients having such wounds were in severe shock, one can generalize with probability of accuracy and say that it is the wounds that are associated with great hemorrhage that cause severe shock. Reasons for laboring this rather obvious point will be discussed later.

In contrast to the rising incidence of severe extremity wounds in progressive shock categories, the percentage of penetrated abdomens, although rather high, shows no such consistent rise. In the severe-shock group, abdominal wounds are definitely less often a cause of the poor condition of the patient than are the combined extremity wounds. (Incidentally, this evidence does not support the view that clostridial infection plays an important part in producing shock in general.)

The question might be raised as to whether the relative importance of abdominal wounds as a cause of shock has heretofore been exaggerated. The poor prognosis often encountered in patients with abdominal wounds probably has a great deal to do with the apprehension felt in the presence of such lesions. The concealed hemorrhage or concealed contamination often present in these cases may lead to subsequent profound shock. So, while on the average abdominal wounds were not as often a cause of severe shock on hospital entry as were serious extremity wounds, the impossibility of accurate preoperative appraisal of the abdominal wound makes it difficult to exaggerate its potentialities.

Shock will be discussed in each of the following sections of this chapter and an attempt will be made to correlate degree of shock with the data under discussion whenever possible.

Cardiovascular System

Electrocardiographic Observations.—Prior to organization of the Board, 58 electrocardiographic records were made on 30 patients in severe shock and after recovery.[5] Since the observations were made on the same type of patients as those studied by the Board and under similar circumstances, electrocardiograms were not made on the Board's cases. The results of that study are summarized here. In 10 patients (one-third of that series) the blood pressure could not be measured on hospital entry. In the other two-thirds the degree of circulatory collapse was somewhat less severe, but even so the systolic blood pressures ranged from 60 to 70 millimeters of mercury and the diastolic from 20 to 40 millimeters.

Definite abnormalities of the electrocardiograms were observed in 5 of the 30 patients. The most striking feature was the normal character of the findings in the remaining twenty-five. In 2 of the 5 patients with abnormal findings, the electrocardiograms showed striking but transient inversion of the T wave in lead 1. In a patient with an intrathoracic injury there was a shift from marked right-axis deviation back to normal following operation. The electrocardiogram in the fourth patient showed bizarre QRS complexes of low voltage, and in the fifth showed evidence of an unusual degree of temporary cardiac irritability with paroxysmal fibrillation and ventricular tachycardia.

[5] Burnett, C. H.; Bland, E. F., and Beecher, H. K.: Electrocardiograms in traumatic shock in man. J. Clin. Investigation **24**: 687–690, September 1945.

This electrocardiographic evidence of abnormality is of some interest but difficult to explain. In no instance were there clinical signs of cardiac weakness, such as abnormal accentuation of the pulmonary second sound, basal râles, gallop rhythm, or congestion of the cervical veins or of the liver. As stated, the majority of the electrocardiographic findings were within normal limits. Several patients in the series were in severe shock, having low blood pressure for a period of hours with no effect upon the electrocardiogram. It may be significant that in both patients with transient inversion of the T wave in lead 1, the wound involved the left side of the chest, although so far as could be determined by roentgenographic examination and clinical findings at the time of operation, the heart and pericardium escaped injury. Furthermore, the transient nature of the inversion was more in accord with a temporary functional disturbance (possible hypoxia) than with lasting tissue injury.

Pulse Rate.—The pulse rates of the patients in the present study were considered in relationship to shock and no significant difference was found between the four categories (Table 8). The pulse rates considered were those taken as close as possible to the time the condition of the patient was evaluated. When the pulse was imperceptible at the time of initial examination, the first recordable rate was used unless the record showed evidence that the patient was well on the way to resuscitation.

TABLE 8.—RELATIONSHIP OF DEGREE OF SHOCK TO PULSE RATE—106 CASES

Pulse Rate	Degree of Shock			
	None (13 cases)	Slight (24 cases)	Moderate (34 cases)	Severe (35 cases)
Minimum	70	88	80	60
Maximum	140	150	160	144
Average	103±7.2	111±3.4	113±3.6	116±3.3

The finding that the average as well as the minimum and maximum pulse rates were about the same in all degrees of shock was surprising. There are two possible explanations for this: 1. The tachycardia in the lesser degrees of shock may have been due in part to excitement. 2. In some cases the elevation of the pulse rate (and the vasoconstriction accompanying it) may have been adequate to ward off the signs of shock. It is interesting that even patients judged to be in severe shock can have a pulse rate as low as 60 beats per minute. Of greater significance than the actual rate of the pulse is its volume, which often was decreased so much in severe shock that the pulse could no longer be felt.

Blood Pressure.—Blood pressures were analyzed in only those 70 cases out of the 186 in which they had been recorded at the time the patient's condition was evaluated. The volume of the circulating blood was also determined in these 70 patients. There was no significant fall in the average systolic blood pressure except in those in moderate or severe shock (Table 9). It will be shown that these patients with considerable shock had lost on the average 33.6 percent of their calculated normal blood volume and nearly 50 percent of the total circulating hemoglobin. In those with severe shock, the systolic blood pressure fell rapidly, the average being 49 millimeters of mercury. This group had lost approximately half the normal blood volume (see Table 22). There was, however, a progressive drop in the average diastolic blood pressure with increasing degrees of shock (Table 9). The average diastolic blood pressure of the patients in severe shock was half that of the patients in moderate shock. As severity of shock increased, there was a significant and progressive decline in the pulse pressure (Table 9). This confirmed the clinical observation that the volume of the pulse was closely correlated with the degree of shock.

TABLE 9.—RELATIONSHIP OF DEGREE OF SHOCK TO BLOOD PRESSURE—70 CASES

Degree of Shock	Systolic Blood Pressure *mm. Hg*			Diastolic Blood Pressure *mm. Hg*			Pulse Pressure *mm. Hg*		
	Lowest	Highest	Average	Lowest	Highest	Average	Lowest	Highest	Average
None (13 cases)	108	150	126±11.9	64	80	75±1.5	30	80	52±4.1
Slight (20 cases)	90	140	109±3.0	40	86	66±2.7	28	80	44±2.7
Moderate (21 cases)	30	136	95±4.9	20	90	58±3.5	10	56	36±2.8
Severe (16 cases)	*0	80	49±7.6	*0	68	25±5.8	*0	58	24±4.7

* When the values were unmeasurable (2 cases) they were considered to be 0.

"Irreversible" Changes in the Cardiovascular System.—Everyone who has treated many patients for shock has encountered some who fail to respond to the transfusion of blood deemed adequate under ordinary circumstances, and this is often attributed to "irreversible" changes that have presumably taken place during prolonged hypotension, ischemia, and anoxia. This problem is

956507 O—52——4

further discussed in the section on Blood Loss. In most instances, adequate explanation can be found for the failure of patients in shock to respond to blood transfusion; some common examples are concealed and continuing hemorrhage, hemothorax, irritant contamination of the peritoneum, peritonitis, clostridial myositis, and fat emboli. Four cases from our series are illustrative.

CASE REPORTS

Case 77.—A patient with a severe thoraco-abdominal wound was received at a forward hospital in severe shock 8¼ hours after he was wounded. Resuscitative measures were continued for nearly 9 hours. During that time he received only 1,500 cc. of whole blood. His condition failed to improve and he was operated upon but did not survive the operation.

Necropsy showed massive collapse of the right lung with a plug of mucus in the right main bronchus. The lower lobe of the left lung was collapsed and about one-third of the left upper lobe was atelectatic. There was gross dilatation of the right ventricle of the heart. On histologic examination minimal evidence of fat embolism in the pulmonary vessels was found but considered of no clinical significance.

Comment.—There was adequate cause for this patient's failure to respond to resuscitation. More aggressive measures should have been taken, including bronchoscopy and the use of more blood in less time. There should have been more concern when no improvement occurred during the first 3 hours after the patient's admission to the hospital.

Case 45.—A patient with a severe abdominal wound was admitted to a forward hospital in severe shock 8 hours after wounding. During the next 3 hours, 2 units (600 cc. total volume) of plasma and 1 liter of whole blood were transfused. The blood pressure during that time changed from imperceptible to 90 millimeters of mercury systolic and 70 diastolic. An additional unit of plasma was administered and an infusion of 500 cc. of 2-percent solution of sodium bicarbonate was given intravenously. Although this was the optimum time for surgery, operation was delayed and 5 hours later the blood pressure was again unmeasurable. It was restored to 86 millimeters of mercury systolic and 60 diastolic after transfusion of 1 liter of whole blood, and operation was performed which lasted 4 hours.

At operation the abdominal cavity was found to be "full of blood." The blood pressure and pulse rate were unmeasurable during much of the operation. The patient never regained consciousness and died 3¾ hours after the end of the operation. Necropsy showed perforation of the inferior vena cava. There was histologic evidence of minimal fat embolism in the pulmonary vessels, probably of no clinical significance.

Comment.—The recurrent hypotension in this patient was probably due to continued extraperitoneal and intraperitoneal hemorrhage. Operation should have been performed while he was responding well to resuscitative measures during the first 3 hours after admission to the hospital.

Case 100.—This patient had multiple wounds involving both arms, the left thigh, and the face. There were compound fractures of the left humerus, radius, and ulna, and of the right ulna. There was also a transection of the right femoral artery with vascular insufficiency in the leg. He was admitted in severe shock to a forward hospital 3½ hours after wounding, and within 90 minutes he received 300 cc. (total volume) of plasma and 2 liters of whole blood. He showed general improvement but his blood pressure was still only 80 millimeters of mercury systolic and 50 diastolic. His pulse rate was 144 beats per minute. Three hours after admission his blood pressure was 90 millimeters of mercury systolic and 58 diastolic. Operation was delayed for 3 additional hours. At no time during operation did the recorded blood pressure fall below 85 millimeters of mercury systolic. The patient had received a total of 4,500 cc. of whole blood before, during, and immediately after operation.

Ten hours after operation the patient's blood pressure was low and he looked pale and "anemic." A transfusion was started, but an hour later he suddenly died. Ten minutes earlier he had carried on an intelligent conversation. Pulmonary embolus was suspected but at necropsy no cause could be found for the sudden death. Microscopically, a moderately severe grade of fat embolism was found in the lungs.

Comment.—The question was raised whether the 5- or 6-hour period of hypotension in this patient could have caused irreversible changes in the cardiovascular system so that it simply "gave out" when it did. This cannot be answered with certainty. The fat embolism in retrospect appears to be the more important consideration.

Case 120.—This patient had a simple penetrating wound of the thigh caused by a shell fragment. The femoral artery below the origin of the profunda femoris was severed. During evacuation the patient had received 4 units (1,200 cc. total volume) of plasma and when he reached the evacuation hospital, about 9 hours after wounding, he must have appeared in good condition for no resuscitation was deemed necessary. At operation, performed 4½ hours after admission, the femoral artery, vein, and nerve were found to be completely transected. The vessels were ligated and the foreign body was removed.

At the conclusion of the operation, the systolic blood pressure was only 70 millimeters of mercury and remained between 70 and 60 throughout the day. Despite this the patient appeared to have good color and his skin was not cold. Transfusion of 1 liter of whole blood did not improve the blood pressure. The right leg looked as though it would not survive. Anuria developed and the patient died 48 hours after operation. Necropsy revealed nothing to account for the postoperative hypotension. There was no concealed hemorrhage and no evidence of clostridial myositis in the involved extremity. There was no histologic evidence of fat embolism.

Comment.—This patient probably had lost more blood than was realized.

Resuscitation

Before admission of the patients in this study to a forward hospital, resuscitative efforts had been limited chiefly to control of pain and hemorrhage and to administration of blood plasma. Relatively little whole blood was given. The 108 patients seen by us on admission had received, on the average, 2 units[6] of plasma before the first blood sample was taken. Plasma administration was distributed in this group as follows:

Number of Patients	*Units of Plasma*	*Number of Patients*	*Units of Plasma*
32	none	1	6
25	1	1	7
17	2	2	8
13	3	1	9
12	4	1	11
3	5		

Thus 69 percent (74) of these patients had received two units (600 cc.) or less of blood plasma before or shortly after arrival at the most forward hospital. Twenty-seven of the 108 patients received transfusions of whole blood prior to withdrawal of the first blood specimen for laboratory analysis. Three of these, or 3 percent, had received whole blood in an aid station before admission to a forward hospital. The blood transfusions were distributed as follows:

Number of Patients	*Units of Blood*
13	1/5 to 1
10	1½ to 2
2	3
1	4
1	6

The following tabulation summarizes the average quantities of blood and of blood plasma used in resuscitating 157 of the very seriously wounded patients in our series (the 108 referred to above and 49 others on whom we had clinical notes):

Blood plasma preoperatively (average of 122 cases)	3.08 units
Blood plasma during operation (average of 10 cases)	1.68 units
Whole blood preoperatively (average of 127 cases)	1,450 cc.
Whole blood during operation (average of 95 cases)	1,160 cc.

[6] 1 unit = 250 cc. of normal plasma diluted to 300 cubic centimeters.

In round numbers, our average patient in this series had just over 3 units (total volume) of blood plasma and 5 blood transfusions (total of about 2,500 cc. of whole blood) to support him from the time of wounding until his operation was completed. It is interesting to observe that plasma was used *during* surgery in only 10 of these 157 patients.

The information concerning the cases referred to here was drawn from the shock tents of most of the hospitals of the Fifth Army and represents a broad sample of current practice in Italy over the last year of the European War. Essentially the same type of case had been studied by two of us earlier at Anzio.[7] In that series the average patient received 1,537 cc. of whole blood (three transfusions) to prepare him for and carry him through surgery. These three transfusions contrast with the five referred to above. A notable difference between the Anzio study and Mediterranean Theater practice in general was in the time elapsed from hospital entry to start of surgery. In the Anzio study this averaged 2 hours, 21 minutes. Reference to an earlier part of this section on Time from Wounding to Hospital Entry and Surgery will show that over the Fifth Army Area as a whole, the average time from hospital entry to surgery varied from 5 hours to 8 hours. Two differing views as to the correct preparation of wounded men for surgery are represented in these figures: the extended, and the rapid. The extended required five transfusions of whole blood; the rapid, three. This has been discussed in a previous publication.[8]

Plasma Protein Concentration and Hematocrit Values On Admission to Forward Hospital

The concentration of protein in the plasma and the blood hematocrit value (both calculated from specific gravities measured by the copper sulfate method[9]) give a clue to the shifts that have taken place between the blood stream and the tissues as well as to blood loss from the body. When considered

[7] BEECHER, H. K., and BURNETT, C. H.: Field experience in use of blood and blood substitutes (plasma, albumin) in seriously wounded men. M. Bull. North African Theat. Op. (no. 1) **2**: 2–7, July 1944.

[8] BEECHER, H. K.: Preparation of battle casualties for surgery. Ann. Surg. **121**: 769–792, June 1945.

[9] PHILLIPS, R. A.; VAN SLYKE, D. D.; DOLE, V. P.; EMERSON, K., JR.; HAMILTON, P. B., and ARCHIBALD, R. M.: Copper sulfate method for measuring specific gravities of whole blood and plasma. BUMED News Letter, U. S. Navy, vol. 1, June 25, 1943.

with quantitative measurements of whole-blood loss, a fairly accurate picture of one consequence of the wound can be obtained. The plasma protein and hematocrit levels were determined in our patients shortly after their admission to the most forward hospital, before resuscitation, anesthetization, or operation had been undertaken.

Relationship to Type of Wound

In Table 10 the relationship of the average plasma protein concentration and the average hematocrit value to the type of wound is shown for 50 patients who, prior to study, had received only 1 unit (300 cc.) of blood plasma or less than 1 unit (in some instances no plasma had been administered). The patients whose wounds were peripheral are grouped and compared with those having nonperipheral wounds; crush cases are not included.

From the table it may be seen that there is no decided difference between the plasma protein levels of patients with peripheral and those with nonperipheral wounds. On the other hand the hematocrit values were significantly higher in the latter group which is consistent with the hemoconcentration sometimes found in such patients. There was also less loss of hemoglobin (as will be discussed in the section on Blood Loss) in those patients with intra-abdominal and thoraco-abdominal wounds than in those having severe wounds of the extremities. Maintenance of a more nearly normal blood volume in patients with such nonperipheral wounds doubtless reduces the need and tendency for blood dilution, although this factor alone would not account for the hemoconcentration when it is found in such cases.

TABLE 10.—RELATIONSHIP OF PLASMA PROTEIN CONCENTRATION AND HEMATOCRIT VALUE ON ADMISSION TO TYPE OF WOUND IN PATIENTS WHO HAD RECEIVED 1 UNIT OR LESS OF PLASMA

Type of Wound (Exclusive of crush)	Average Plasma Protein Concentration *Gm. per 100 cc. (normal: 6.5)*	Average Hematocrit Value *cc. cells in 100 cc. (normal: 47)*
Peripheral (25 cases)	**6.2±0.1**	**37.4±1.0**
Nonperipheral (Abdominal, thoracic, and thoraco-abdominal) (25 cases)	**6.5±0.1**	**42.0±1.0**

Relationship to Blood Loss

When average plasma protein concentrations and average hematocrit values in patients with peripheral and nonperipheral wounds are compared with loss of blood volume (39 cases), it may be seen from Table 11 that the hematocrit values were significantly lower in all patients who had lost more than 30 percent of their calculated normal blood volume. The hematocrit level of 36 is 23.4 percent below the normal of 47 (Wintrobe method).

In the case of the plasma proteins, however, even when there was a loss of 30 percent or more of the normal blood volume, the average concentration was 6.1 Gm. per 100 cc. (only 6.1 percent below the normal of 6.5). In other words, the hematocrit level fell proportionately about four times as much as that of the plasma proteins. The blood appears to have been diluted by protein-rich fluid (6.1 Gm. per 100 cc. of blood). The evidence is too meager to justify much speculation here. However, as pointed out by Evans,[10] the axial stream of corpuscles is surrounded by a plasma envelope. This varies in thickness and total volume, depending upon certain hydraulic principles. It might be possible that the alterations in the circulation caused by the loss of 30 percent or more of the normal volume of blood (slowing of the peripheral circulation, for example) resulted in dragging an appreciable volume of plasma with normal protein content into

TABLE 11.—RELATIONSHIP OF PLASMA PROTEIN CONCENTRATION, HEMATOCRIT VALUE, AND TYPE OF WOUND TO BLOOD LOSS IN PATIENTS WHO HAD RECEIVED 1 UNIT OR LESS OF PLASMA

Blood Volume	Loss of Less than 30 Percent			Loss of 30 Percent or More		
Type of Wound (Exclusive of crush)	Peripheral (10 cases)	Non-peripheral[1] (17 cases)	All Types (27 cases)	Peripheral (8 cases)	Non-peripheral[1] (4 cases)	All Types (12 cases)
Average Plasma Protein Concentration[2] . . . . (Gm. per 100 cc.)	6.4±0.1	6.5±0.1	6.5±0.1	6.0±0.1	6.4	6.1±0.1
Average Hematocrit Value[2] . . (cc. cells in 100 cc.)	39.0±1.7	43.0±1.0	41.5±1.0	35.0±1.3	37.8	36.0±1.1

[1] Abdominal, thoracic, and thoraco-abdominal.
[2] Determinations made on hospital admission.

[10] EVANS, ROBLEY: Personal communication.

the circulating blood. Or it might be possible that protein was brought into the circulation from the liver.

Influence of Plasma Therapy

The influence of previous administration of blood plasma upon the concentration of plasma protein and the hematocrit value was considered, and the findings in different types of wounds are shown in Table 12 and Charts 1 and 2. Only three of the patients had had blood transfusions; these will be ignored. It is clear from the table and charts that plasma therapy did not influence the plasma protein level, but it did have an important effect on the hematocrit level.

The plasma protein concentration and hematocrit value were also analyzed in regard to shock, the data being broken down into two categories in which "no shock" and "slight shock" were grouped together, as were "moderate shock" and "severe shock." No important differences were found between the two categories.

TABLE 12.—EFFECT OF PLASMA THERAPY ON AVERAGE PLASMA PROTEIN AND HEMATOCRIT ADMISSION LEVELS IN 89 PATIENTS WITH VARIOUS TYPES OF WOUNDS

Type of Wound (Crush excluded)	Number of Cases	Units of Plasma Received	Plasma Protein Concentration *Gm. per 100 cc.*	Hematocrit Value *cc. cells in 100 cc.*	Time from Wounding to Determination *hours*
Peripheral	25	0 to 1	6.2±0.1	37.4±1.0	8.5±1.2
	17	2 to 3	5.9±0.1	31.9±1.5	*8.1±1.5
	13	4 to 6	6.1±0.1	*28.6±1.9	9.8±1.2
Total . . .	55	0 to 6	6.1±0.1	33.7±0.9	8.7±0.7
Abdominal	11	0 to 1	6.6±0.2	44.1±1.8	6.3±1.4
	5	2 to 4	6.7±0.3	40.2±4.3	7.8±3.1
	3	5 to 11	6.1	*32.2	*12.2
Total . . .	19	0 to 11	6.6±0.1	41.6±1.9	6.8±1.3
Thoracic	8	0 to 1	6.5±0.2	40.0±1.2	7.9±2.6
	7	2 to 5	6.6±0.2	35.4±1.8	7.2±1.7
Total . . .	15	0 to 5	6.5±0.1	37.8±1.2	7.6±1.4

* No determination made in one case. (Determinations made on hospital admission.)

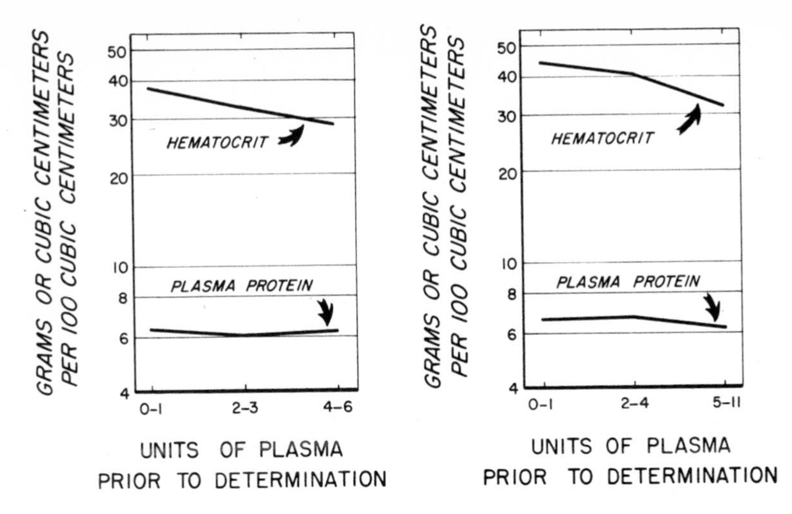

CHART 1. Influence of plasma therapy on plasma protein and hematocrit levels in peripheral wounds

CHART 2. Influence of plasma therapy on plasma protein and hematocrit levels in abdominal wounds

Relationship to Shock

Plasma protein and hematocrit levels were also studied in relation to the clinical condition of about 100 badly wounded patients (crush cases excluded) on admission to the forward hospital. The fall in average plasma protein concentration is probably significant as the cases are grouped in Table 13 and Chart 3; the fall in hematocrit value is definitely significant. There was no evidence of hemoconcentration. When the patients were grouped according to

TABLE 13.—PLASMA PROTEIN AND HEMATOCRIT LEVELS ON ADMISSION IN RELATION TO SHOCK*

Degree of Shock	None	Slight	Moderate	Severe	All Cases
Average Plasma Protein Concentration . . . . . (Gm. per 100 cc.)	6.6±0.1 (15 cases)	6.4±0.1 (26 cases)	6.2±0.1 (34 cases)	6.0±0.1 (25 cases)	6.3±0.1 (100 cases)
Average Hematocrit Value (cc. cells in 100 cc.)	42.5±1.7 (15 cases)	38.4±1.5 (26 cases)	34.6±1.0 (33 cases)	31.5±1.5 (24 cases)	36.1±0.8 (98 cases)

* All types of wounds, exclusive of crush cases.

TABLE 14.—PLASMA PROTEIN AND HEMATOCRIT LEVELS ON ADMISSION IN RELATION TO SHOCK IN PATIENTS WITH ABDOMINAL WOUNDS

Degree of Shock	None—Slight	Moderate—Severe
Average Plasma Protein Concentration . . . (Gm. per 100 cc.)	6.9±0.1 (10 cases)	6.1±0.2 (9 cases)
Average Hematocrit Value . . . . (cc. cells in 100 cc.)	47.0±1.6 (10 cases)	34.9±1.8 (8 cases)
Average Hours after Wounding	7.0±1.5 (10 cases)	11.6 (9 cases)

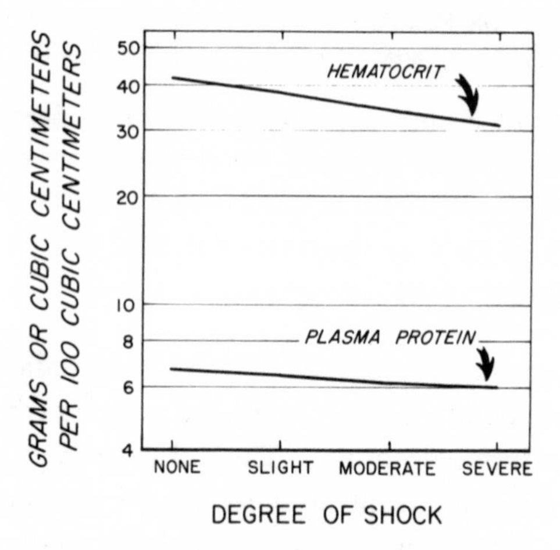

CHART 3. Plasma protein and hematocrit levels in relation to shock—all types of wounds

location of the major wound, there was no significant fall in the concentration of plasma protein in those with peripheral wounds in relation to the degree of shock. The findings in patients with abdominal wounds showed up differently (Table 14). In the group with minimal shock, the plasma protein concentration may possibly be accounted for by weeping of the irritated peritoneal surfaces, fluid being released which contained less protein than the plasma. As shock became moderate or severe, probably due to greater blood loss, the plasma protein concentration fell to a figure like that for extremity wounds, with hemodilution overcoming the effects of exudation. These data indicate that the plasma protein and hematocrit values can vary independently.

Blood Loss

Volume and Hemoglobin

The quantity of blood a wounded man can lose and yet recover has generally been underestimated. One indication that this is so was the fact, well shown in the prolonged campaigns of the Mediterranean Theater, that robust young soldiers tolerated surgery well, long before the blood volume or even the blood pressure had been restored to normal. Actually the concept of restoration of the patient in shock to normal prior to surgery is based upon a false premise. Full organic restoration probably requires days to achieve. A good response of a young wounded man to treatment is by no means admissible evidence that his circulatory system has been restored to normal; it is evidence of the existence of safety factors in human physiology. These points have been discussed elsewhere.[11]

In the belief that measurement of the blood loss that had been sustained by these severely wounded men by the time of their arrival at a forward hospital would clarify the matter of the importance of whole blood for the wounded, such a study was carried out. The direct relationship between quantity of blood lost and degree of shock had long been recognized, but further evidence of this relationship was desirable in view of the ever-recurring suggestions that the cause of shock is mysterious and to be explained by the presence of toxins in the body or by the breakdown of some vague but vital force.

The blood volume and the hemoglobin concentration were determined in 67 patients[12] shortly after their arrival at the most forward hospital (which in most instances was a field hospital). The blood volume loss and the total hemoglobin loss, expressed as percentages of a calculated normal for each patient, were then determined on the basis of these findings. Normal blood volume was considered to be 8.5 percent of the body weight, after Gregersen. (See Appendix C for the method used.) Peters[13] has commented on the loss of the dye T–1824 from the blood stream. Such loss of dye would of course

[11] See footnote 8. Also see section on Resuscitation in volume on general surgery of the series: *The Medical Department of the United States Army*. To be published.

[12] The blood studies were actually made in 71 cases (see Table 15), but one case was discarded because of a probable technical error and three others are excluded from the present discussion since they represent types not common to the group; namely, two crush injuries (Cases 93 and 124) and a head injury (Case A–7).

[13] PETERS, J. P.: Role of sodium in production of edema. New England J. Med. **239**: 353–362, Sept. 2, 1948.

TABLE 15.—INITIAL BLOOD CHANGES IN 71 SEVERELY WOUNDED MEN

Case No.	Blood Pressure at Time of Blood Volume Determination	Degree of Shock	Blood Sugar	Time after Wounding	Blood Volume Deviation from Normal (percent)			Circulating Hemoglobin	
					From Observed Value	By Correction		Hemoglobin Present	Hemoglobin Deviation from Normal by Correction B
						A	B		
	mm. Hg		*mg. per 100 cc.*	*hours*				*grams*	*percent*
53	80/40	Moderate	106	3¼	−10.6	−22.9	−22.9	689.2	−37.8
83	130/70	Slight	....	5¼	+13.1	−3.3	−0.8	941.1	−16.1
91	108/78	None	....	2¾	−26.0	−37.7	−37.7	464.3	−52.9
[1]93	(0)	Severe	....	14½	−11.7	−34.0	−30.3	1,203.8	+2.6
100	80/50	....do....	....	4½	−28.4	−69.0	−65.0	551.3	−76.6
102	150/80	None	....	3¼	−21.3	−36.9	−29.1	702.8	−39.0
107	80/50	Moderate	374	3	−20.7	−78.6	−68.9	419.2	−77.6
108	58/0	Severe	372	3½	−25.5	−38.9	−30.0	341.9	−64.1
110	(0)	....do....	....	¾	−35.7	−37.6	−37.6	553.5	−47.4
111	120/80	Slight	157	14½	−2.7	−7.1	−7.1	851.8	−5.1
113	94/58	....do....	149	3¼	−14.9	−20.2	−20.2	573.1	−28.2
122	50/30	Severe	87	4	−34.4	−55.0	−48.2	632.3	−58.4
[1]124	120/64	None	....	10¼	+15.3	−2.8	−2.8	1,012.5	−1.6
125	72/58	Severe	125	23	−21.3	−33.0	−29.1	562.2	−52.7
126	100/60	Moderate	183	2¾	−30.9	−32.3	−32.3	666.6	−44.4
127	90/40	Slight	....	11	−39.8	−59.4	−44.2	331.2	−65.9
128	110/80	....do....	184	6½	+6.2	−49.8	−32.6	837.8	−39.8
129	120/64	Moderate	191	5½	−21.7	−30.9	−21.7	485.6	−44.2
130	60/20	Severe	272	5	−31.3	−51.6	−40.5	410.9	−62.0
131	40/20	....do....	177	5¾	−29.8	−43.6	−39.0	477.5	−54.3
134	120/76	None	....	15¼	−7.8	−11.3	−7.8	1,098.9	−3.8
139	(0)	Severe	....	9	−19.3	−75.7	−23.3	491.0	−54.5
140	100/60	Slight	141	4½	+16.8	−1.1	−1.1	1,002.2	−5.8
141	100/60	....do....	131	7	−20.2	−25.5	−25.5	648.5	−39.1
142	110/70	Moderate	210	6¾	−25.7	−31.9	−27.0	521.3	−43.0
143	80/54	....do....	203	6	+3.4	−13.9	+1.8	790.8	−24.0
144	90/62	Slight	....	12¼	+8.8	−6.7	−1.5	542.8	−36.6
145	100/50	....do....	....	9	−8.4	−15.7	−12.1	785.0	−30.7
147	80/48	Severe	165	13¾	−6.5	−24.1	−14.3	510.4	−42.7
148	74/20	Moderate	175	12	−5.2	−24.8	−14.9	493.2	−45.8
149	48/?	Severe	115	17¾	−2.3	−31.3	−9.8	693.3	−32.7
A-1	116/60	Slight	155	2¾	−9.3	−17.4	−14.0	967.2	−22.6
A-2	114/62	....do....	170	4¼	−2.3	−2.3	−2.3	922.0	−9.6
A-3	136/90	Moderate	185	4	+5.4	+2.9	+2.9	896.6	−8.3
A-4	132/72	None	93	4¼	−8.2	−8.2	−8.2	639.0	−31.1
A-5	120/86	Slight	106	8	−25.3	−25.3	−25.3	604.4	−35.6
A-6	118/64	Moderate	208	3¼	−24.2	−29.8	−24.2	479.7	−38.4

[1] Case of crush injury.
(0): Not measurable.

TABLE 15.—INITIAL BLOOD CHANGES IN 71 SEVERELY WOUNDED MEN—*Continued*

Case No.	Blood Pressure at Time of Blood Volume Determination	Degree of Shock	Blood Sugar	Time after Wounding	Blood Volume Deviation from Normal (percent)			Circulating Hemoglobin	
					From Observed Value	By Correction		Hemoglobin Present	Hemoglobin Deviation from Normal by Correction B
						A	B		
	mm. Hg		*mg. per 100 cc.*	*hours*				*grams*	*percent*
[2] A-7	(0)	?	315	½	−31.6	−31.6	−31.6	540.6	−47.0
A-8	108/70	Slight	....	10	−14.8	−14.8	−14.8	667.4	−23.3
A-9	112/70	Moderate	....	7½	−25.9	−35.0	−25.9	449.9	−49.1
A-10	108/74	Slight	....	11	−3.7	−3.7	−3.7	842.5	−28.4
A-11	110/76	....do....	79	5¼	−29.9	−33.4	−29.9	716.4	−37.4
A-12	104/70	Moderate	164	2¾	−11.3	−20.4	−20.4	676.2	−35.6
A-13	150/70	None	121	18¾	−18.4	−18.4	−18.4	555.0	−36.2
A-14	100/80	Moderate	93	5¼	−32.6	−40.2	−32.6	522.7	−50.3
A-15	104/70	....do....	143	7	−29.2	−44.4	−29.2	488.3	−53.5
A-16	130/70	None	139	5¼	−8.2	−10.5	−8.2	895.8	−12.2
A-17	140/60	Slight	201	3½	−41.5	−63.9	−49.0	411.6	−69.1
A-18	30/20	Moderate	134	8¼	−42.7	−46.6	−42.7	398.4	−61.7
A-19	116/78	None	167	8¼	−31.9	−31.9	−31.9	579.3	−42.5
A-20	92/50	Slight	145	13¼	−34.1	−37.9	−34.1	429.1	−56.6
A-21	68/50	Severe	234	4¼	−46.7	−71.0	−54.8	240.4	−83.8
A-22	140/80	None	110	1½	−2.8	−2.8	−2.8	1,200.6	+11.5
A-23	128/80	....do....	127	4½	+17.0	+17.0	+17.0	1,120.7	+13.3
A-24	110/70	....do....	140	4½	−0.3	−10.3	−10.3	832.5	−6.4
A-25	126/80	Slight	140	3¼	−18.7	−22.3	−18.7	923.5	−15.1
A-26	110/70	....do....	196	4	−7.4	−7.4	−7.4	711.6	−23.1
[3] A-27	114/80	None	125	5¼	+32.7	+32.7	+32.7	1,170.6	+48.4
A-28	64/20	Severe	218	6¾	−9.2	−28.0	−9.2	522.7	−38.7
A-29	80/38	....do....	382	5¾	−28.2	−54.9	−37.1	407.0	−63.6
A-30	88/40	Moderate	198	5¼	−31.8	−54.1	−40.7	378.7	−66.7
A-31	80/52	....do....	180	10	−10.2	−17.8	−10.2	778.8	−26.9
A-32	80/40	....do....	115	7½	−25.4	−37.9	−29.5	549.8	−46.8
A-33	90/50	....do....	175	5¼	−2.9	−28.4	−25.3	585.5	−40.6
A-34	80/68	Severe	125	26¾	+12.8	−16.6	−8.2	952.8	−19.0
A-35	86/66	Moderate	159	?	−37.5	−41.9	−37.5	415.2	−55.1
A-36	108/88	....do....	163	20½	−34.1	−38.6	−38.6	388.1	−56.8
A-37	120/68	....do....	136	3	−41.6	−52.4	−52.4	418.2	−62.4
A-38	(0)	Severe	133	?	−24.6	−58.3	−48.7	482.2	−66.1
A-39	124/72	None	184	4	−7.1	−7.1	−7.1	786.4	−20.5
A-40	100/64	Slight	126	3½	+3.5	+3.5	+3.5	899.4	−5.5

[2] Case of head injury.
[3] Probable technical error in this case.
(0): Not measurable.

TABLE 16.—BLOOD CHANGES IN 69 SEVERELY WOUNDED MEN CLASSIFIED ACCORDING TO DEGREE OF SHOCK

A. No Shock—12 Patients

Case No.	Blood Volume and Total Hemoglobin Determinations *Percent deviation from normal*						Blood Pressure at Time of Blood Volume Determination *mm. Hg*	Time after Wounding *hours*	Blood Sugar *mg. per 100 cc.*
	Blood Volume			Hemoglobin					
	From Observed Value	By Correction A	By Correction B	From Observed Value	By Correction A	By Correction B			
91	−26.0	−37.7	−37.7	−43.1	−52.9	−52.9	108/78	2¾	—
102	−21.3	−36.9	−29.1	−31.1	−39.0	−39.0	150/80	3¼	—
*124	+15.3	−2.8	−2.8	+14.7	−1.6	−1.6	120/64	10¼	—
134	−7.8	−11.3	−7.8	−3.8	−3.8	−3.8	120/76	15¼	—
A-4	−8.2	−8.2	−8.2	−31.1	−31.1	−31.1	132/72	4¼	93
A-13	−18.4	−18.4	−18.4	−36.2	−36.2	−36.2	150/70	18¾	121
A-16	−8.2	−10.5	−8.2	−12.2	−12.2	−12.2	130/70	5¼	139
A-19	−31.9	−31.9	−31.9	−42.5	−42.5	−42.5	116/78	8¼	167
A-22	−2.8	−2.8	−2.8	+11.5	+11.5	+11.5	140/80	1½	110
A-23	+17.0	+17.0	+17.0	+13.3	+13.3	+13.3	128/80	4½	127
A-24	−0.3	−10.3	−10.3	+4.1	−6.4	−6.4	110/70	4½	140
A-39	−7.1	−7.1	−7.1	−20.5	−20.5	−20.5	124/72	4	184

* Case of crush injury.

give a falsely high value for blood volume. Our blood-loss values were estimated by difference, difference between an average normal blood volume (8.5 percent of body weight) and the value found. Therefore the losses we report are lower than the fact; they are minimal rather than maximal.

To compensate for the effect on his blood volume of the blood and plasma received by the patient, certain corrections were applied to our blood volume determinations. The majority of patients had received some plasma prior to hospital admission and a few had received whole blood. Although blood volume determinations were made as soon after hospital admission as possible, resuscitative procedures had likewise been initiated. Actually, in most cases, determinations and resuscitation proceeded concurrently. Two methods of correcting blood volume findings were therefore utilized: Correction A and Correction B.

Correction A was the subtraction of the total quantity of blood and blood plasma received by the patient from the time of wounding until

TABLE 16.—BLOOD CHANGES IN 69 SEVERELY WOUNDED MEN CLASSIFIED ACCORDING TO DEGREE OF SHOCK

B. Slight Shock—20 Patients

Case No.	Blood Volume and Total Hemoglobin Determinations *Percent deviation from normal*						Blood Pressure at Time of Blood Volume Determination *mm. Hg*	Time after Wounding *hours*	Blood Sugar *mg. per 100 cc.*
	Blood Volume			Hemoglobin					
	From Observed Value	By Correction A	By Correction B	From Observed Value	By Correction A	By Correction B			
83	+13.1	−3.3	−0.8	−3.9	−16.1	−16.1	130/70	5¼	—
111	−2.7	−7.1	−7.1	−5.1	−5.1	−5.1	120/80	14½	157
113	−14.9	−20.2	−20.2	−23.4	−28.2	−28.2	94/58	3¼	149
127	−39.8	−59.4	−44.2	−63.1	−65.9	−65.9	90/40	11	—
128	+6.2	−49.8	−32.6	−9.7	−39.8	−39.8	110/80	6½	184
140	+16.8	−1.1	−1.1	+11.7	−5.8	−5.8	100/60	4½	141
141	−20.2	−25.5	−25.5	−34.7	−39.1	−39.1	100/60	7	131
144	+8.8	−6.7	−1.5	−30.0	−36.6	−36.6	90/62	12¼	—
145	−8.4	−15.7	−12.1	−27.8	−30.7	−30.7	100/50	9	—
A-1	−9.3	−17.4	−14.0	−17.8	−22.6	−22.6	116/60	2¾	155
A-2	−2.3	−2.3	−2.3	−9.6	−9.6	−9.6	114/62	4¼	170
A-5	−25.3	−25.3	−25.3	−35.6	−35.6	−35.6	120/86	8	106
A-8	−14.8	−14.8	−14.8	−23.3	−23.3	−23.3	108/70	10	—
A-10	−3.7	−3.7	−3.7	−28.4	−28.4	−28.4	108/74	11½	—
A-11	−29.9	−33.4	−29.9	−37.4	−37.4	−37.4	110/76	5¼	79
A-17	−41.5	−63.9	−49.0	−61.6	−69.1	−69.1	140/60	3½	201
A-20	−34.1	−37.9	−34.1	−56.6	−56.6	−56.6	92/50	13¼	145
A-25	−18.7	−22.3	−18.7	−15.1	−15.1	−15.1	126/80	3¼	140
A-26	−7.4	−7.4	−7.4	−23.1	−23.1	−23.1	110/70	4	196
A-40	+3.5	+3.5	+3.5	−5.5	−5.5	−5.5	100/64	3½	126

completion of the test.

Correction B was the subtraction of only the quantity of blood and plasma received from the time of the patient's hospital admission until completion of the test.

Correction A was applied for the purpose of correlating the patient's clinical condition on arrival at the hospital with the amount of blood (the percentage of his estimated normal blood volume) that he had actually lost due to his wounds, regardless of the amount that may have been replaced. Correction B was for correlation between the patient's clinical condition on arrival and the blood deficit existing at that time. The same corrections were applied in calculating the total hemoglobin loss. However, in the case of hemoglobin

TABLE 16.—BLOOD CHANGES IN 69 SEVERELY WOUNDED MEN CLASSIFIED ACCORDING TO DEGREE OF SHOCK

C. Moderate Shock—21 Patients

Case No.	Blood Volume and Total Hemoglobin Determinations *Percent deviation from normal*						Blood Pressure at Time of Blood Volume Determination *mm. Hg*	Time after Wounding *hours*	Blood Sugar *mg. per 100 cc.*
	Blood Volume			Hemoglobin					
	From Observed Value	By Correction A	By Correction B	From Observed Value	By Correction A	By Correction B			
53	−10.6	−22.9	−22.9	−29.6	−37.8	−37.8	80/40	3¼	—
107	−20.7	−78.6	−68.9	−49.5	−77.6	−77.6	80/50	3	374
126	−30.9	−32.3	−32.3	−43.0	−44.4	−44.4	100/60	2¾	183
129	−21.7	−30.9	−21.7	−44.2	−44.2	−44.2	120/64	5½	191
142	−25.7	−31.9	−27.0	−41.9	−43.0	−43.0	110/70	6¾	210
143	+3.4	−13.9	+1.8	−22.5	−24.0	−24.0	80/54	6	203
148	−5.2	−24.8	−14.9	−39.6	−45.8	−45.8	74/20	12	175
A-3	+5.4	+2.9	+2.9	−5.8	−8.3	−8.3	136/90	4	185
A-6	−24.2	−29.8	−24.2	−38.4	−38.4	−38.4	118/64	3¼	208
A-9	−25.9	−35.0	−25.9	−49.1	−49.1	−49.1	112/70	7½	—
A-12	−11.3	−20.4	−20.4	−23.5	−35.6	−35.6	104/70	2¾	164
A-14	−32.6	−40.2	−32.6	−50.3	−50.3	−50.3	100/80	5¼	93
A-15	−29.2	−44.4	−29.2	−53.5	−53.5	−53.5	104/70	7	143
A-18	−42.7	−46.6	−42.7	−61.7	−61.7	−61.7	30/20	8¼	134
A-30	−31.8	−54.1	−40.7	−57.8	−66.7	−66.7	88/40	5¼	198
A-31	−10.2	−17.8	−10.2	−26.9	−26.9	−26.9	80/52	10	180
A-32	−25.4	−37.9	−29.5	−42.6	−46.8	−46.8	80/40	7½	115
A-33	−2.9	−28.4	−25.3	−21.7	−40.6	−40.6	90/50	5¼	175
A-35	−37.5	−41.9	−37.5	−55.1	−55.1	−55.1	86/66	?	159
A-36	−34.1	−38.6	−38.6	−56.8	−56.8	−56.8	108/88	20½	163
A-37	−41.6	−52.4	−52.4	−62.4	−62.4	−62.4	120/68	3	136

there was essential agreement between calculation A and calculation B because, with rare exceptions, whole blood had not been administered before the patient reached the most forward hospital.

Tables 15 through 22 show blood and hemoglobin loss in relation to other findings for patients individually and by groups. The loss is given as the percentage difference between a calculated normal and the observed value, or between the calculated normal and the observed value modified by Corrections A and B. For blood all three determinations are shown. For hemoglobin only the estimated loss derived by Correction B is shown. It will be noted that a few entries (shown as plus values in the tables) seem to indicate that the blood volume was greater than normal despite loss of blood. Several factors, indi-

TABLE 16.—BLOOD CHANGES IN 69 SEVERELY WOUNDED MEN CLASSIFIED ACCORDING TO DEGREE OF SHOCK

D. Severe Shock—16 Patients

Case No.	Blood Volume and Total Hemoglobin Determinations *Percent deviation from normal*						Blood Pressure at Time of Blood Volume Determination *mm. Hg*	Time after Wounding *hours*	Blood Sugar[1] *mg. per 100 cc.*
	Blood Volume			Hemoglobin					
	From Observed Value	By Correction		From Observed Value	By Correction				
		A	B		A	B			
[2]93	−11.7	−34.0	−30.3	+12.0	+2.6	+2.6	(0)	14½	—
100	−28.4	−69.0	−65.0	−44.1	−76.6	−76.6	80/50	4½	—
108	−25.5	−38.9	−30.0	−61.8	−64.1	−64.1	58/0	3½	372
110	−35.7	−37.6	−37.6	−45.7	−47.4	−47.4	(0)	¾	—
122	−34.4	−55.0	−48.2	−45.9	−58.4	−58.4	50/30	4	87
125	−21.3	−33.0	−29.1	−44.9	−52.7	−52.7	72/58	23	125
130	−31.3	−51.6	−40.5	−51.6	−62.0	−62.0	60/20	5	272
131	−29.8	−43.6	−39.0	−45.1	−54.3	−54.3	40/20	5¾	177
139	−19.3	−75.7	−23.3	−50.5	−70.7	−54.5	(0)	9	—
147	−6.5	−24.1	−14.3	−37.5	−42.7	−42.7	80/48	13¾	165
149	−2.3	−31.3	−9.8	−26.1	−32.7	−32.7	48/?	17¾	115
A-21	−46.7	−71.0	−54.8	−75.6	−83.8	−83.8	68/50	4¼	234
A-28	−9.2	−28.0	−9.2	−38.7	−38.7	−38.7	64/20	6¾	218
A-29	−28.2	−54.9	−37.1	−54.7	−63.6	−63.6	80/38	5¾	382
A-34	+12.8	−16.6	−8.2	(0)	−19.0	−19.0	80/68	26¾	125
A-38	−24.6	−58.3	−48.7	−42.0	−66.1	−66.1	(0)	?	133

[1] Blood sugar was determined in another patient in severe shock (Case 112) 11¾ hours after wounding and found to be 216 mg. per 100 cc. of blood.

[2] Case of crush injury.

(0): Not measurable.

vidually or collectively, might have brought about this apparent discrepancy: 1. In the case of uncorrected entries, blood and plasma administered may have been in excess of blood loss. 2. Entries are from calculations based upon an *average* normal which may have been too low for some patients. 3. There may have been errors in technique in blood volume determination.

Relationship of Blood Loss to Type of Wound

Fifty-nine of the patients listed in Tables 15 and 16 suffered primarily from a single major wound (abdominal, chest, or peripheral) and could therefore be more readily studied as to the relationship of blood loss to type of wound.

956507 O—52——5

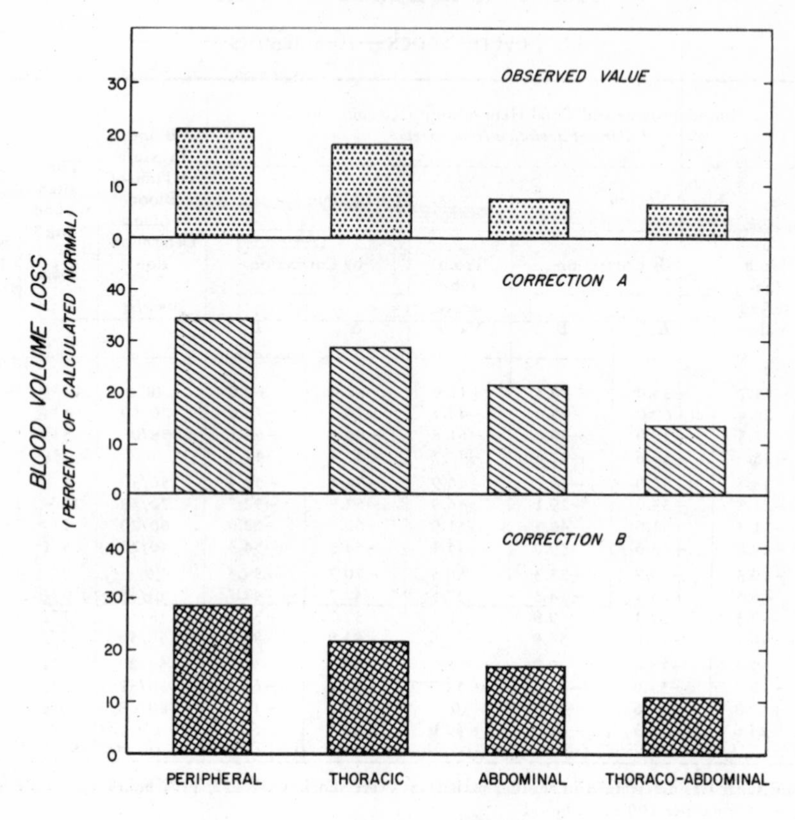

CHART 4. BLOOD VOLUME LOSS IN RELATION TO LOCATION OF WOUND

The findings in these 59 patients, and in 6 others who had combined thoraco-abdominal wounds, are presented in Tables 17 and 18, and in Charts 4 and 5. The huge standard errors present in several instances indicate the wide variations in the results found. From the table it would appear that loss of blood volume was greatest in the patients with peripheral wounds (Table 17). However the number of cases was small, the variability in the data was wide, and the true state of affairs possibly was masked by dilution of the blood volume after wounding by movement of fluid from the tissues to the blood stream.

The data on hemoglobin loss are probably more revealing. There is a significantly greater loss of hemoglobin in men with peripheral wounds than in those with abdominal wounds (Table 18) and in this case the situation is not

CHART 5. HEMOGLOBIN LOSS IN RELATION TO LOCATION OF WOUND

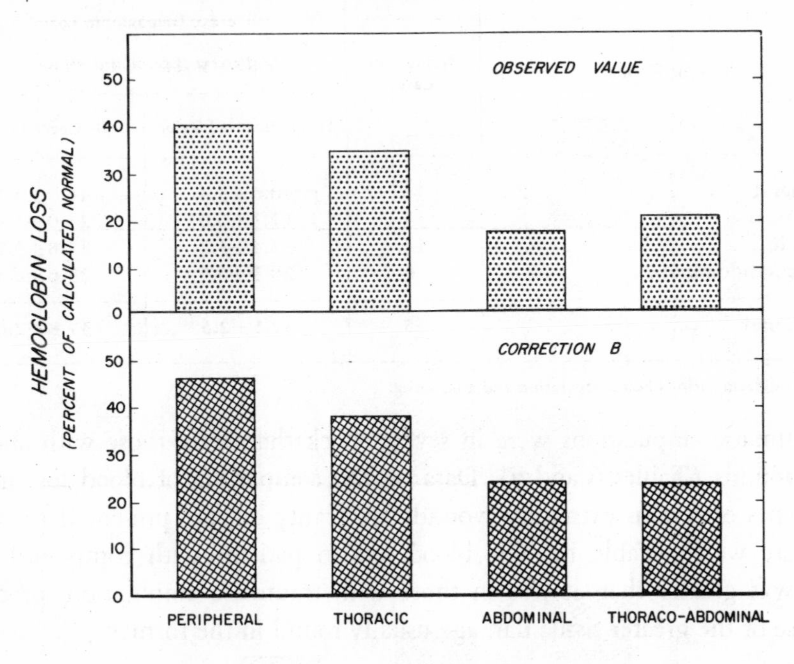

obscured by the factor of hemodilution. This difference is in agreement with the previous finding that more patients with compound fractures of long bones

TABLE 17.—RELATIONSHIP OF BLOOD VOLUME LOSS TO TYPE OF WOUND

Type of Wound	Number of Cases	Average Blood Volume Loss * Percent of calculated normal		
		From Observed Value	By Correction A	By Correction B
Peripheral	32	20.8±3.0	34.2±3.2	28.2±3.1
Abdominal	13	7.6±3.6	21.3±6.2	16.4±5.5
Thoracic	14	17.9±2.6	28.6±4.6	21.4±2.3
Thoraco-abdominal . .	6	6.6±6.8	13.7±5.5	10.3±6.2
Total	65	16.2±1.9	28.5±2.5	22.7±2.1

* All determinations before operation and anesthesia.

TABLE 18.—RELATIONSHIP OF HEMOGLOBIN LOSS TO TYPE OF WOUND

Type of Wound	Number of Cases	Average Hemoglobin Loss * *Percent of calculated normal*	
		From Observed Value	By Correction B
Peripheral	32	40.0±3.4	46.0±3.1
Abdominal	13	17.3±6.0	24.0±6.4
Thoracic	14	34.4±3.2	37.8±3.2
Thoraco-abdominal	6	20.3±6.5	23.6±6.3
Total	65	32.5±2.5	37.8±2.6

* All determinations before operation and anesthesia.

or traumatic amputations were in severe shock than were those with abdominal wounds (Tables 6 and 7). Data on the comparison of blood loss in the two types of serious extremity wounds are scanty but are presented for what they are worth, Table 19. The blood loss in patients with compound fractures was greater than it was in those with traumatic amputation, probably because of the greater tissue damage usually found in the former.

TABLE 19.—LOSS OF BLOOD VOLUME AND TOTAL HEMOGLOBIN IN 31 PATIENTS WITH SEVERE EXTREMITY WOUNDS

Type of Wound	No Fracture	Compound Fracture	Traumatic Amputation
Average Blood Volume Loss * (By Correction A)	21.9±8.1 (7 cases)	40.8±4.2 (19 cases)	27.0±3.2 (5 cases)
Average Hemoglobin Loss * (By Correction B)	32.8±7.0 (7 cases)	51.6±4.2 (19 cases)	43.0±3.9 (5 cases)

* Percent of calculated normal.

Table 20 shows the average blood volume and hemoglobin losses in 40 patients with all types of wounds who had received either none or small amounts of plasma but in no instance more than 1 unit before the determinations were made. The losses here are less than those shown in Tables 17 and 18 because the group includes fewer of the patients in severe shock. Again a greater average loss of hemoglobin than of blood volume is shown. This is explained by hemodilution which normally takes place after blood loss. Red blood cells are not replaced appreciably during the interval from wounding to arrival at a forward hospital except by transfusion.

TABLE 20.—LOSS OF BLOOD VOLUME AND TOTAL HEMOGLOBIN IN 40 PATIENTS WHO HAD RECEIVED 1 UNIT OR LESS OF PLASMA

Relationship to Type of Wound

Type of Wound	Number of Cases	Average Blood Volume Loss * (By Correction A) *Percent of calculated normal*	Average Hemoglobin Loss * (By Correction B) *Percent of calculated normal*
Peripheral	18	23.9±3.9	38.0±4.3
All Other	22	15.2±2.9	22.5±3.8
Total	40	19.1±2.4	29.5±3.1

* All determinations before operation and anesthesia.

Relationship of Blood Loss to Time from Wounding

There was no important *average* increase in blood volume loss or in hemoglobin loss with increased time elapsing between wounding and hospital entry (Table 21). However, those men who were suffering from continuing blood loss were probably given priority of evacuation. Somewhat greater blood losses were usually found in those who arrived at the hospital soon after wounding than in those who were brought in later.

TABLE 21.—RELATIONSHIP OF BLOOD LOSS TO TIME FROM WOUNDING IN 67 CASES (ALL TYPES OF WOUNDS)

Time from Wounding *Hours*	Number of Cases	Average Blood Volume Loss (By Correction A) *Percent of calculated normal*	Average Hemoglobin Loss (By Correction B) *Percent of calculated normal*
None to 6	41	29.0	37.5
7 to 12	17	31.9	42.3
13 and Over	9	24.7	35.8

Relationship of Blood Loss to Degree of Shock

It is well known that individuals do not respond alike to a given blood loss; even previously healthy, normal young soldiers vary greatly in their response. This fact, together with the inexactness inherent in any clinical appraisal of the degree of shock plus the errors of the experimental method used, might have tended to obscure a real relationship between shock and blood loss. However this relationship was so striking that, even with the relatively small number of cases, the positive correlation of blood loss to the severity of shock was statistically significant (Table 22 and Chart 6).

TABLE 22.—RELATIONSHIP OF BLOOD LOSS TO DEGREE OF SHOCK IN 67 CASES (ALL TYPES OF WOUNDS)

Degree of Shock	Number of Cases	Average Blood Loss — *Percent of calculated normal* — From Observed Value		By Correction A	
		Volume	Hemoglobin	Volume	Hemoglobin
None	11	10.5±4.1	17.4±6.4	14.4±4.9	20.0±6.7
Slight	20	11.2±6.5	25.0±4.4	20.7±4.1	29.7±4.2
Moderate	21	21.7±3.1	41.7±3.3	34.3±3.7	46.1±3.3
Severe	15	22.0±3.9	44.3±4.3	45.9±4.6	55.5±4.5

The degree of wound shock as we saw it in men injured in battle precisely paralleled the quantity of blood actually lost. Conversely, recovery from shock resulted promptly from administration of whole blood. Although we made intensive search at the bedside of thousands of wounded men throughout the shock tents in Italy, we never found a clear case of "irreversible shock," mentioned so frequently in the literature. It is true that there were wounded men in whom the loss of blood was so rapid and so great that it was impossible to transfuse them with blood fast enough to save their lives. (For example, we were unable, in the case of the soldier who had both thighs blown off by a shell burst just outside our door at Anzio to get blood into him fast enough to save his life; he died in a very few minutes.) Nor were we able to resuscitate patients who had had inadequate circulation in the central nervous system

CHART 6. RELATIONSHIP OF BLOOD LOSS TO DEGREE OF SHOCK

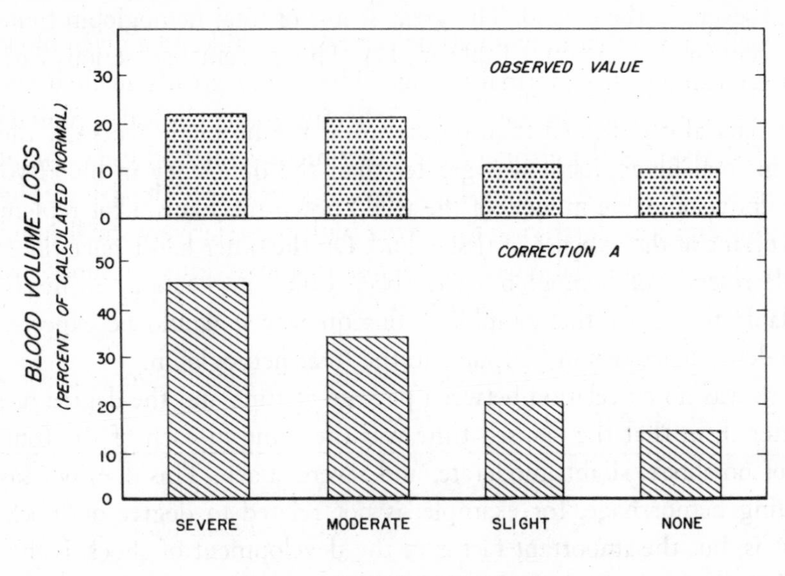

so long that nearly all centers except the respiratory appeared to be dead; we were not able to overcome death of organs or of nervous tissue by resuscitative effort. But we believe that application of the term "irreversible shock" to either type of case is to use a definition that has no place at the bedside, however interesting it may be as a concept, and that may do real harm by providing an excuse for limiting resuscitative effort.

In short, if "irreversible shock" in the accepted sense was present, we missed it. If toxins caused any of the shock we saw, with the exception of that due to overwhelming and clinically apparent bacterial infections, we failed to recognize it. The shock we saw was caused by loss of blood (or of fractions of the blood). It was relieved by administration of whole blood.

From our data it may be said that, in general, when a third of the blood volume is lost, clinical shock of more than slight degree will result, and when half is lost, severe shock will result. It was also shown that in individual cases as much as 75 percent of the blood could be lost and the patient survive. Cases A–17, A–21, A–29, A–37, A–38, 127, and 139 are examples of severe blood loss and survival. The greatest blood volume losses found were 78.6 percent in Case 107 and 75.7 percent in Case 139 (Table 16, C and D). Both determinations were obtained by Correction A. Shock was moderate in the first case and severe in the second. The greatest loss of total hemoglobin found was 83.8 percent in Case A—21 (Table 16, D). This patient had serious extremity wounds and was in severe shock.

Our data also indicated that, on arrival at the hospital, generally the deficiency in total hemoglobin was greater than the deficiency in blood volume. This is understandable in view of the well-known mechanism for replenishing blood volume at the expense of tissue fluid. On the other hand, once the readily available reserves of hemoglobin have been called into action, no mechanism is available to replace them rapidly; consequently it would be expected that greater deficiencies would be found in the total hemoglobin.

There was no correlation between passage of time and the degree of shock encountered, in that the elapsed time was the same in each of the four categories of no shock, slight, moderate, and severe shock. This does not say that continuing hemorrhage, for example, is not related to degree of shock; certainly it is, but the important factor in the development of shock is the character of the wound, particularly as it indicates the quantity of blood lost, not the passage of time per se.

We have tried various ways of handling the data on shock. Some investigators have attempted to separate the effects of blood loss alone from the effects supposedly accounted for by "sympathico-adrenal activity." Practically, this is impossible. Moreover, the validity of any such separation even if possible must be questioned. For example there is the matter of increased glycogenolysis in shock. Following all the recent advances in knowledge of carbohydrate metabolism, it seems to be too great a simplification to hang the explanation on the rather shaky peg of "sympathico-adrenal activity," so we take refuge in our purpose of merely stating our findings, with little conjecture, and leaving to future study the search for their significance.

One great consequence of blood loss is the intense vasoconstriction, the shrinkage of the capacity of the vascular bed to accommodate the decreased blood volume. Contraction of the spleen probably plays a relatively small role in compensating for the blood lost in battle. Other body adjustments to blood loss do, however, take place, such as the entry of fluid into the blood vessels in an attempt at compensation. The greatest extravascular store of readily available fluid in the body is that in the extracellular space. Dehydration and oligemia may make quite early demands, not only on this extracellular but also on the intracellular supply.

Biochemic Changes Encountered

The clinical appearance of the newly wounded man, as well as his subsequent course, offers abundant evidence that profound changes have occurred in his internal state by the time he is admitted to a hospital. To be reported here are chiefly the changes found in the blood although certain urinary findings also are recorded. These changes are significant not only because they reveal the problem at hand, but also because they offer some basis for reasonable therapy. Several factors influence the presence or extent of the abnormalities found. These are discussed in the following sections.

Blood Chemistry Findings

Relationship to Location of Wound.—No significant relationship was found between the location or type of the wound and the plasma nonprotein nitrogen, creatinine, uric acid, phosphorus, or magnesium (See Table 24, page 60). Average values for serum sodium, plasma chlorides, and plasma carbon-dioxide combining power also were determined and likewise failed to show any significant relationship to the type of wound.

Relationship to Delay in Hospital Arrival.—With increased passage of time following wounding, the average plasma nonprotein nitrogen level rose (Table 23). This upward swing of the nonprotein nitrogen offers a basis for some inter-

TABLE 23.—RELATIONSHIP OF PLASMA NONPROTEIN NITROGEN LEVEL TO TIME FROM WOUNDING IN 92 PATIENTS WITH ALL TYPES OF WOUNDS

Time from Wounding *hours*	Average Nonprotein Nitrogen * *mg. per 100 cc.*	Type of Wound	Percent of Cases
1 to 7 (48 cases)	34.2±1.1	Peripheral	48
		Abdominal and thoraco-abdominal	33
		Thoracic	19
7 to 13 (26 cases)	41.2±1.7	Peripheral	73
		Abdominal and thoraco-abdominal	12
		Thoracic	15
13 or More (18 cases)	46.3±3.2	Peripheral	67
		Abdominal	22
		Thoracic	11

* Averages based on determinations made before operation and anesthesia.

TABLE 24.—BIOCHEMIC FINDINGS[1] IN RELATION TO TYPE AND LOCATION OF WOUND

Type of Wound	Nonprotein Nitrogen *mg. per 100 cc.*	Creatinine *mg. per 100 cc.*	NPN / Creatinine x 10	Uric Acid *mg. per 100 cc.*	Phosphorus *mg. per 100 cc.*	Magnesium *mg. per 100 cc.*
Peripheral (Without fracture)	39.0±3.7 (11 cases)	1.7±0.16 (11 cases)	2.6±0.20 (11 cases)	5.0 (5 cases)	4.5±0.65 (6 cases)	2.3 (5 cases)
Peripheral (With fracture)	41.0±1.8 (32 cases)	1.6±0.10 (31 cases)	2.7±0.13 (31 cases)	4.4±0.50 (19 cases)	4.9±0.50 (24 cases)	2.3±0.13 (20 cases)
Peripheral (With traumatic amputation)	47.0±4.3 (6 cases)	1.5±0.30 (6 cases)	3.7±0.65 (6 cases)	5.5 (2 cases)	4.9 (4 cases)	2.0 (3 cases)
Abdominal[2]	34.0±2.2 (19 cases)	1.4±0.15 (19 cases)	2.7±0.12 (19 cases)	4.9±0.59 (16 cases)	3.9±0.30 (17 cases)	2.0±0.10 (16 cases)
Thoraco-abdominal	38.0±3.1 (7 cases)	1.5±0.28 (7 cases)	3.0±0.37 (7 cases)	6.1 (5 cases)	4.5±0.55 (7 cases)	2.0 (5 cases)
Kidney Injury	35.0±2.9 (9 cases)	1.5±0.25 (9 cases)	2.6±0.29 (9 cases)	6.5±0.99 (6 cases)	4.0±0.50 (9 cases)	2.0±0.12 (7 cases)
Liver Injury	37.0±3.0 (10 cases)	1.3±0.10 (10 cases)	3.0±0.23 (10 cases)	5.8±0.98 (6 cases)	3.9±0.40 (9 cases)	2.0±0.10 (6 cases)
Thoracic	36.0±2.5 (14 cases)	1.3±0.15 (14 cases)	2.9±0.26 (14 cases)	4.1±0.63 (8 cases)	4.2±0.28 (13 cases)	1.9±0.10 (11 cases)

[1] Averages based on determinations made before operation and anesthesia.
[2] With and without kidney and liver injury.

esting speculation, out of place here, but one might ask in passing: Is this rise a reflection of decreased renal blood flow? Does this rise mean that renal impairment is initiated by the wound and continues, with accumulation of nonprotein nitrogenous waste products? Does this presumed malfunction set the stage for later trouble with the kidneys? The plasma creatinine level did not rise significantly with the passage of time preceding hospital entry, nor did that of uric acid, phosphorus, or magnesium (Table 25). Also no correlation was found between passage of time and levels of plasma chlorides, serum sodium, or plasma carbon-dioxide combining power.

TABLE 25.—RELATIONSHIP OF SEVERAL PLASMA CONSTITUENTS* TO TIME FROM WOUNDING

Time from Wounding *hours*	Creatinine *mg. per 100 cc.*	Uric Acid *mg. per 100 cc.*	Phosphorus *mg. per 100 cc.*	Magnesium *mg. per 100 cc.*
1 to 7	1.3±0.1 (50 cases)	4.5±0.4 (38 cases)	4.4±0.3 (49 cases)	2.1±0.1 (41 cases)
7 to 13	1.6±0.1 (26 cases)	4.7±0.5 (15 cases)	4.8±0.3 (19 cases)	2.1±0.1 (15 cases)
13 to 24	1.7±0.2 (19 cases)	5.9±0.7 (7 cases)	4.2±0.5 (11 cases)	1.8±0.1 (9 cases)

* Averages based on determinations made before operation and anesthesia.

Relationship to Clinical Condition.—The interesting relationships of the plasma nonprotein nitrogen, creatinine, phosphorus, and magnesium to the degree of shock are shown in Table 26. Statistically significant rises occurred for nonprotein nitrogen, phosphorus, creatinine, and magnesium in progressive categories from "no shock" to "severe shock," with the chief difference occurring between the moderate- and severe-shock groups. The rise in uric acid was not statistically significant. When these substances were compared with blood loss, the same positive correlation was found for the nonprotein nitrogen, creatinine, phosphorus, and magnesium, as would be expected. Again the correlation in the case of uric acid was not significant. These comparisons are shown in Table 27; blood loss was divided into five categories from no loss to loss of more than 40 percent of the calculated normal blood volume.

Data relevant to acid-base balance are presented in Tables 28 and 29 and Chart 7. An acidosis was present in those patients with severe shock and is

TABLE 26.—BIOCHEMIC FINDINGS* IN RELATION TO SHOCK

Degree of Shock	Nonprotein Nitrogen *mg. per 100 cc.*	Creatinine *mg. per 100 cc.*	NPN / Creatinine x 10	Uric Acid *mg. per 100 cc.*	Phosphorus *mg. per 100 cc.*	Magnesium *mg. per 100 cc.*
No Shock	34.0±1.5 (18 cases)	1.0±0.05 (18 cases)	3.3±0.12 (18 cases)	4.0±0.62 (10 cases)	3.3±0.24 (14 cases)	1.7±0.05 (11 cases)
Slight Shock	35.0±1.8 (24 cases)	1.3±0.09 (24 cases)	2.9±0.17 (24 cases)	4.5±0.41 (16 cases)	3.8±0.18 (20 cases)	1.9±0.06 (17 cases)
Moderate Shock	37.0±1.6 (32 cases)	1.4±0.08 (32 cases)	2.8±0.15 (32 cases)	4.8±0.61 (17 cases)	4.3±0.23 (24 cases)	2.0±0.09 (20 cases)
Severe Shock	44.0±2.1 (24 cases)	2.1±0.15 (23 cases)	2.3±0.15 (23 cases)	5.2±0.56 (16 cases)	5.8±0.52 (21 cases)	2.5±0.16 (16 cases)

* Averages based on determinations made before operation and anesthesia.

TABLE 27.—BIOCHEMIC FINDINGS* IN RELATION TO BLOOD LOSS

Blood Volume Loss (By Correction A) *Percent of calculated normal*	Nonprotein Nitrogen *mg. per 100 cc.*	Creatinine *mg. per 100 cc.*	NPN / Creatinine x 10	Uric Acid *mg. per 100 cc.*	Phosphorus *mg. per 100 cc.*	Magnesium *mg. per 100 cc.*
0 to 5	31.0±3.1 (9 cases)	1.0±0.07 (9 cases)	3.1±0.19 (6 cases)	4.4±0.76 (6 cases)	3.2±0.34 (8 cases)	1.8±0.07 (8 cases)
5 to 15	36.0±2.4 (9 cases)	1.1±0.05 (9 cases)	3.2±0.20 (9 cases)	4.8±0.73 (9 cases)	3.7±0.18 (9 cases)	1.9±0.07 (9 cases)
15 to 25	37.0±2.3 (12 cases)	1.3±0.14 (12 cases)	3.0±0.17 (12 cases)	3.9±0.42 (9 cases)	4.0±0.28 (12 cases)	1.8±0.08 (11 cases)
25 to 40	38.0±2.3 (19 cases)	1.7±0.18 (19 cases)	2.6±0.17 (19 cases)	5.0±0.53 (16 cases)	4.2±0.33 (17 cases)	2.1±0.10 (17 cases)
Over 40	41.0±2.2 (18 cases)	1.8±0.13 (18 cases)	2.5±0.18 (18 cases)	4.8±0.60 (16 cases)	5.5±0.58 (18 cases)	2.4±0.18 (18 cases)

* Averages based on determinations made before operation and anesthesia.

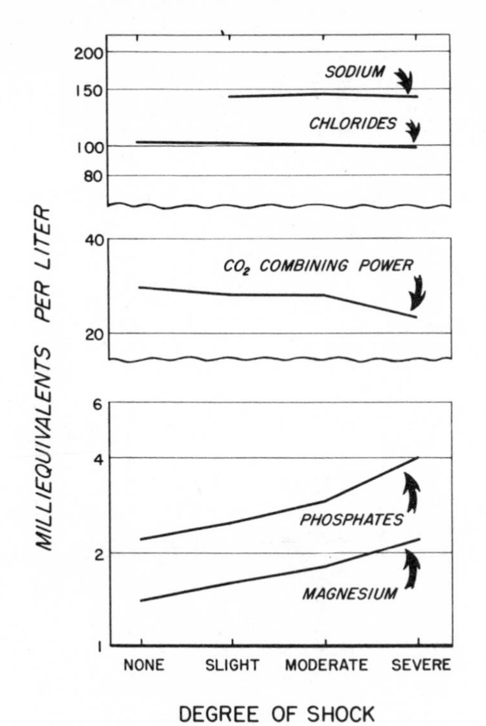

CHART 7. Plasma electrolytes (on hospital admission) in relation to shock

reflected in the carbon-dioxide combining power. A significant fall of carbon-dioxide combining power was correlated with shock (Table 28). Evidence that these low values are due to a metabolic acidosis will be presented in the discussion of azotemia in Chapter IV. Plasma chlorides were uniformly normal in all shock categories (Table 28); likewise, urinary chlorides were essentially normal although they showed wide variations in concentration (Table 29). There was, then, no evidence of salt deprivation on hospital entry. Phosphates, although significantly higher in terms of total anions in those in severe shock than in those with no clinical evidence of shock, could have had little effect on the acid-base balance. Plasma proteins are not included in Table 28, but they showed insufficient variation in terms of electrolyte concentration to have affected acid-base balance.

The plasma was examined for lactic acid in 5 patients shortly after they were wounded. The findings were compared with those in 7 normal, active

TABLE 28.—PLASMA ELECTROLYTES ON ADMISSION IN RELATION TO SHOCK

Average Electrolytes *mEq./L.*	All Cases *	No Shock	Slight Shock	Moderate Shock	Severe Shock
Carbon-dioxide Combining Power	25.3±0.5 (93 cases)	27.9±1.0 (13 cases)	26.1±0.7 (22 cases)	26.1±0.9 (31 cases)	22.1±0.9 (25 cases)
Chlorides	100.5±0.6 (96 cases)	102.0±3.0 (13 cases)	101.0±0.7 (24 cases)	100.0±0.5 (33 cases)	99.5±0.9 (24 cases)
Phosphates	3.0±0.2 (78 cases)	2.2±0.3 (13 cases)	2.5±0.2 (20 cases)	2.9±0.3 (25 cases)	4.0±0.5 (20 cases)
Magnesium	1.8±0.07 (64 cases)	1.4±0.05 (11 cases)	1.6±0.06 (18 cases)	1.8±0.10 (19 cases)	2.2±0.16 (16 cases)
Sodium **	144.3 (15 cases)	....	142.1 (6 cases)	147.1 (4 cases)	144.7 (5 cases)

* Crush cases not included.
** On blood serum.
mEq./L. = milliequivalent levels.

TABLE 29.—PREOPERATIVE URINARY FINDINGS IN RELATION TO SHOCK

Degree of Shock	Average pH	Average Chlorides *mg. per 100 cc. as NaCl*	Average Sodium Received since Wounding * *grams*	No Sodium since Wounding *number of cases*
No Shock	6.3±0.2 (7 cases)	1,128±185 (5 cases)	1.0 (4 cases)	3
Slight Shock	5.7±0.1 (6 cases)	945±169 (8 cases)	0.8 (5 cases)	2
Moderate Shock	5.7±0.1 (6 cases)	423±185 (5 cases)	3.7 (4 cases)	2
Severe Shock	5.7±0.2 (7 cases)	704±241 (5 cases)	3.2 (7 cases)	None
All Cases	5.9±0.1 (26 cases)	819±105 (23 cases)	2.2 (20 cases)	7

Note: Specific gravity of urine: 1.027±0.001 (26 cases).

* 10 grams of sodium citrate furnish 2.3 grams of sodium. 10 grams of sodium bicarbonate furnish 2.7 grams of sodium.

soldiers and in 10 bed patients convalescing from severe wounds. The results are recorded in Table 30. They show a twofold increase in the concentration of lactic acid in the wounded when compared with normal, active soldiers and with convalescent bed patients.

TABLE 30.—CONCENTRATION OF LACTIC ACID IN PLASMA IN SEVERELY WOUNDED SUBJECTS AND CONTROLS

Subjects	Lactic Acid Concentration in the Plasma *mg. per 100 cc.*		
	Minimum	Maximum	Average
Normal Controls (7 active soldiers)	17	24	21
Wounded Examined 6 to 19 Hours (average 10 hours) after Wounding (5 cases)	29	46	38
Patients in third to fifth Week of Convalescence from War Wounds (10 cases)	14	21	16

TABLE 31.—AVERAGE PLASMA BILIRUBIN AND HEMOGLOBIN LEVELS IN PATIENTS WITH VARIOUS TYPES OF WOUNDS

Type of Wound	Liver	Kidney	Intra-abdominal	Thoraco-abdominal	Thoracic	Peripheral	
						With Fracture	Without Fracture
Van den Bergh Index (mg. of bilirubin per 100 cc.)	0.36±0.04 (9 cases)	0.42±0.07 (8 cases)	0.43±0.11 (15 cases)	0.39±0.04 (7 cases)	0.58±0.07 (15 cases)	0.57±0.05 (36 cases)	0.49±0.12 (6 cases)
Plasma Hemoglobin (mg. per 100 cc.)	10.7±1.4 (10 cases)	12.8±2.3 (8 cases)	10.1±1.8 (15 cases)	12.7±2.2 (7 cases)	10.1±1.6 (15 cases)	10.9±1.1 (42 cases)	11.3±2.9 (10 cases)

TABLE 32.—AVERAGE PLASMA BILIRUBIN AND HEMOGLOBIN LEVELS IN RELATION TO TIME FROM WOUNDING

Time from Wounding until Blood Sample Drawn *hours*	Van den Bergh Index *mg. of bilirubin per 100 cc.*	Plasma Hemoglobin *mg. per 100 cc.*
1 to 6	0.45±0.05 (47 cases)	11.4±0.9 (48 cases)
7 to 12	0.64±0.07 (23 cases)	9.4±1.4 (27 cases)
13 to 24	0.69±0.07 (13 cases)	11.1±2.1 (18 cases)

Plasma Bilirubin (van den Bergh Index) and Plasma Hemoglobin Levels

Relationship to Type of Wound.—On comparison of the type of wound with the plasma bilirubin and hemoglobin, no impressive relationships were found (Table 31).

Relationship to Time from Wounding.—The van den Bergh index rose significantly with increases in time from wounding to examination (Table 32). This may have been due to the absorption of breakdown products from hematomas, and to impaired liver function (see Chapter II). The situation was simpler at this time (when most of these patients had not yet been transfused with blood) than it would be later when large volumes of blood had been given which might tend to elevate the bilirubin level. The plasma hemoglobin level appeared to rise with the passage of time, but this was not significant so far as the data at hand are concerned.

Relationship to Clinical Condition.—There was no clear relationship between degree of shock and the plasma bilirubin or hemoglobin levels (Table 33). However, when the bilirubin level was compared with the blood loss (Correction A), a significant relationship seemed to emerge, although the values were all at a rather low level (Table 34). Presumably the rise is to be accounted for by hemolysis of blood in damaged tissues, followed by absorption into the blood stream. There was no apparent correlation of blood loss with plasma hemoglobin levels.

TABLE 33.—AVERAGE PLASMA BILIRUBIN AND HEMOGLOBIN LEVELS IN RELATION TO DEGREE OF SHOCK*

Degree of Shock	Van den Bergh Index *mg. of bilirubin per 100 cc.*	Plasma Hemoglobin *mg. per 100 cc.*
None	0.43±0.08 (11 cases)	12.1±1.8 (14 cases)
Slight	0.68±0.10 (23 cases)	11.3±1.6 (23 cases)
Moderate	0.54±0.06 (27 cases)	10.8±1.4 (33 cases)
Severe	0.47±0.05 (21 cases)	8.8±0.9 (24 cases)

* Averages based on determinations made before operation and anesthesia. Crush cases not included.

956507 O—52——6

TABLE 34.—AVERAGE PLASMA BILIRUBIN AND HEMOGLOBIN LEVELS IN RELATION TO BLOOD LOSS*

Blood Loss (By Correction A) *Percent of calculated normal*	None to 5%	5 to 15%	15 to 25%	25 to 40%	Over 40%
Plasma Bilirubin . . (mg. per 100 cc.)	0.31±0.07 (6 cases)	0.56±0.10 (8 cases)	0.50±0.10 (10 cases)	0.52±0.05 (20 cases)	0.64±0.11 (18 cases)
Plasma Hemoglobin (mg. per 100 cc.)	15.5±2.6 (7 cases)	11.2±3.6 (8 cases)	9.8±2.0 (11 cases)	14.3±1.6 (20 cases)	10.0±1.2 (18 cases)

* Averages based on determinations made before operation and anesthesia. Crush cases not included.

TABLE 35.—AVERAGE PLASMA GLUCOSE LEVELS IN SEVERELY WOUNDED MEN

A. Relationship to Degree of Shock

Degree of Shock	None	Slight	Moderate	Severe
Glucose Level * . . . . (mg. per 100 cc.)	134±9 (9 cases)	149±9 (14 cases)	178±13 (19 cases)	202±26 (13 cases)

B. Relationship to Blood Loss

Blood Loss (By Correction A) *Percent of calculated normal*	None to 5	6 to 15	16 to 25	26 to 40	Over 40
Glucose Level * . . . . (mg. per 100 cc.)	143±12 (6 cases)	159±15 (7 cases)	153±7 (9 cases)	177±18 (17 cases)	194±23 (15 cases)

C. Relationship to Time from Wounding

Time from Wounding	None to 6 Hours	7 to 12 Hours	13 to 24 Hours
Glucose Level * . . . . (mg. per 100 cc.)	182±13 (36 cases)	161±10 (13 cases)	144±7 (8 cases)

* Normal: from 80 to 90 mg. per 100 cc. of plasma.

CHART 8. PLASMA GLUCOSE LEVELS

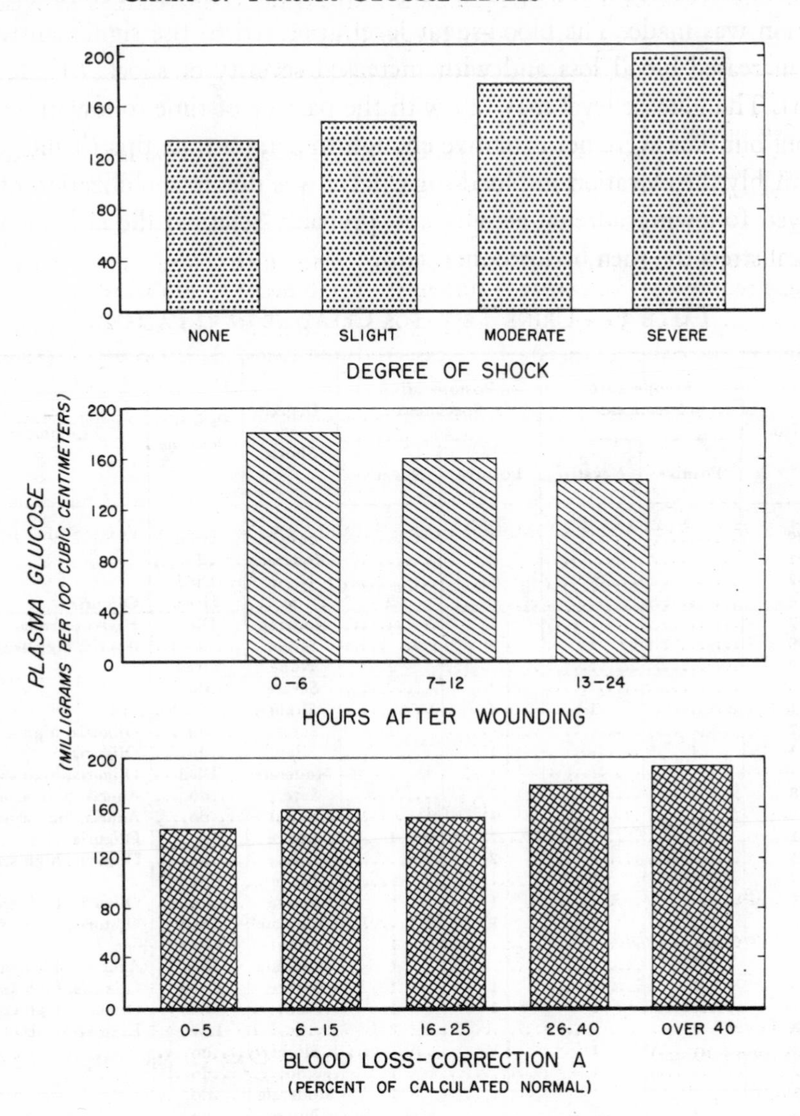

Blood Sugar

The blood-sugar level was determined in 57 severely wounded men as they arrived at the forward hospital and was found to be above normal in all of them (Table 35 A and Chart 8). Normal by the method used was considered to be from 80 to 90 mg. per 100 cc. of plasma. Some of the men had received plasma but none had had a significant quantity of whole blood before the determination was made. The blood-sugar level appeared to rise significantly both with increased blood loss and with increased severity of shock (Table 35 A and B). The glucose level may fall with the passage of time following wounding, but our data were not extensive enough to demonstrate this (Table 35 C). Presumably the elevation in blood-sugar level was due to mobilization of liver glycogen following adrenal activity and probably reflected the emotional and physical stress the men had experienced.

TABLE 36.—URINE TESTS FOR CREATINE IN 32 PATIENTS

Case No.	Preoperative Specimens		Postoperative Specimens		Degree of Shock	Patient's Outcome	Comment *
	Positive	Negative	Positive	Negative			
89	....	....	1	....	Severe	Lived	
101	....	....	3	....	Moderate	....do....	
102	....	....	6	....	None	Died	
106	....	....	....	2	....do....	Lived	Oliguria.
107	....	....	1	....	Moderate	Died	High azotemia.
108	....	1	3	....	Severe	....do....	Anuria, high azotemia.
109	....	....	....	2	None	Lived	
110	....	....	3	....	Severe	....do....	
111	....	1	4	....	Slight	....do....	
112	....	....	....	1	Severe	....do....	Oliguria, high azotemia.
113	1	....	1	....	Slight	....do....	Oliguria.
117	....	....	1	1	Moderate	Died	Oliguria, high azotemia.
118	....	....	2	....	Severe	....do....	Anuria, high azotemia.
120	....	....	1	....	Slight	....do....	Anuria, high azotemia.
121	....	....	....	1	Severe	....do....	Oliguria.
123	....	....	2	....	....do....	....do....	Oliguria, high azotemia.
124	....	1	....	....	None	Lived	
125	....	....	1	1	Severe	....do....	Oliguria, high azotemia.
126	....	1	1	....	Moderate	Died	Oliguria.
127	....	....	....	1	Slight	Lived	
129	1	....	....	1	Moderate	Died	Anuria, high azotemia.
130	2	....	1	1	Severe	Lived	Oliguria, high azotemia.
131	....	1	2	1	....do....	Died	Oliguria, high azotemia.
133	....	....	....	2	....do....	Lived	High azotemia.
A-1	....	1	1	....	Slight	....do....	
A-2	....	1	....	1	....do....	....do....	
A-3	....	1	....	1	Moderate	....do....	
A-4	1	....	....	....	None	....do....	
A-5	1	....	1	....	Slight	....do....	
A-6	1	....	1	....	Moderate	....do....	NPN to 60.
A-16	....	1	....	....	None	....do....	NPN to 63.
A-40	....	....	1	....	Slight	....do....	
Total	7	9	37	16	....	L:21 D:11	

* Anuria: urinary output of less than 100 cc. daily; oliguria: 24-hour urinary output of 100-600 cc. for at least 1 day in the posttraumatic period; high azotemia: plasma nonprotein nitrogen over 65 mg. per 100 cc.

Urinary Findings

Acid-Base Relationship.—Sodium in the urine was measured in too few cases for reliable averages. Most of the values found were within the normal range. Magnesium, like phosphates on the acid side, was increased but not sufficiently so to affect total acid-base equilibrium. Urinary pH and specific gravity indicate that these men had essentially normal renal function at the time they were wounded, in that they could make both an acid and a concentrated urine. The acid-base relationship will be discussed further in Chapter III.

Creatinuria.—The appearance of creatine in the urine of adult males is abnormal. On the assumption that there might be some abnormality in the metabolism of creatine and creatinine in shock, the urine was examined for creatine in 32 patients (Table 36). In all, 69 urine specimens were tested; the results are summarized in Table 37. Creatine was found in the urines of 26 of the 32 patients. It was present in 6 out of 15 of the patients examined preoperatively, and in 20 out of 29 patients whose urines were examined postoperatively. In 13 of the 32 patients urine tests yielded only positive results, in 11 patients only negative, and in the remaining 9, different specimens tested yielded both positive and negative results.

With one exception (Case 121) all patients who died showed creatinuria at one time or another. It was also present in approximately half the patients who survived. In relation to shock, 14 of 18 patients who had been in moderate or severe shock showed creatinuria. This tendency for creatine to be excreted in the urine in cases of moderate and severe shock and in fatal cases might indicate that it is the result of metabolic changes which accompany shock.

Table 37.—Summary of Results in 69 Urine Specimens Tested for Creatine

Source	Positive (44 specimens)	Negative (25 specimens)
Preoperative	7	9
Postoperative	37	16
From Patients with No Shock or Slight Shock	18	11
From Patients with Moderate or Severe Shock	26	14
From Patients Who subsequently Died	20	7
From Patients Who Lived	24	18

Liver Function in the Newly Wounded Man

As will be discussed in Chapter II, the only direct laboratory test of liver function carried out here was that of the bromsulfalein excretion. The van den Bergh index and uric acid levels have also been considered as being in part at least related to liver function.

Bromsulfalein Retention

On Arrival at the Most Forward Hospital.—In 59 severely wounded patients the average bromsulfalein retention on forward hospital arrival was 12.4 ± 1.2 percent (standard error of the mean) 45 minutes after 5 mg. of dye per Kg. of body weight had been injected intravenously. This is well above the normal of 1.0 ± 0.1 percent (as established in a control group of 45 subjects), and above our arbitrarily chosen upper limit of normal of 3 percent (see Chapter II).

Relationship to Time from Wounding.—There was no difference between the average bromsulfalein retention in 29 men examined within the first 6 hours after wounding (14.4 ± 1.8 percent) and in 19 men examined after the first 6 hours (13.1 ± 1.6 percent).

Relationship to Location of Wound.—In 22 patients with serious extremity wounds there was 13.3 ± 2.3-percent average retention, and in 18 patients with abdominal wounds there was an average of 14.7 ± 2.1-percent retention—no difference. In 11 men with penetrating chest wounds, however, the average retention was only 7.0 ± 1.8 percent, which is significantly lower than that found in the other groups.

Relationship to Shock.—In 57 patients separated into the 4 shock categories (no shock, slight, moderate, and severe shock) no significant correlation with bromsulfalein excretion could be found; neither was there any correlation with blood volume or hemoglobin loss.

Relationship to Plasma Administration.—Curiously enough, there was a great increase in average bromsulfalein retention (14.0 ± 2.0 percent) in 25 men who had had one or two units of plasma, over the average retention (8.0±2.0 percent) in 15 men who had had none. Three or more units of plasma did not increase the effect beyond that produced by one or two units. The effect was transient and disappeared between the first and second day following operation.

Plasma Bilirubin and Uric Acid

The bilirubin and uric acid concentrations in the blood have been discussed earlier in this chapter in relation to other factors studied.

SUMMARY

In the past, battle wounds have been described chiefly in terms of organic damage or tissue loss. The purpose of this chapter has been to describe, shortly after the soldier arrived at the forward hospital, the latent consequences of his wounds as they influenced organic function and produced changes in blood volume and chemistry, and abnormalities in the urine. These matters were studied, before vigorous resuscitative efforts had yet been made, in 108 patients. Altogether, 186 patients were studied in the course of the work carried out by the Board for the Study of the Severely Wounded.

In considering patients who had received not more than one unit of plasma, or none at all, it was observed that the hematocrit level was higher in those with abdominal wounds than it was in those with peripheral wounds, but even in the patients with abdominal wounds the average hematocrit values were somewhat below normal. While severe hemoconcentration can occur in cases of burns, crush, and abdominal wounds, this was infrequent in our series and was by no means a general characteristic of shock as we saw it.

When the patients who had received little or no plasma or blood therapy at the time of first examination were divided into two groups, depending upon whether more or less than 30 percent of the blood volume had been lost, a puzzling situation was apparent: the average concentration of protein in the plasma in the more severely bled-out group was 6.1 grams per 100 cubic centimeters. This is 6.1 percent below normal. On the other hand, the average hematocrit value in this same group had fallen to 36 from the normal of 47, a reduction of 23.4 percent. The hematocrit level thus fell about four times as much as that of the plasma proteins. One implication of this is that the blood had been diluted with protein-rich fluid. Its possible source is discussed.

Evidence is presented that the plasma protein level was not influenced by plasma therapy, although the hematocrit level was. There was a sharp fall in hematocrit value with increasing severity of shock. Other examples of the independent variation of these two factors are given.

It is shown that men can lose about 75 percent of their blood and yet recover—more than had been generally supposed. Blood loss in various types of wounds is discussed. Data presented show that there was a quantitative relationship between loss of blood volume or hemoglobin and the degree of shock met clinically. This supports the view that the major cause of the shock we encountered was hemorrhage.

No important differences in blood volume or hemoglobin loss were encountered with the passage of time from wounding to examination. This was possibly to be accounted for by the high priority and consequent rapid evacuation given to patients with bleeding wounds.

The clinical condition of the newly wounded man offers abundant evidence that his internal state has been profoundly altered by the time he enters a forward hospital. In addition to the matters already mentioned, this was studied in terms of nitrogenous waste products, electrolytes, bilirubin, and blood sugar. In general, these substances were found not to be influenced by the location of the wound. The plasma nonprotein nitrogen level rose rather strikingly with delay following wounding. The full significance of this is not clear, but it offers grounds for some interesting speculation. Examination of the four shock categories in sequence from "no shock" to "severe shock" shows significant rises in nonprotein nitrogen, creatinine, phosphorus, and magnesium.

Acidosis was present in the patients in severe shock. They showed a considerable fall in carbon-dioxide combining power as compared with that of patients with no clinical evidence of shock. The acidosis appeared to be of the "metabolic" type.

No evidence of salt deprivation was found on hospital entry. Examination of the admission urine specimen with regard to hydrogen ion concentration and specific gravity indicated that the men studied had essentially normal renal function at the time they were wounded.

The van den Bergh index rose significantly with increasing time from wounding to examination. This is discussed briefly. No clear relationship of shock to bilirubin or plasma hemoglobin levels was found. The blood-sugar level was found to be above normal. It was particularly high in the patients with severe shock.

Definite depression of liver function, as measured by bromsulfalein retention, was found on hospital arrival. We found no correlation between liver function and the degree of shock. The administration of one or two units of plasma appeared to impair liver function still further. This was a transitory effect and was not increased by giving three or four units of plasma.

CHAPTER II

Liver Function in the Severely Wounded

Methods

The only specific laboratory test of liver function used in this study was that of bromsulfalein excretion, although the van den Bergh index and uric acid levels were also considered in conjunction with liver activity. The test was selected because of facilities available and on the basis of experience of the group studying infectious hepatitis in the Mediterranean Theater of Operations.

Procedures

The standard procedure for the determination of bromsulfalein dye retention, using the Hynson, Westcott and Dunning Comparator Block, was abandoned for the following reasons: Various degrees of hemolysis in the samples of plasma would result in readings that indicated as much as 5-percent retention when no bromsulfalein was present. Therefore low-retention figures could not be accurately determined, as results were often not reproducible to within ± 5-percent retention. Furthermore the method was time-consuming.

The test was set up on the Coleman Junior Spectrophotometer Model No. 6, using a 1: 6 dilution of plasma, and reading the color of the alkalinized bromsulfalein at 575 millimicrons. Five milligrams of bromsulfalein dye per kilogram of body weight were injected intravenously and 45 minutes later a blood sample was drawn from a different vein. In brief, the procedure (fully described in Appendix C) was as follows:

1. To 1 cc. of plasma in a cuvette were added 5 cc. of a 0.9-percent solution of sodium chloride. These ingredients were well mixed and the spectrophotometer was set to read 100-percent transmission at 575 millimicrons.

2. Three drops of a 10-percent solution of sodium hydroxide were added to the same tube; the tube was inverted once and was read in the spectrophotometer.

3. The transmission percentage was observed and the percentage of dye retention recorded from the standard curve.

Standards of Normal and Abnormal Function (Controls)

In order to establish a standard of liver function that would be normal for our particular subjects who were all combat soldiers, 50 apparently healthy men on active duty in the combat zone were selected at random as a control group. The men selected were hospital personnel, ranging in age from 19 to 45 years, the average age being twenty-nine. Forty-five minutes after injection of bromsulfalein, 45, or 90 percent of the subjects, had less than 3-percent retention of the dye, with an average retention of 1.0±0.1 percent (standard error of the mean) for the group.

Five subjects, or 10 percent of the group, had more than 3-percent retention of the dye after 45 minutes, as shown in Table 38. It seems reasonable that the first three (Subjects A, B, and C) and possibly all five of these men may be considered to have had abnormal liver function of some degree, since the percentage of dye retention persisting after 45 minutes was "abnormally" high for this group. In any case, since 90 percent of men with apparently normal liver function had less than 3-percent bromsulfalein retention 45 min-

TABLE 38.—HIGH RETENTION OF BROMSULFALEIN IN 5 SUBJECTS* OF CONTROL GROUP

Subject	Percentage of Retention after 45 Minutes		Comments
	First Test	Second Test (1 month later)	
A	16.0	4.0	Improvement indicates that impaired function was present at time of first test.
B	3.5	4.3	Subject had had jaundice 2 ½ years previously. Palpable liver, 3 fingers below costal margin on inspiration. Liver disease present.
C	15.2	15.6	Persistent high retention. Liver definitely abnormal.
D	7.2	3.9	Possibly abnormal function.
E	5.8	7.6	Weight of subject 105 Kg. Possibly abnormal liver function.

* None of these 5 subjects had any definite clinical symptoms of poor liver function.

utes after 5 mg. per Kg. of body weight were injected, we arbitrarily chose 3-percent dye retention as the upper limit of normal.

Liver Function in Severely Wounded Patients on Entry to the Most Forward Hospital

The average severely wounded battle casualty showed considerable impairment of liver function as measured by bromsulfalein retention on hospital entry. The average dye retention in 59 severely wounded patients was 12.4 percent±1.2 percent, which is well above the arbitrary normal limit of 3 percent. This finding was considered in connection with several factors. As in the entire study, the number of patients on whom various combinations of findings are shown represent the maximum number available for that particular comparison.

Relationship to Time from Wounding

Forty-eight patients were divided into two groups according to whether liver function was measured (a) within the first 6 hours following wounding or (b) more than 6 hours after wounding. The average percentage of dye retention was found to be: for (a), 14.4±1.8 percent (29 patients); for (b), 13.1±1.6 percent (19 patients). It was therefore concluded that there was no relationship between time from wounding and bromsulfalein retention.

Relationship to Location of Major Wound

Twenty-two patients with severe extremity wounds had an average retention of 13.3±2.3 percent; 18 patients with abdominal wounds 14.7±2.1 percent, and 11 patients with chest wounds 7.0±1.8 percent. If a conclusion may be drawn from this small number of patients, those with chest wounds appeared to have significantly less dye retention than those with wounds of the extremities or of the abdomen. Patients with direct injury to the liver had a somewhat higher average retention (18.4 percent) than those with abdominal wounds without direct liver injury (14.7 percent). However there was such a wide spread in the data, particularly in the patients with direct liver damage, that the difference between the two groups cannot be considered significant.

CHART 9. COMPARISON OF DEGREE OF SHOCK, BLOOD LOSS, AND LIVER FUNCTION

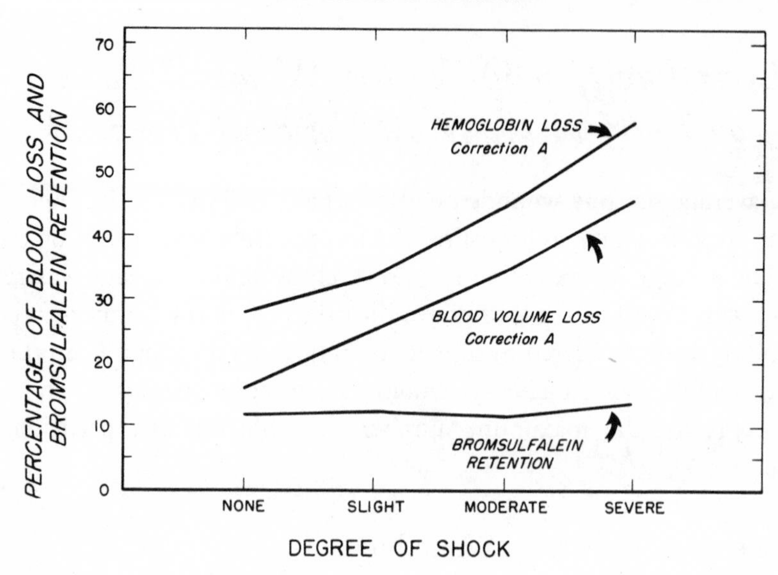

Relationship to Shock and Blood Loss

Whether liver malfunction increases with the presence and severity of shock was considered. Bromsulfalein retention was measured in 57 patients classified according to degree of initial shock, and the mean values are shown in Table 39. The test was made, on the average, from 6 to 8 hours after wounding. No significant increase in bromsulfalein retention was found with increased severity of shock; in fact dye retention was just as high in the patients without shock as it was in those with slight or moderate degrees of shock. Although a slight increase in retention is shown for patients in severe shock, there was considerable spread in the bromsulfalein data, as indicated by the large standard errors of the mean, and this increase is not significant. It is possible that a larger series might have shown some correlation with severe shock. As might be expected, there was also no correlation of bromsulfalein retention with blood volume loss or total hemoglobin loss (Table 40). Chart 9 compares this lack of correlation with the high correlation between degree of shock and blood loss (volume and hemoglobin) which was brought out in Chapter I.

Liver function was clearly impaired in these severely wounded patients. It

TABLE 39.—BROMSULFALEIN RETENTION AND SHOCK

Degree of Shock	Number of Patients	Time from Wounding to Test	Brom-sulfalein Retention
		hours	*percent*
None	10	5.9±1.5	11.6±2.3
Slight	17	6.0±1.8	11.9±2.2
Moderate	17	6.5±0.6	11.1±2.7
Severe	13	* 8.1±1.7	13.5±1.7

* Known in only 11 cases.

was just as much affected in those without shock as it was in those with severe shock. Shock therefore was evidently not the key to this condition. The great deterioration of the circulation found with increasing degrees of shock did not appear to strain liver function measurably insofar as can be judged from these data. The main cause of the impaired function must be sought elsewhere.

Before it is assumed from these findings, however, that there was no more impairment of liver function in those patients who had severe shock than in patients without shock, the question should be raised as to whether the degree of liver impairment could be masked by the given dose of bromsulfalein in a patient who, for example, had lost 50 percent of his normal blood volume. In this instance the given dose of dye would be abnormally concentrated, since it would be less diluted in the abnormally small volume of blood present. Per-

TABLE 40.—BROMSULFALEIN RETENTION AND BLOOD LOSS

Number of Patients	Hemoglobin Loss (By Correction A*)	Average Bromsulfalein Retention	Number of Patients	Blood Volume Loss (By Correction A*)	Average Bromsulfalein Retention
	percent of calculated normal	*percent*		*percent of calculated normal*	*percent*
11	0 to 25	12.2±3.2	22	0 to 25	11.1±1.9
17	26 to 45	11.2±2.1	18	26 to 45	13.8±2.3
22	Over 45	14.3±2.1	12	Over 45	14.8±3.3

* Observed value less all blood or plasma administered from time of wounding to completion of the determination.

haps an *impaired* liver would be able to excrete a greater absolute quantity of such unusually concentrated dye (unusually concentrated because of the abnormally small total volume of blood diluting it) than it would if the usual dilution of the dye had occurred. If so, this conceivably could mask liver impairment. Moreover, if normal circulation is preserved longer in the liver than it is in other organs, then good excretion of the dye might occur even in the presence of abundant blood loss and severe clinical shock. While it seems unlikely that these factors could account for the apparent masking of liver impairment as a consequence of severe shock, they must be considered.

Effect of Blood Plasma Therapy on Liver Function

There seemed to be a significant increase in bromsulfalein retention following administration of one or two units (250-500 cc. total volume) of plasma (Table 41). However, there was no further increase after administration of

TABLE 41.—EFFECT OF BLOOD PLASMA THERAPY ON BROMSULFALEIN RETENTION

Average Bromsulfalein Retention *percent*	No Plasma Administered	Plasma Administered *units**	
		1 or 2	3 or more
On Admission	8.0±2.0 (15 cases)	14.0±2.0 (25 cases)	13.7±2.0 (16 cases)
First Postoperative Day	7.2±2.2 (10 cases)	9.7±2.1 (16 cases)	6.6±1.7 (7 cases)

* 1 unit = 300 cc. total volume.

three or more units. Whole blood, on the other hand, showed an opposite effect. At the time these bromsulfalein determinations were made, only negligible quantities of whole blood had been transfused. By the first day following operation, large quantities of blood, up to several liters in given cases, had been transfused, yet dye retention was less than it had been on the patients' hospital entry. The whole picture is puzzling and one would like to see more data. If the increase in dye retention following administration of plasma was a real effect, it was a transient one, and if real, might it have been due to the preservative used in the plasma, or to the foreign protein in pooled plasma?

CHART 10. BROMSULFALEIN RETENTION AND PATIENTS' OUTCOME

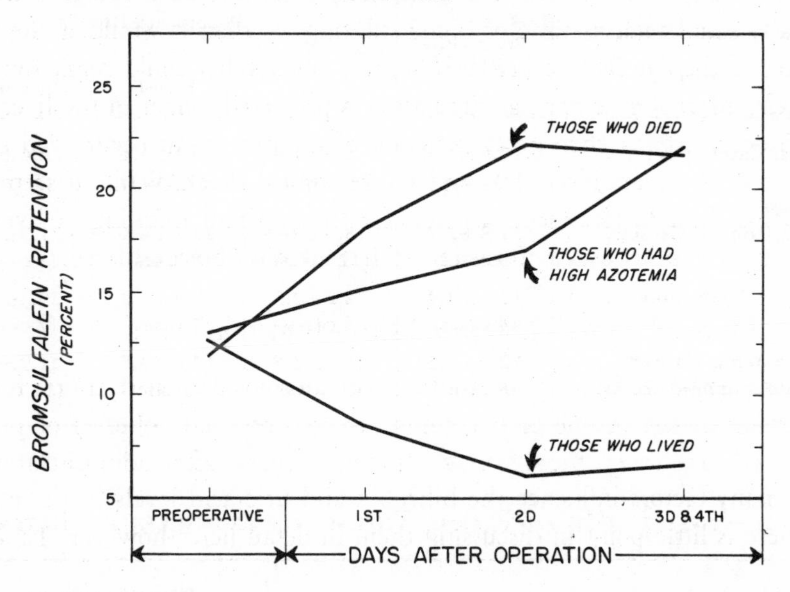

Postoperative Course and Liver Function

In Table 42 liver function is considered in relation to the patient's outcome. Average bromsulfalein retention, measured during the preoperative period and the first 4 postoperative days, is shown for those who lived and those who, either in the period covered or subsequently, died, as well as those who at this time or later developed "high azotemia."[1] The first group, showing bromsulfalein retention in those who lived, is the only one in which the data can be considered in any satisfactory quantitative sense (Chart 10). Not only are the cases relatively few in the other groups, but since death had not occurred nor had uremia or high azotemia appeared in many instances until considerably later than the time interval covered by this table, the high bromsulfalein retentions of those who died in the first four or five days are masked by patients whose values were normal at this time but later became abnormal. The data shown in Table 42 are given, however, because they do show qualitatively a typical trend.

[1] In this study "high azotemia" was defined as a plasma nonprotein nitrogen level of 65 mg. per 100 cc. or higher at any time in the posttraumatic period.

TABLE 42.—BROMSULFALEIN RETENTION AND PATIENTS' OUTCOME

Average Bromsulfalein Retention *percent*	Preoperative Period	Postoperative Day		
		First	Second	Third and Fourth
Nonfatal Cases	12.6±1.4 (45 cases)	8.6±1.4 (40 cases)	6.1±1.1 (32 cases)	6.6±1.2 (15 cases)
Fatal Cases—				
Death from all Causes . . .	11.8±2.7 (9 cases)	18.0±2.9 (12 cases)	22.1±4.4 (8 cases)	21.5±7.4 (8 cases)
Uremic Deaths only . . .	12.5±1.4 (4 cases)	12.2±2.3 (5 cases)	17.4±5.2 (7 cases)	29.4±6.8 (7 cases)
High Azotemia Cases . . . . (Includes uremic deaths)	12.9±2.3 (8 cases)	15.1±3.8 (9 cases)	17.0±3.5 (12 cases)	21.9±5.7 (11 cases)

So many factors influence the bilirubin and uric acid levels in the plasma that there is little point in discussing them in detail here; however, Tables 43

TABLE 43.—PLASMA URIC ACID LEVELS IN RELATION TO PATIENTS' COURSE

Patients	Average Uric Acid Levels (*mg. per 100 cc.*)			
	Preoperative	Postoperative Day		
		First	Second	Third or Later
All Patients	5.0±0.3 (55 cases)	6.6±0.7 (19 cases)	6.6±1.1 (17 cases)	8.1±1.5 (14 cases)
Good Postoperative Course . (Does not include high azotemia or fatalities)	4.4±0.3 (39 cases)	4.7±0.7 (9 cases)	4.5±0.7 (9 cases)	3.3±0.4 (8 cases)
Postoperative Course not Good . . . . (Includes high azotemia and fatalities)	6.5±0.7 (14 cases)	8.2±1.0 (10 cases)	10.7±1.9 (6 cases)	12.2±1.6 (8 cases)

and 44, Charts 11 and 12 are presented to show the trend of these substances in the postoperative course of patients. One must assume that the transfused blood had a considerable influence.

TABLE 44.—PLASMA BILIRUBIN LEVELS IN RELATION TO PATIENTS' COURSE

Patients	Average Plasma Bilirubin Levels (*mg. per 100 cc.*)				
	Preoperative	Postoperative Day			
		First	Second	Third and Fourth	Fifth or Later
All Patients	0.59±0.04 (77 cases)	1.63±0.33 (27 cases)	1.55±0.26 (29 cases)	1.69±0.35 (22 cases)	2.55±0.81 (19 cases)
Good Postoperative Course . . . . (Does not include high azotemia or fatalities)	0.61±0.06 (58 cases)	1.36±0.27 (17 cases)	1.31±0.27 (18 cases)	0.91±0.15 (8 cases)	0.84±0.24 (7 cases)
Postoperative Course not Good . . . . (Includes high azotemia and fatalities)	0.43±0.04 (17 cases)	2.04±0.62 (12 cases)	1.98±0.62 (9 cases)	2.50±0.66 (10 cases)	2.98±1.0 (15 cases) or *2.22±0.7 (14 cases)

* One value of 13.6 omitted to get this average.

956507 O—52——7

CHART 11. PLASMA URIC ACID LEVELS IN RELATION TO PATIENTS' COURSE

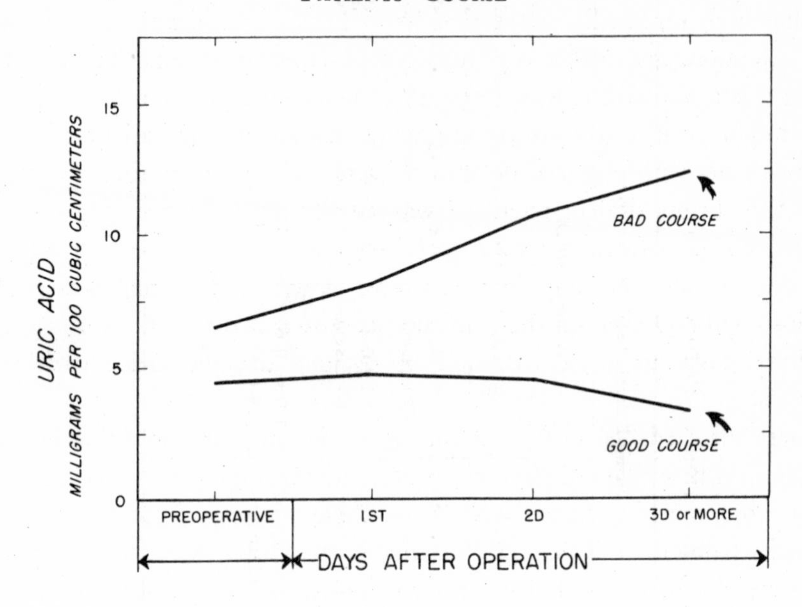

CHART 12. PLASMA BILIRUBIN LEVELS IN RELATION TO PATIENTS' COURSE

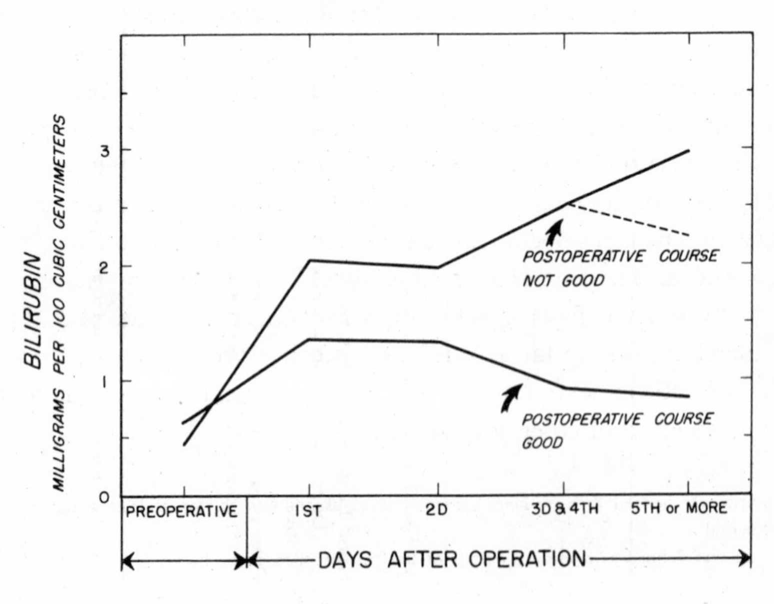

Effect of Ether Anesthesia on Liver Function

It has been repeatedly stated that liver function, as measured by bromsulfalein retention, is considerably impaired by ether anesthesia. Tentatively accepting this statement, it was necessary to determine just how important this factor might be in causing bromsulfalein retention in our patients, for many of the patients with oliguria[2] or anuria[3] were not seen until after operation at which time bromsulfalein retention was usually high. Accordingly data were obtained on 42 patients prior to operation and again on the first day after administration of ether anesthesia. In most of the cases the test was repeated on the second and even on the third postoperative day. The findings in the 42 individual cases are presented in Table 45 and the averages are shown in Table 46.

It was observed that in the patients who were in grave condition following operation, as proved by their early deaths, the average percentage of dye retention rose sharply. There were 8 of these moribund patients; they are grouped separately on Table 46. Presumably the failing liver function in these 8 cases was due to anoxia, but whatever its cause, the moribund patients reacted so differently from the others that the findings when these 8 are eliminated from the total of 42 are also shown. Surely this grouping gives a more accurate picture of the effect, or lack of it, of ether on liver function. Since there was a decrease in average bromsulfalein retention following ether anesthesia in both the entire group and the patients who survived, the point of whether or not the moribund patients should be included need not be labored.

The failure of ether to produce an increase in bromsulfalein retention was of considerable surprise to us, and we are at a loss to explain why our findings are the opposite of those reported by others. It must be taken into account, however, that our first postoperative examination of liver function was 24 hours after anesthesia. The intervening time should be studied, as healthy young soldiers may respond more quickly than average civilian patients. It may be stated, therefore, that so far as this study is concerned, evidence of poor liver function in patients seen for the first time postoperatively is not to be explained as an effect of ether anesthesia.

[2] Oliguria was defined as a 24-hour urinary output of 100-600 cc. for at least 1 day in the post-traumatic period.

[3] Anuria was defined as a urinary output of less than 100 cc. in 24 hours.

TABLE 45.—ETHER ANESTHESIA IN RELATION TO BROMSULFALEIN RETENTION AND PLASMA NONPROTEIN NITROGEN LEVELS IN 42 PATIENTS

Case No.	Age	Major Wounds	Degree of Shock	On Admission		Duration of Anesthesia	First Postoperative Day		Second Postoperative Day	
				Dye Retention	NPN		Dye Retention	NPN	Dye Retention	NPN
	yrs.			percent	mg. per 100 cc.	minutes	percent	mg. per 100 cc.	percent	mg. per 100 cc.
91	27	Traumatic amputation, thigh	None	15	33	90	5	....	....	—
106	21	Transection, femoral artery	......do......	8	30	180	7	24	1	—
125	34	Perforating, chest; fracture, humerus; gas gangrene	Severe	15	64	150	26	89	6	136
130	27	Compound comminuted fractures, tibia, ilium (with penetrating, chest)	......do......	3	27	240	3	49	18	60
134	33	Penetrating, abdomen, chest	None	10	35	50	17	....	12	46
139	26	Penetrating, chest; fracture, femur	Severe	15	53	150	8	36	....	—
140	23	Penetrating, abdomen	Slight	10	37	175	8	....	11	41
141	19	Penetrating, abdomen, chest	......do......	15	36	135	7	29	4	—
142	24	Penetrating, chest	Moderate	5	26	75	6	29	6	—
144	32	Perforating, face with compound fractures	Slight	10	33	135	8	....	6	24
145	41	Penetrating, arm, thigh, chest	......do......	14	43	120	13	....	8	34
148	25	Traumatic amputation, both lower legs	Moderate	6	46	60	....	40	....	—
A-1	23	Penetrating, chest	Slight	6	26	210	1	30	....	—
A-2	21	Perforating, abdomen	......do......	7	29	225	2	26	3	—
A-3	25	Penetrating, abdomen	Moderate	7	27	160	22	46	6	60
A-5	17	Traumatic amputation, foot	Slight	6	30	50	0	28	2	21
A-6	22	Penetrating, abdomen	Moderate	31	38	180	34	45	30	46
A-11	?	Penetrating, chest	Slight	14	27	70	6	29	2	31

A-16	23	Penetrating, chest, abdomen	None	6	47	90	10	63	....	—
A-17	21	Traumatic amputation, lower arm; penetrating, abdomen	Slight	30	31	180	16	34	9	26
A-18	35	Traumatic amputation, leg (with fracture, other leg)	Moderate	40	53	120	12	69	8	43
A-19	26	Compound fracture, tibia	None	23	42	90	17	53	4	36
A-20	29	Traumatic amputation, foot	Slight	15	30	77	1	27	1	23
A-21	21	Near traumatic amputation, midthigh	Severe	9	58	90	7	58	2	51
A-22	21	Perforating, liver, kidney	None	23	31	140	10	29	12	—
A-27	25	Penetrating, abdomen	.......do.......	0	29	145	0	27	0	26
A-28	20	Compound fractures, femur, humerus	Severe	24	41	195	3	37	2	25
A-29	20	Severed femoral artery	.......do.......	22	44	70	4	34	2	29
A-31	20	Perforating, chest	Moderate	11	48	180	6	49	6	25
A-32	19	Penetrating, chest	.......do.......	8	37	100	4	46	5	—
A-35	25	Near traumatic amputation, lower leg	.......do.......	34	31	60	5	34	....	—
A-37	19	Compound fracture, humerus	.......do.......	4	36	85	2	29	2	28
A-38	19	Compound comminuted fracture with severe mangling, lower leg	Severe	6	48	215	3	44	3	40
A-40	25	Penetrating, back, abdomen, chest	Slight	0	36	182	1	29	1	26
*122	22	Perforating, chest, abdomen	Severe	19	42	300	30	63	....	—
*126	23	Thoraco-abdominal	Moderate	0	49	110	30	51	....	—
*129	20	Penetrating wounds, lumbar region, compound comminuted fractures	.......do.......	15	32	125	4	82	6	104
*131	27	Penetrating, chest, abdomen	Severe	10	39	253	16	104	7	116
*143	28	Perforating, chest, abdomen	Moderate	26	38	120	28	66	27	62
*147	23	Penetrating, abdomen	Severe	10	47	163	20	105	....	—
*A-30	24	Severed femoral artery	Moderate	12	39	120	30	61	39	90
*A-36	21	Multiple soft-tissue wounds, both thighs	.......do.......	1	53	210	42	77	....	—

* Patient died.

TABLE 46.—EFFECT OF ETHER ANESTHESIA ON AVERAGE BROMSULFALEIN RETENTION AND NONPROTEIN NITROGEN LEVELS[1]

Patients	All Patients (42 cases)	Patients not Moribund [2] (34 cases)	Moribund Patients Only (8 cases)
Age of Patient (years)	24.5	24.8±0.9	23.4
Bromsulfalein Retention on Hospital Entry (percent)	12.8	13.3±1.7	11.6
Nonprotein Nitrogen Level (mg. per 100 cc.)	*38.6*	*37.7 ±1.7*	*42.4*
Ether Anesthesia Duration (minutes)	140.0	132.0±6.0	175.0
Bromsulfalein Retention, First Postoperative Day (percent)	11.6	8.3±1.4	25.0
Nonprotein Nitrogen Level (mg. per 100 cc.)	*47.8*	*39.7 ±3.0*	*76.2*
Bromsulfalein Retention, Second Postoperative Day (percent)	7.8	6.1±1.2	19.8
Nonprotein Nitrogen Level (mg. per 100 cc.)	*48.0*	*39.9 ±5.0*	*93.0*

[1] Since there is a possibility that the liver plays a larger role than is now recognized in nonprotein nitrogen levels, the effect of ether anesthesia on the plasma nonprotein nitrogen was also investigated. It has been stated that ether anesthesia produces a rise in the nonprotein nitrogen level. No evidence to substantiate this was found in our patients, if those who are moribund are excluded. It is well-known and confirmed here that the nonprotein nitrogen level rises rapidly in moribund patients.

[2] Standard errors of the mean are shown for this series to indicate the spread encountered.

SUMMARY

Liver function in the severely wounded was measured by bromsulfalein retention. In 90 percent of 50 apparently healthy soldiers, the average bromsulfalein retention was found to be 1.0±0.1 percent 45 minutes after intravenous injection of 5 mg. of the dye per Kg. of body weight. On the basis of the findings in this control group, the upper limit of normal retention was arbitrarily fixed at 3 percent.

Considerable impairment of liver function was observed in the newly wounded at the time of their arrival at a most forward hospital, the average impairment in 59 patients being 12.4±1.2 (standard error of the mean) percent as measured by bromsulfalein retention. This finding has been considered in connection with several factors:

Time from Wounding.—No relationship could be found between time from wounding and bromsulfalein retention.

Location of Wound.—Patients with extremity wounds had the same average retention (13.3±2.3 percent) as those with abdominal wounds (14.7±2.1 percent). Curiously, those with chest wounds seemed to have less retention of the dye (7.0±1.8 percent) than those in the previous categories. Patients with direct injury to the liver showed 18.4-percent average retention. It is doubtful if this is significantly higher than that found in other abdominal wounds, since there was considerable spread in the data.

Shock.—No correlation between presence or degree of shock and liver function was shown, and, as might be expected, no correlation of bromsulfalein retention with blood-volume loss or hemoglobin loss. The great deterioration of the circulation found in patients in the more severe shock categories does not appear to strain liver function measurably insofar as can be judged from these data.

Plasma.—It was surprising that one of the great stresses placed upon the body, such as that due to shock, had little if any effect on liver function as measured by bromsulfalein retention, yet the administration of one or two units of blood plasma produced a considerable, although transient, increase in retention.

POSTOPERATIVE FINDINGS

Liver function during the postoperative course of the severely wounded, as determined by bromsulfalein retention and bilirubin and uric acid levels, is recorded.

The statement has been made repeatedly in the past that liver function as measured by bromsulfalein retention is considerably impaired by ether anesthesia. In order properly to assess patients seen for the first time postoperatively, liver function studies were carried out in 42 patients before and after prolonged ether anesthesia. Contrary to other reports, we found in these patients at least a decrease in bromsulfalein retention postoperatively, except in those who were moribund. There is generally a sharp increase in bromsulfalein retention in patients whose condition is deteriorating rapidly.

CHAPTER III

Renal Function in the Severely Wounded

The desirability of measuring renal function as accurately as possible in the severely wounded was clear at the outset of the study. In the majority of cases this was done by determination of phenolsulfonphthalein excretory capacity and by urine concentration tests, in conjunction with routine urine and blood chemistry analyses. Mannitol and sodium para-amino hippurate did not become available for clearance measurements until the last weeks of the Italian campaign. Results of the phenolsulfonphthalein, urine concentration, and the few renal clearance tests performed will be described.

Phenolsulfonphthalein Excretory Capacity

Because of practical considerations, the phenolsulfonphthalein excretion test was made postoperatively except on one patient who had no surgery, when it was done after transference from the shock ward, but in all cases it was some hours after the patient had been adequately resuscitated. Fifty-seven patients were tested, all of them within 72 hours after wounding, and some of them were tested again after the third day in order to follow their rate of improvement. The latter group comprised 12 patients available for retesting out of 37 in whom dye excretion had been found low in the first test and 3 patients on whom the first tests had been made later than the third day after wounding, but in whom the quantity of dye excreted was still low (Cases 125, 104, and 29 on Table 48).

Technique of Test.—The following technique of performing this test[1] was commonly employed. Six milligrams of phenolsulfonphthalein were injected

[1] See Appendix C for details of performing the test.

intravenously and urine was collected 15, 30, 60, and 120 minutes later. It was necessary to use an indwelling catheter in almost every instance to insure accurate collection. Oral intake of fluid was restricted in most patients at the time the test was performed; therefore, in order to promote urine flow, infusion of 1 liter of 5-percent dextrose in isotonic saline solution, or 10-percent dextrose in distilled water, was frequently started about 30 minutes before the dye was injected.

Excretory Capacity in the First 3 Days after Wounding.—The average results of the test made on 57 patients[2] during this period, together with other pertinent data, are shown in Table 47 and Chart 13.

The most striking finding was the difference in the average percentage of dye excreted by the 20 patients who had not been in shock and that excreted by the 37 who had had slight, moderate, or severe shock. At all test periods the *average* excretion was normal for the group that had not been in shock. (See also section to follow on the effect of anesthesia on these patients.) During the first 30 minutes, the average excretion was low for the group that had been in shock, and decreased progressively with increasing severity of initial shock. Although standard errors of the mean are rather large, and although there are no significant differences between the three groups with slight, moderate, or severe initial shock, the qualitative variations are evident. After the first 30 minutes, average dye excretion became normal for all patients except the 14 who had been in severe shock at hospital admission. In them the average excretion was significantly less than normal even after 2 hours.

The table shows that as phenolsulfonphthalein excretory capacity diminished, not only did the severity of initial shock increase but also, as would be expected, there was a rise in the number of patients who had had hypotension on admission and the number who subsequently developed urinary suppression and/or high azotemia.

Effect of Anesthesia.—One might argue that the diminished ability to excrete phenolsulfonphthalein in these patients might have been largely or partially an effect of the anesthetics employed, especially ether. Our data indicate that this is not true. Nineteen of the 20 patients shown in Table 47 and Chart 13, who had neither initial shock nor hypotension, received ether anesthesia, either

[2] Twenty-one of these are not included in the total series of 186 patients. They were added merely to enlarge the series of phenolsulfonphthalein tests without attempting to do complete studies. Seventeen of the 21 had no initial shock; 1 slight shock, and 3 moderate shock. Data on these additional cases were obtained from the 8th Evacuation Hospital.

TABLE 47.—AVERAGE PHENOLSULFONPHTHALEIN EXCRETORY CAPACITY OF 57 PATIENTS WITHIN 72 HOURS AFTER WOUNDING

Relationship to Degree of Shock on Hospital Admission

Degree of Shock on Admission	Number of Patients (Total: 57)	Average Phenolsulfonphthalein Excretion, *percentage increments*[1]: 15 minutes (*min. n.*: 25)	30 minutes (*min. n.*: 35)	60 minutes (*min. n.*: 45)	120 minutes (*min. n.*: 50)	Time from Wounding to Test (*hours*)	NPN on Day of Test (*mg. per 100 cc.*)	High Azotemia[2] (*number of patients*)	Oliguria or Anuria[3] (*number of patients*)	Hypotension[4] on Admission[5] (*number of patients*)
None	20	31.6±2.47	50.5±2.57	64.9±2.86	73.3±2.82	19.05±1.55 (maximum 44)	28±1.2	0	1	0
Slight	11	16.86±3.43	34.55±4.66	51.45±5.68	61.0±5.8	30.64±4.54 (maximum 66)	31.18±2.04	0	3	2
Moderate	12	12.75±2.77	33.25±5.56	49.08±7.12	66.08±7.73	31.25±3.22 (maximum 46)	43.08±4.44	3	4	11
Severe	[5] 14	9.66±3.42	25.22±6.42	36.38±8.66	43.62±9.6	37.4±3.05 (maximum 60)	47.8±4.2	7	8	14

[1] Minimum normals from Stitt.
[2] NPN level of 65 mg. per 100 cc. or higher at any time during posttraumatic period.
[3] Oliguria: 24-hour urinary output of 100–600 cc. for at least 1 day during posttraumatic period. Anuria: 24-hour urinary output of less than 100 cc.
[4] Systolic blood pressure of 80 mm. Hg or less.
[5] Includes one crush case without operation; all other P.S.P. tests were done postoperatively.

CHART 13. PHENOLSULFONPHTHALEIN EXCRETORY CAPACITY IN RELATION TO INITIAL SHOCK

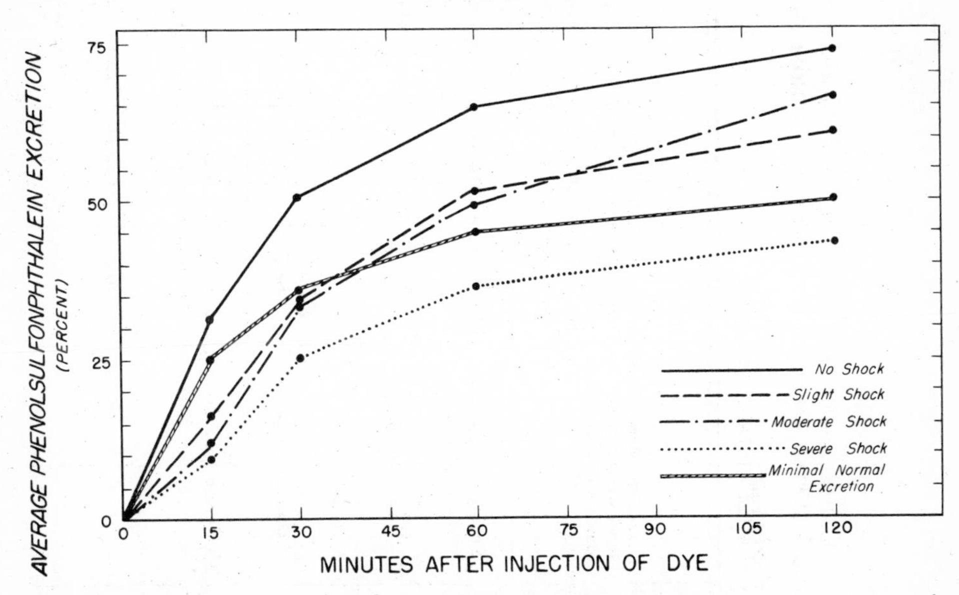

INCREMENTS of the percentage of phenolsulfonphthalein excreted are represented. Findings are discussed in the text. (Minimum normal excretion from Stitt, E. R.; Clough, P. W., and Clough, M. C.: Practical Bacteriology, Haematology, and Animal Parasitology. 9th ed. Philadelphia, Blakiston, 1938, p. 733.)

alone or with sodium pentothal, and none showed any diminution of their excretory capacity. If ether per se had any marked effect on dye excretion, it should have been evident in this group. Moreover, the average interval between wounding and performance of the test (and thus between operation and performance of the test) in these 20 patients was much less than it was in those who had been in shock and there was less time in which to recover from the effects of anesthesia had there been any. Another observation in support of the conclusion that anesthesia did not affect the ability of the kidneys to excrete phenolsulfonphthalein was that excretion was greatly diminished in the crush case in which no anesthetic had been administered.

Rate of Improvement in Excretory Capacity.—The test was repeated one or more times on 15 patients who showed a low rate of excretion when first tested. Pertinent data on each of them are given in Table 48. Thirteen of these patients recovered (3 had the syndrome of recovery diuresis to be described in

TABLE 48.—PHENOLSULFONPHTHALEIN EXCRETION AND RELATED DATA IN 15 PATIENTS ON WHOM THE TEST WAS REPEATED

Case No.	Time from Wounding to Test	Phenolsulfonphthalein Excretion *percentage increments*				NPN on Day of Test *mg. per 100 cc.*	Degree of Shock on Admission	Hypotension[1] on Admission	High Azotemia	Output of Urine (Classification)	Patient's Outcome
		15 min.	30 min.	60 min.	120 min.						
81	39 hours	0.3	2.0	14.0	25.0	77	Severe	Present	Present	Oliguria	Uneventful recovery.
	5 days	4.0	19.0	33.0	55.0	56					
60	24 hours	0.3	1.3	2.0	3.5	58	....do....	....do....	....do....	....do....	Recovery diuresis.
	4 days	1.0	2.0	3.0	5.0	108					
	9 days	6.0	18.0	25.0	34.0	46					
	12 days	21.0	31.0	43.0	52.0	33					
[2] 125	4 days	3.0	6.0	10.0	15.0	108	....do....	....do....	....do....	....do....	Do.
	14 days	3.0	7.0	18.0	27.0	65					
[2] 104	5 days	23.0	33.0	47.0	57.0	44	Moderate	....do....	....do....	....do....	Do.
	7 days	5.0	9.0	14.0	30.0	29					
	11 days	42.0	56.0	69.0	78.0	29					
107	23 days	6.0	15.0	21.0	28.0	41	....do....	....do....	....do....	Normal	Death, 6 days after wounding. Alkalosis, uremia contributory.
	5 days	0.8	1.2	3.0	17.0	73					

63	24 hours	3.0	18.0	38.0	63.0	43	....do....	....do....	Absent	Oliguria	Uneventful recovery.
	4 days	2.0	6.0	31.0	39.0	31					
	8 days	21.0	44.0	62.0	73.0	25					
1	37 hours	0.0	0.0	2.0	16.0	54	....do....	....do....	....do....	....do....	Do.
	4 days	43.0	56.0	69.0	79.0	36					
[2] 29	4 days	0.0	11.0	40.0	59.0	49	....do....	....do....	Present	....do....	Stormy course. Probable blood stream infection.
	5 days	25.0	41.0	61.0	75.0	46					
53	31 hours	8.0	15.0	27.0	56.0	37	....do....	....do....	Absent	....do....	Uneventful recovery.
	4 days	34.0	48.0	63.0	73.0	27					
15	24 hours	23.0	42.0	55.0	70.0	36	Slight	....do....	....do....	....do....	Do.
	4 days	47.0	63.0	73.0	77.0	31					
83	23 hours	6.5	23.0	36.0	44.0	26	....do....	Absent	....do....	Normal	Do.
	4 days	55.0	69.0	78.0	89.0	24					
111	14 hours	7.0	34.0	68.0	74.0	30	....do....	....do....	....do....	....do....	Do.
	5 days	41.0	43.0	71.0	74.0	48					
128	30 hours	16.0	19.0	39.0	40.0	31	....do....	....do....	....do....	....do....	Do.
	5 days	22.0	23.0	43.0	45.0	39					
106	16 hours	20.0	47.0	67.0	73.0	24	None	....do....	....do....	....do....	Do.
	4 days	40.0	57.0	73.0	81.0	....					
102	15 hours	18.0	28.0	48.0	53.0	43	....do....	....do....	....do....	....do....	Death, 19 days after wounding, from causes unrelated to renal insufficiency.
	5 days	42.0	64.0	76.0	84.0	....					

[1] 80 mm. Hg or less, systolic.
[2] Patients tested for the first time on the fourth or fifth day after wounding.

Chapter V). One patient died with alkalosis and renal failure, and the other died of peritonitis.

Inspection of this table shows that of 15 patients tested on the fourth or fifth day after wounding, 7 had normal excretion; in all 7 excretion had been low during the first 3 days after wounding. Three had had moderate initial shock, 2 slight shock, and 2 none. Of the 8 patients in whom excretion was low on the fourth or fifth day after wounding, 3 had been tested for the first time during this period, and 5 are known to have had diminished excretion during the first 3 days. The degree of shock on hospital admission in the 8 patients had been severe in 3, moderate in 3, and slight in two.

Four patients were retested between the seventh and fourteenth days. One had normal excretion by the eleventh day; another had slightly diminished excretion only during the first 15 minutes of the test on the eighth day, and two who had recovery diuresis (Cases 60 and 125) still had abnormal excretion on the twelfth and fourteenth days after wounding, respectively.

With the exception of one patient (Case 107) who died with alkalosis and renal failure, all patients in whom excretion was low on initial tests showed improvement in excretory capacity, reflected chiefly in ability to excrete increased quantities of dye during the first 30 minutes, although the total quantities excreted also increased with passage of time.

The time required for phenolsulfonphthalein excretory capacity to return to normal was well correlated with urinary output, nonprotein nitrogen retention, and degree of initial shock and hypotension (Table 48). In general, those patients with a normal output of urine or only slight suppression, with minimal nitrogen retention, and only slight initial shock regained renal function, as measured by phenolsulfonphthalein excretion, most rapidly.

Summary, P.S.P. Test

Phenolsulfonphthalein excretory capacity was determined during the first 3 days after wounding in 57 patients. The test was made after resuscitation had been effected and, with the exception of 1 patient who was not operated upon, after surgery had been completed. In 20 of these patients who had had neither initial shock nor hypotension, the average dye excretion was normal. In the remaining 37, all of whom had been in various degrees of shock, with hypotension occurring in 27, the average dye excretion was low, especially during the first 30 minutes. The amount of dye cleared decreased as severity of previous shock increased. In patients who had had slight and moderate shock, average excretion was abnormal only in the first 30 minutes; in those who had had severe shock it was low throughout the 2-hour period.

The test was repeated one or more times between the fourth and fourteenth postoperative days on 15 of 37 patients in whom initial excretion had been found low. In 14 of them dye excretion returned to normal during this time. In those patients in whom impairment was only mild, kidney function was apparently normal by the fourth or fifth day. In patients in whom it was more severe (e.g., in recovery diuresis) renal insufficiency, as gaged by phenolsulfonphthalein excretory capacity, persisted much longer.

Renal Clearance Studies

The majority of the severely wounded patients who died exhibited evidence of renal insufficiency (see Chapter V). Histologic examination of the kidneys of these patients showed damage predominantly in the lower nephron and relatively little evidence of glomerular damage (see Chapter IX). The anatomic findings immediately raised the question of how closely functional impairment corresponded with anatomic alterations. One obvious approach to solution of this problem was utilization of clearance methods of measuring renal function. This was done in 11 patients—a small series but the largest we could obtain after the materials necessary for performance of the tests became available.

Mannitol was used for measurement of glomerular filtration rate (C_M), sodium para-amino hippurate for effective renal plasma flow (C_{PAH}) and maximum tubular excretory capacity (Tm_{PAH}). Analysis of these substances is discussed in Appendix C. Quantities given and rates of administration were essentially those suggested by Goldring and Chasis.[3] Indwelling, multiple-eyed catheters were routinely employed. The bladder was washed with 10 to 30 cc. of isotonic salt solution at the end of each collection period, followed by 10 to 20 cc. of air to insure complete emptying.

Renal clearance findings together with other pertinent data on the 11 individual patients are shown in Table 49. Five patients were studied within the first 31 hours after wounding, but not until resuscitation had been effected and operation completed. One of them had had no shock, 1 slight, 2 moderate, and

[3] GOLDRING, W., and CHASIS, H.: Hypertension and Hypertensive Disease. New York, The Commonwealth Fund, 1944.

1 severe initial shock. None of them had high azotemia (a plasma nonprotein nitrogen level of 65 mg. per 100 cc. or higher) while we observed them. Output of urine was normal in 4 patients; one was listed as having had oliguria for 1 day (Case 142), but it was slight and can be disregarded.

The remaining six patients were first studied between 3 and 30 days after wounding. All of them had high azotemia at some time during their course. One had no initial shock, two moderate, and three severe shock. In three patients clearances were first measured while renal failure was severe and repeated after recovery diuresis had taken place. A fourth had had severe renal failure, but clearance tests were not made until 30 days after wounding, by which time he had recovery diuresis and his plasma nonprotein nitrogen was normal. The remaining two patients died 16 hours and 5 days, respectively, after clearance studies were done; in both uremia was present at the time of death but in neither was it an immediate or contributory cause of death.

Results

Charts 14 through 16, in each of which all 11 cases are included, were constructed from mean normals[4 5 6] and average values listed in Table 49. The 5 patients who did not have high azotemia are represented by open symbols; the 6 who had renal failure by solid or semi-solid symbols. For Cases 138, 150, and 133—those with the lowest renal clearance values—only the initial observation is shown. Chart 17 shows these initial values in addition to results when the tests were repeated on 1 of these 3 patients.

Glomerular Filtration Rate and Effective Plasma Flow $\left(\frac{C_M}{C_{PAH}}\right)$*—Table 49 and Chart* 14.—These were definitely below normal in one patient (Case 139) 20 hours after wounding; he was the only one of the five studied during the early postoperative period who had had severe initial shock. In two of these five glomerular filtration rate and effective plasma flow were in the low normal ranges. Marked diminution of both components in the three patients (Cases 133, 138, 150) with severe renal failure is evident. There were lesser degrees of impairment in the two in whom renal failure was only coincident in death

[4] Ibid.

[5] BERGER, E. Y.; FARBER, S. J., and EARLE, D. P., JR.: Renal excretion of mannitol. Proc. Soc. Exper. Biol. & Med. 66: 62–66, Oct. 1947.

[6] CHASIS, H.; REDISH, J.; GOLDRING, W.; RANGES, H. A., and SMITH, H. W.: Use of sodium p-amino hippurate for functional evaluation of human kidney. J. Clin. Investigation 24: 583–588, July 1945.

Chart 14. Relationship between Average Effective Plasma Flow and Glomerular Filtration Rate in 5 Patients Without and 6 Patients With Renal Failure

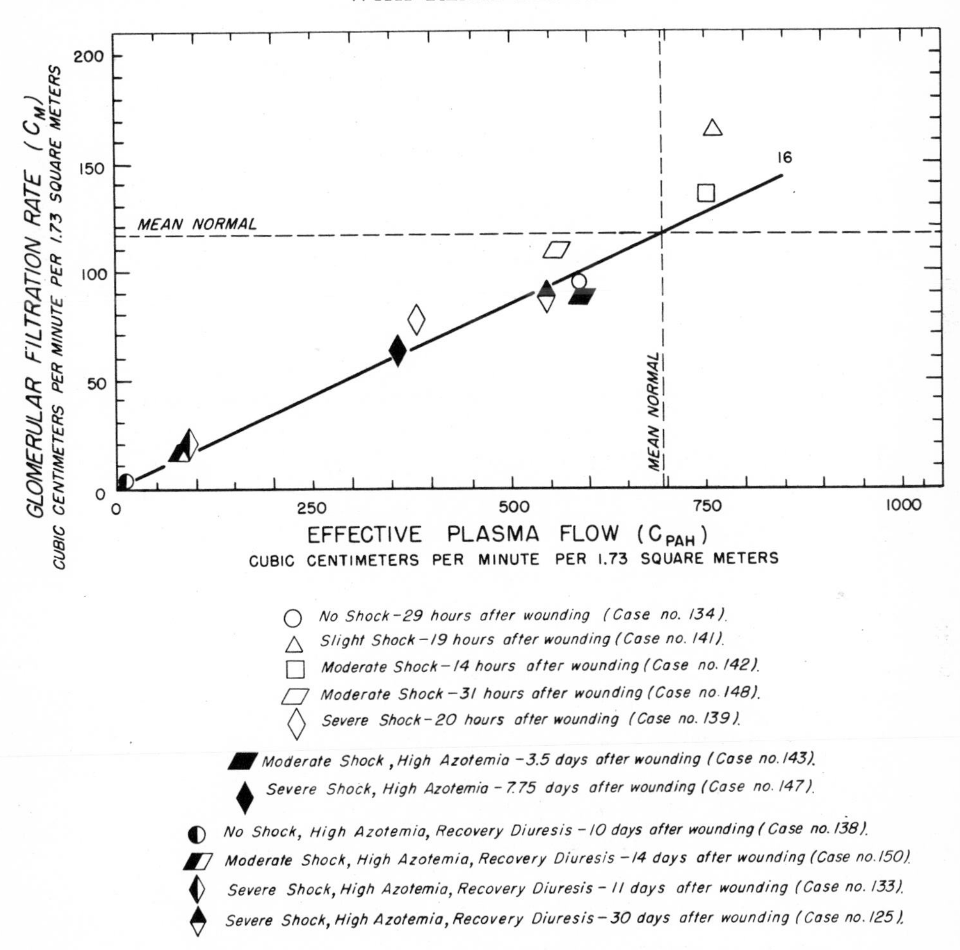

THE VALUES represented in this and in the succeeding two charts were obtained from average values shown in Table 49. The diagonal line shows normal filtration fraction $\left(\frac{C_M}{C_{PAH}}\right)$. The solid and semisolid symbols represent patients with high azotemia and various degrees of renal failure; the open figures patients who at no time had azotemia.

(Cases 143 and 147), and in the one (Case 125) who had fairly well recovered from renal failure. The tendency of glomerular filtration rate and effective

956507 O—52——8

TABLE 49.—SUMMARY OF RENAL CLEARANCE STUDIES IN 11 PATIENTS

Case No.	Urine Flow *cc. per min.* (all periods)	Glomerular Filtration Rate (C_M) *cc. per min.*	Effective Plasma Flow (C_{PAH}) *cc. per min.*	Effective Blood Flow *cc. per min.*	Maximal Tubular Excretory Capacity (Tm_{PAH}) *mg. per min.*	Time after Wounding	Degree of Shock on Admission	High Azotemia	NPN on Day of Test *mg. per 100 cc.*	Output of Urine *Classification*	Output of Urine on Day of Test *cc.*	Blood Pressure on Day of Test	Patient's Outcome
134	3.6	95	588	1,071	84	29 hrs.	None	No	43	Normal	1,635	114/65	Recovery.
141	4.8	167	762	1,093	56	19 hrs.	Slight	No	41	......do......	2,420	120/80	Do.
142	4.8	135	754	1,136	91	14 hrs.	Moderate	No	27	Oliguria	1,693	130/70	Do.
148	3.8	109	567	816	63	31 hrs.	......do......	No	40	Normal	1,787	130/70	Do.
139	5.2	79	381	556	97	20 hrs.	Severe	No	[1] 36	......do......	3,762	114/78	Do.
	2.34	20	99	163	7	11 days	......do......	Yes	108	Un-known; probable oliguria	[2] 1,270	150/110	Recovery diuresis.
	4.0	26	....	....	....	13 days			112		2,380	140/110	
133	3.42	58	342	499	....	28 days			36		over 1,000	122/96	
	4.33	157	688	1,146	....	47 days			24		over 1,000	120/70	
	9.14	107	....	....	90	49 days			20		over 1,000	120/70	

125	5.72	89	544	870	80	30 days	......do......	Yes	26	Oliguria	1,550	130/91	Do.
150	4.42	15	87	131	12	14 days	Moderate	Yes	123	Anuria	3,350	170/100	Do.
	4.74	100	414	686	67	26 days			24		[2] 3,000	130/70	
138	3.0	3	20	28	4	10 days	None	Yes	217	Unknown; probable oliguria	[2] 1,500	140/68	Do.
	5.54	64	431	676	43	26 days			44		[2] 4,500	128/70	
143	3.8	89	598	1,037	108	3 days, 14 hrs.	Moderate	Yes	57	Normal	1,986	110/60	Died 5 days later. Uremia coincident at death.
147	4.1	64	356	630	70	7 days, 18 hrs.	Severe	Yes	99	......do......	1,558	110/60	Died 16 hrs. later. Uremia coincident at death.
Mean normal with standard deviation [3]		116± 28.6	697± 135.9	1,204± 255.9	77.5± 12.9								

Values in columns 3 through 6 corrected to 1.73 square meters of body surface; each represents average values for 2 to 4 periods in all cases except Case 134 where effective plasma and blood flow were determined during 1 period only.

[1] 1 day later.

[2] Approximate.

[3] Normals and standard deviations: See footnote 3 in text.

plasma flow each to diminish proportionately was demonstrated by the relatively normal filtration fractions $\left(\frac{C_M}{C_{PAH}}\right)$ in most cases.

Maximum Tubular Excretory Capacity (Tm_{PAH})—*Table* 49 *and Chart* 15.—There is wide variation in this measurement which may represent the actual amount of actively functioning tubular tissue, and is hence related to the functional size of the kidneys. It was significantly low in only the three patients with severe renal failure (Cases 133, 138, 150). It is of interest that the one patient with severe initial shock, who was studied 20 hours after wounding, had a low filtration rate and effective plasma flow but normal Tm (Case 139). Relating plasma flow to maximum excretory capacity $\left(\frac{C_{PAH}}{Tm_{PAH}}\right)$ provides substantially an expression of the quantity of plasma cleared per unit of functionally active tubular tissue. The diagonal line in the chart is the normal ratio. Ratios significantly

CHART 15. RELATIONSHIP BETWEEN AVERAGE EFFECTIVE PLASMA FLOW AND MAXIMAL TUBULAR EXCRETORY CAPACITY

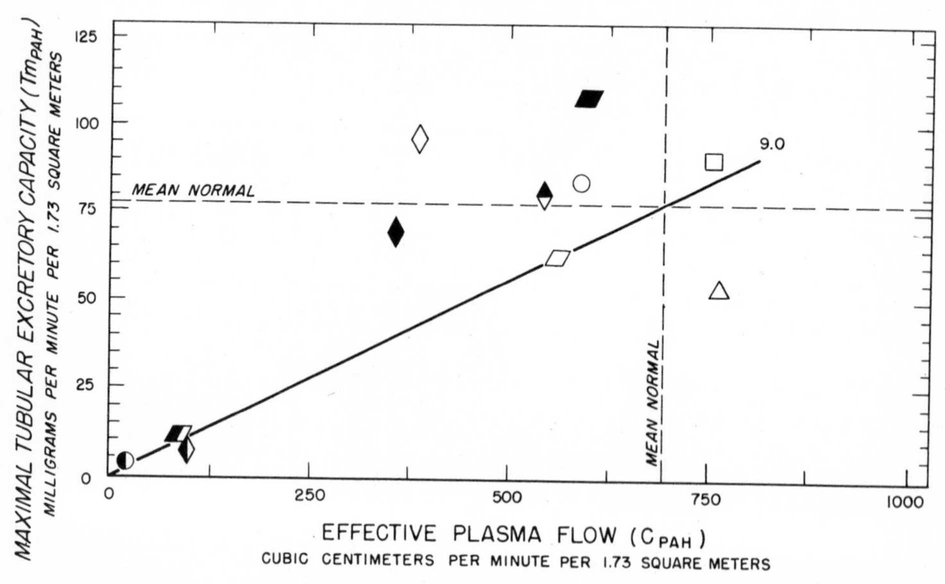

THE SYMBOLS for the individual cases represented are explained on Chart 14. The diagonal line represents $\frac{C_{PAH}}{Tm_{PAH}}$. Variation is wide, but noteworthy perhaps is the fact that all but two patients had normal ratios or ratios less than normal.

CHART 16. RELATIONSHIP BETWEEN AVERAGE GLOMERULAR FILTRATION RATE AND MAXIMAL TUBULAR EXCRETORY CAPACITY

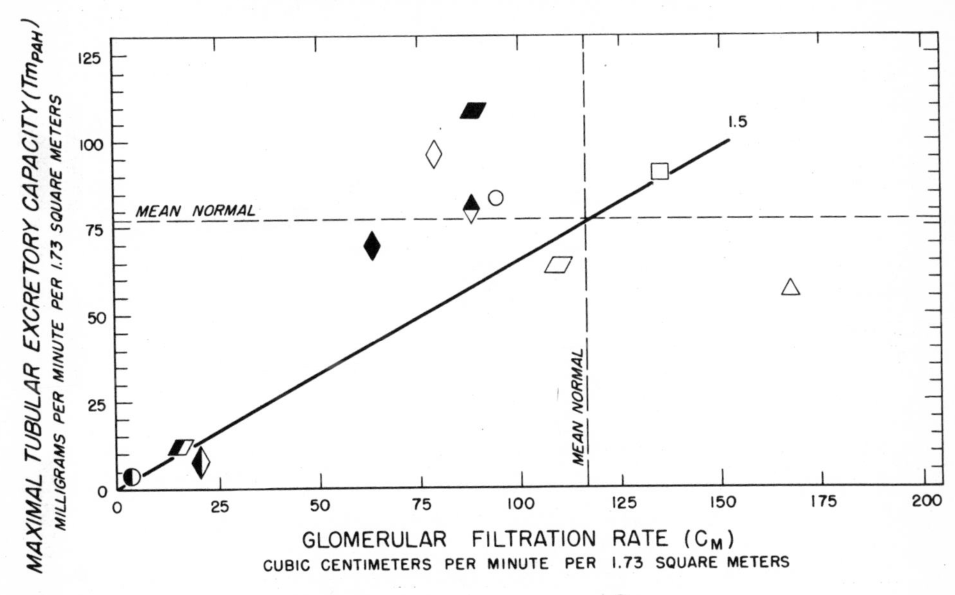

THERE IS an unexpected tendency for the ratio of $\frac{C_M}{Tm_{PAH}}$ to be below normal. The symbols used for individual cases are the same as those of Charts 14 and 15.

below normal presumably indicate relative renal ischemia. It may be significant that this ratio was normal or below normal in nine patients, and that it was lowest in the patient tested shortly after he had recovered from severe shock (Case 139).

Relating filtration rate to maximal tubular excretory capacity $\left(\frac{C_M}{Tm_{PAH}}\right)$ (normal ratio: the diagonal line in Chart 16) gives an expression of glomerular function per unit of functioning tubular tissue. Ratios below normal presumably indicate greater relative impairment of glomerular function than tubular, and high ratios the reverse. Nine of the 11 patients had either a normal or low ratio, a fact which, if significant, is difficult to explain in view of the anatomic lesion in this type of case.

Rate of Recovery as Gaged by C_M, C_{PAH}, *and* Tm_{PAH}—*Table* 49 *and Chart* 17.—Findings in three patients (Cases 133, 138, and 150) who had severe renal failure but recovered (see discussion of recovery diuresis in Chapter V) are

CHART 17. SEVERE RENAL FAILURE AND SUBSEQUENT RECOVERY DIURESIS; RATE OF RECOVERY (CASE 133)

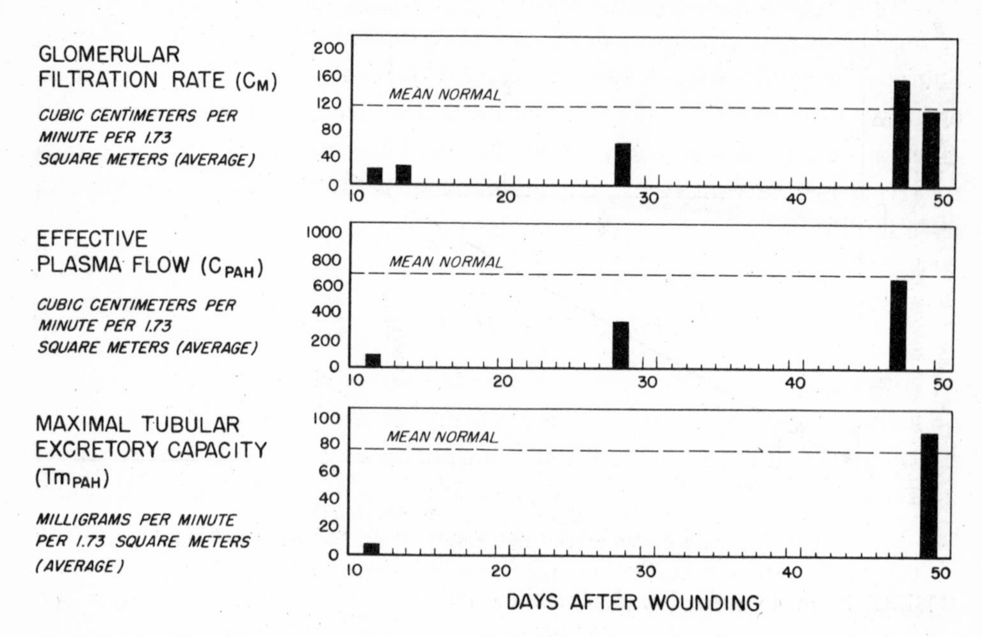

NOTE (1) the relatively proportionate reduction in glomerular filtration rate, effective plasma flow, and maximum tubular excretory capacity, and (2) similar recovery rates for all three.

shown in Table 49 and Chart 17 (Case 133). Initial observations were made during periods of maximum failure, subsequent ones after recovery had largely taken place. In general, on the basis of clearance measurements, all portions of the nephron were about equally affected; recovery likewise occurred at about an even rate in all portions. Function was apparently completely restored in one patient (Case 133) 49 days after wounding and partially so in another patient 26 days after wounding.

Summary, Renal Clearance

Renal clearance was measured in 11 patients in this study. Of 5 tested within 31 hours after wounding, findings were essentially normal in four. The fifth patient showed significantly low rates of glomerular filtration and effective plasma flow, but normal maximum tubular excretory capacity. He was the only one studied in the early postoperative period who had had severe initial shock.

Six patients in whom high azotemia (a plasma nonprotein nitrogen level of 65 mg. per 100 cc. or higher) developed were studied in various stages of renal failure. The results suggest that in this type of renal insufficiency all portions of the nephron suffer functional impairment, and that all portions regenerate at about an equal rate if recovery ensues. Evidence has been presented that a relative renal ischemia may exist, but the number of cases is too small for this to be of significance.

Urine Concentration Test

Although the value of the urine concentration test was self-evident, practical difficulties prevented our using it as a measure of renal function in many cases. Restriction of fluids during the first few postoperative days was almost always inadvisable for the patients' welfare. Pituitrin was therefore employed, using the accepted method of administering 0.5 cc. of posterior pituitary extract (10 units) subcutaneously and collecting urine specimens 1 and 2 hours afterward. However, many of the patients in whom we should like to have known concentrating ability were daily receiving considerable quantities of sodium chloride intravenously. Since the antidiuretic hormone may be ineffective during saline administration, there was concern that in a large number of cases the pituitrin test would be complicated by recent administration of isotonic saline solution, but in most instances we did not feel justified in requesting that the saline solution be withheld.

A compromise regimen was therefore established in which all parenteral fluids were withheld for 7 or 8 hours before the pituitrin was administered whenever such restriction clearly would not be harmful in any way to the patient. Under these conditions a value for normal concentrating ability is difficult to state; we have assumed that a specific gravity of 1.025 or higher represents normal integrity of tubular reabsorptive capacity for water. Data on the 32 patients in whom concentrating ability of the kidneys was tested in this manner during the postoperative days indicated are shown in Table 50.

Of the 17 patients in whom we assumed there was no impairment of concentrating ability (that is, the specific gravity of one hourly specimen was 1.025 or higher) during the first week after wounding, 8 had had moderate or severe

TABLE 50.—RESULTS OF URINE CONCENTRATION TESTS EMPLOYING PITUITRIN—32 CASES

Specific Gravity of Urine[1]	Time from Wounding to First Test	Other Related Factors — Number of Patients: Degree of Initial Shock							Total Patients
	Days	None	Slight	Moderate	Severe	Hypotension on Admission	Oliguria or Anuria	High Azotemia Developed	
1.025 or Higher . .	2 to 7	3	6	5	3	8	6	2	17
1.018 to 1.025 . .	2 to 8	0	1	8	0	5	5	1	9
Under 1.018 . . .	1 to 17	1	1	1	3	4	[2] 5	5	6
Total . . .		4	8	14	6	17	16	8	32

[1] Normal by the method used: 1 hourly specimen of 1.025 or higher.
[2] Actual output unknown in 2 cases, but good presumptive evidence of oliguria.

shock and hypotension on admission. In 2 of these 17, high azotemia subsequently developed. Of the 9 patients with slightly decreased ability to reabsorb water from the kidney tubules (specific gravity of urine 1.018 to 1.025), 8 had been in moderate shock, 5 had hypotension on admission, in 5 oliguria or anuria developed, and in 1 high azotemia. In the 6 patients with marked impairment of concentrating ability, 4 had had moderate or severe shock, and 4 hypotension. Severe and prolonged azotemia developed in 5 of these 6; they are discussed in the section on recovery diuresis in Chapter V.

The urine concentration test was made more than once in eight patients. In two of them the specific gravity, which was 1.018 at the time of the first test, rose to 1.020 two and seven days later, respectively. In one it increased from 1.017 to 1.022 in three days. One of these three patients also had high azotemia and oliguria, and two had normal output of urine and a plasma nonprotein nitrogen level under 65 mg. per 100 cubic centimeters. The remaining five patients had recovery diuresis, and after periods of from 14 to 40 days still were unable to produce a concentrated urine.

Although the series was small, it suggests that the concentrating ability of the kidneys may follow somewhat the same pattern as ability to excrete phenolsulfonphthalein, mannitol, and sodium para-amino hippurate. Ability to make a concentrated urine appeared to diminish within 2 days following shock, and improve over a period of from 3 to 7 days, unless renal failure was severe (recovery diuresis) in which case maximum tubular reabsorption of water remained diminished for many days or even weeks. In two patients (Cases 125 and 133) specific gravity remained fixed even after clearance of mannitol and sodium para-amino hippurate had returned to normal.

COMMENT

It has been demonstrated by Lauson, Bradley, and Cournand[7] that during shock glomerular filtration rate and effective plasma flow are reduced. These workers have also advanced evidence that reduction in renal blood flow is partially explained by active vasoconstriction of the renal blood vessels as well as by reduction of arterial pressure.

[7] Lauson, H. D.; Bradley, S. E., and Cournand, A.: Renal circulation in shock. J. Clin. Investigation 23: 381–402, May 1944.

None of our studies were carried out while the patients were in shock. Those performed in the first few days after trauma suggest that the impairment in kidney function may persist for some days after shock is relieved, even though the usually accepted signs of renal failure (suppression of urinary output, nitrogen retention) may be meager. These patients probably rapidly regain normal kidney function.

If the initial insult, whatever it might have been, was great, the resulting renal insufficiency was much more severe and prolonged, and in a significant proportion of cases resulted in death in uremia. A few patients, however, did recover, with gradually increasing function over a period of days to weeks, as indicated by their progress in restoration of ability to excrete phenolsulfonphthalein, improvement in the glomerular filtration rate, and by increased effective plasma flow, maximum tubular excretory capacity, and concentrating capacity of the urine.

Although the histologic picture in fatal cases might suggest a selective functional impairment of the lower nephron, our studies indicated that all functional components of the kidneys were about equally impaired. Glomerular filtration rate and effective plasma flow were reduced in essentially proportionate degrees in most of the patients we studied. That there may have been some relative renal ischemia in these cases is suggested by the fact that in the few patients on whom clearance tests were done, the ratio of $\frac{C_{PAH}}{Tm_{PAH}}$ tended to be low. One bit of evidence in favor of greater relative insult in the lower nephron may be cited from the two patients in whom ability to concentrate urine was still much impaired after clearances had returned to normal. Mannitol measures glomerular filtration; sodium para-amino hippurate is believed to be excreted by the proximal tubules. Urine concentration takes place primarily in the distal tubule. The question arises whether this lag in recovery of concentrating capacity is a manifestation of greater relative damage to the lower nephron. The discrepancies between the physiologic and anatomic findings could perhaps be explained by the production in these patients of renal vascular shunts, such as Trueta[8] and his associates have recently demonstrated in animals. It is impossible to state from our data whether such a mechanism was operative.

[8] TRUETA, J.; BARCLAY, A. E.; DANIEL, P. M.; FRANKLIN, K. J., and PRICHARD, M. M. L.: Studies in the Renal Circulation. Springfield, Ill., Charles C Thomas, 1948.

SUMMARY

Renal function in the wounded man was studied by measuring phenolsulfonphthalein excretory capacity in 57 patients; glomerular filtration rate, effective plasma flow, and maximal tubular excretory capacity of para-amino hippuric acid in 11 patients, and urine concentration, employing pituitrin, in 32 patients. All studies were made after resuscitation had been effected, and in all surgical cases after operation had been completed. The results were qualitatively similar and indicated that functionally all portions of the nephron were about equally impaired for a period of a few to many days, depending on the severity of the initial insult which in most patients paralleled the degree of shock on admission. Similarly, diminished renal function, as indicated by these tests, was associated with corresponding increases in the level of plasma nonprotein nitrogen and with decreases in urinary output. When recovery occurred, improvement of most of these functions proceeded at about an equal rate.

These physiologic findings do not correspond with the histologic findings in fatal cases, where the lesion was observed predominantly in the lower nephron. The fact that ability to produce a concentrated urine was impaired in a few patients long after phenolsulfonphthalein excretion, glomerular filtration rate, effective plasma flow, and maximum tubular excretion of PAH had returned to normal might suggest greater relative damage to the lower nephron.

CASES OF SPECIAL INTEREST IN THIS CHAPTER

P.S.P. Re-test

1 29 60 81 102 106 111

128

15 53 63 83 104 107 125

Renal Clearance Test

125 134 139 142 147

150

133 138 141 143 148

CHAPTER IV

Diagnosis of Lower Nephron Nephrosis Resulting from Trauma and Shock ("Shock Kidney")

As Derived from Clinicopathologic Correlation

The clinical syndrome of renal insufficiency following traumatic shock had not yet, to our knowledge at the time of this study, been defined in the medical literature. In the interval preceding publication Lucké[1] has described, from both clinical and pathologic points of view, a group of similar cases under the term "lower nephron nephrosis." The present study, though now no longer novel, was done independently before his publication and therefore offers unbiased confirmation which seems worthy of record. Since civilian practice brings so few apposite cases under the observation of any single group of investigators, one of our clearest obligations was to attempt definition of this syndrome.

In exploration of a new syndrome the first necessity is establishment of a base of departure; that is, an apparently new combination of symptoms, signs, laboratory observations, or distinctive morphologic lesions. With widening experience, additions to and subtractions from this combination are made until the pattern becomes stabilized, the diagnostic importance of each feature or group of features being assessed by the frequency with which it occurs in the disease in question as compared with its infrequency in other conditions.

Since the case fatality rate of this condition was high, there is little risk of distorting the picture by using the fatal cases to establish the base of departure. In 38 of 60 cases in which necropsy material was available, pigment nephropathy,

[1] Lucké, B.: Lower nephron nephrosis. Mil. Surg. 99: 371–396, November 1946.

the characteristic renal lesion of "shock kidney" which will be described in Chapter IX, was present. In the following discussion the symptomatology in these cases will be presented, comparing the findings as we proceed with the control group of 22 cases in which pigment nephropathy was proved absent at necropsy. To determine whether diagnosis of renal injury can be established beyond reasonable doubt, the fatal cases will be further compared with nonfatal cases in which there was evidence of kidney dysfunction.

Objective Evidence of Renal Insufficiency in Cases of Histologically Proved Nephropathy

Oliguria and Anuria

For purposes of this study, oliguria was defined as a 24-hour output of urine greater than 100 cc. and less than 600 cc.; anuria as an output not exceeding 100 cc. per day. Urine output, known in 35 of the above-mentioned 38 patients with the characteristic renal lesion, had been subnormal for one or more days in all, 15 patients remaining in the oliguric and 20 reaching the anuric level. Oliguria or anuria was present from the onset of shock in all but one case, and in this case the delay was apparent rather than real. The initial shock had been mild, but secondary shock of greater severity occurred after operation and was promptly followed by anuria. The majority of patients showed progression from oliguric to anuric levels, but occasionally anuria was present from the start. In 15 patients with clinical uremia and histologically proved nephropathy, the urine output never declined below the oliguric level. It is worth emphasis that these individuals, often casually referred to as "anuria cases," may never in fact become anuric. Unless 24-hour outputs are carefully measured, significant oliguria may easily be missed.

Nine patients with oliguria (or anuria) failed to show a significant renal lesion at necropsy. This is not surprising, considering the variety of conditions from which these severely wounded men suffered which would tend to lower urine output, such as deficient blood volume, prolonged hypotension, paralytic ileus, infection, and exudation into traumatized areas and into infected serous cavities. In two of the nine oliguria or anuria was intermittent; in both the clinical picture was dominated by severe peritonitis.

Azotemia

"High azotemia," arbitrarily defined as a nonprotein nitrogen level in the plasma of 65 mg. per 100 cc. or higher, was found in 36 of the 38 proved nephrotic cases; in 1 case no determination was available, and in the remaining 1, death occurred within 35 hours of injury. In this patient the nonprotein level had already climbed to 63 mg. per 100 cc., only 2 points below our arbitrary limit, and there can be no reasonable doubt that this limit would have been passed had he lived a few hours longer. Like oliguria, nitrogen retention was evident from the outset. The retention level climbed steadily, usually from 30 to 40 points a day, the maximal level depending solely on the length of time elapsing before death ensued or, in those who survived, before onset of diuresis. Nitrogen retention, like oliguria, was also observed in the absence of a renal lesion (7 instances) and is explainable on similar grounds.

Hypertension

We defined hypertension for purposes of this study as an elevation of the systolic blood pressure to or above 135 mm. Hg and of the diastolic to 90 mm. Hg or higher. By civilian standards these figures must seem low, but it is to be remembered that we were dealing primarily with a homogeneous group of young men between 18 and 30 years of age who had recently suffered severe trauma usually associated with the loss of considerable amounts of blood. By this standard, 20 of 32 patients with the renal lesion whose blood pressures had been recorded were judged to have significant elevations of systolic or diastolic pressure or both. Hypertension rarely appeared within the first 48 hours; it was frequent by 72 hours, and was the rule by 96 hours.

Of the remaining 12 patients with the characteristic renal lesion who failed to show an elevation of blood pressure, 3 died within 2 days of injury and 6 on the third day. In only 3 patients living beyond the 3-day period did hypertension fail to develop. One died on the fourth, 1 on the fifth, and 1 on the seventh day respectively. The last 2 patients also had a severe progressive peritonitis. It seems reasonable to conclude that hypertension is a characteristic if not constant symptom of the syndrome.

The importance of hypertension is increased when viewed from the converse point of view. No patient in this series whose kidneys failed to show pigment nephropathy at necropsy had a sustained elevation of blood pressure, although an occasional determination might have been above the arbitrary limit. It must be remembered, however, that no cases of cerebral injury were included in our series. In such cases hypertension secondary to increased intracranial pressure is of course frequent.

Pigment Excretion in the Urine

As part of the routine urine examination of all patients included in this study, the supernatant urine after centrifugation was tested with benzidine for the presence of dissolved heme-containing pigments,[2] which, as will be discussed fully in Chapter VIII, were largely hemoglobin and myoglobin.

All patients with morphologic evidence of renal damage excreted benzidine-positive material in the urine. In 11 patients (exclusive of those in whom there was direct trauma to the urinary tract) enough pigment was excreted to make the urine grossly red or brown. In some cases descriptions such as "dark amber" suggest a pigment element, but in the majority amber and yellow were the colors recorded, and only the benzidine test revealed the pigment element. Pigment excretion, furthermore, was in most instances transitory and usually disappeared on the third or fourth day. On the other hand, pigment excretion was observed in 6 patients whose kidneys did not show significant lesions at necropsy.

Other Urinary Findings

Other chapters of this volume contain complete discussions of the chemical abnormalities found in the blood and urine and the results of renal function tests performed during the course of the studies. Repetition would be pointless, especially since these factors have little diagnostic value. However, three urinary abnormalities, determination of which lies within the realm of routine clinical pathology, are worthy of mention since, although of limited diagnostic value, they were constant features of the syndrome.

1. *Proteinuria.*—All patients with proved renal lesions showed proteinuria. However, since proteinuria was absent in only 14 of the entire series of casualties studied and was present in 51 patients without clinical or anatomic evidence of nephropathy, its diagnostic import is negligible.

[2] See Appendix C, section on routine urinalyses, for technique of performing the test.

2. *Persistent Acidity.*—The urine of all patients manifesting nephropathy at necropsy was acid on initial examination. The range of pH was from 5.0 to 6.9 with an average value of 5.8. The urines of the control group ranged from 5.0 to 8.4 with an average of 6.2, overlapping too much to give the figures any diagnostic value. In succeeding specimens the urine from the nephropathic group remained persistently acid with few exceptions, occasionally even despite a therapeutically-induced alkalosis.

3. *Fixation of Specific Gravity.*—The specific gravities of the initial specimens varied from 1.009 to 1.032, though the majority of specimens fell within the range of 1.020 to 1.026. No significant difference was found in patients with and without nephropathy. Diversity in these initial specimens is not surprising, since it is probable that in many instances part of the urine may have been excreted by the kidney before the patient was wounded. With the passage of time the specific gravity of subsequent specimens declined in the nephropathic group, despite oliguria, and a tendency to fixation between 1.010 and 1.015 became apparent in all the patients with proved renal lesions. Evidence of continued power of urine concentration occasionally helped to distinguish cases of "extrarenal" oliguria and azotemia from the true nephropathies.

Summary: Diagnosis of Lower Nephron Nephrosis ("Shock Kidney")

Seven phenomena have been described which are characteristic of the renal lesion following traumatic shock. One of these, proteinuria, has no diagnostic value because of its frequency in non-nephropathic cases. Two others, persistent acidity of the urine and fixation of specific gravity at a low level despite oliguria, are of great interest in defining the physiologic abnormality, but proved of limited diagnostic value since therapeutic emergencies frequently prevented verification by suitable test. A tetrad of findings—*oliguria, azotemia, pigment excretion,* and *hypertension*—were of practical diagnostic value.

Each of these may be present singly in patients with normal kidneys. So may any pair. The combination of oliguria and azotemia, for instance, was found five times; even the triad of oliguria, azotemia, and pigment excretion was found twice in patients with morphologically normal kidneys. The complete tetrad, however, was never found in this series in patients with normal kidneys. Barring the complication of a head injury, it was concluded that this tetrad might be considered reliable evidence of renal damage.

Uremic Symptomatology

Subjective symptoms of the type commonly to be expected in uremia were conspicuous primarily by their absence. In the initial stages of the disorder minor symptoms might well have been masked by the greater discomforts of recent trauma, surgery, and anesthesia, or been suppressed by postoperative narcosis. As the days pass, these distractions cease to be of importance, yet again and again statements such as "patient comfortable" and "no complaints" appeared in the records. A brief review of the usual symptoms of renal insufficiency, noting their frequency in this material, is in order.

Headache.—Headache was not mentioned in any case record. Minor complaints might not have been recorded, but even so headache could not have been a conspicuous feature.

Nausea and Vomiting.—Many of our patients had abdominal wounds with subsequent gastric and intestinal surgery complicated by various grades of peritoneal irritation. They were often treated by Wangensteen drainage, making interpretation of gastro-intestinal symptoms difficult. Nausea appeared in three of the crush-syndrome cases and also in three others not complicated by abdominal wounds. In only two of these was it associated with vomiting, once on the seventh and once on the thirteenth day. Persistent hicupping was twice recorded.

Vision.—No patient complained of visual difficulties. Eyeground examinations were recorded in nine cases. In six patients the eyes were found to be normal when examined at intervals of from 3 to 10 days, and in three patients were found to be abnormal. Two of the latter patients showed retinal hemorrhages on the fifth and tenth days of disease, respectively, and one showed papilledema on the ninth day.

Consciousness.—Drowsiness was the most frequent cerebral symptom and was noted in 17 instances. Its onset was recorded as early as the second day, as late as the ninth. Very frequently the notation was accompanied by a statement such as "patient drowsy but when aroused answers questions clearly and intelligently." One patient was frankly disoriented, and two were irrational. In 11 patients drowsiness progressed to stupor; in 6 of these the condition was described as coma. This stage seldom antedated death by many hours. Onset of coma was recorded as early as the third and as late as the tenth day. At the time of onset, the nonprotein nitrogen levels ranged from 89 to 305 mg. per 100 cc. of plasma. One patient regained consciousness after a lapse of 2 hours at a time when the

956507 O—52——9

nonprotein nitrogen level was 339 mg. per 100 cc. of plasma.

Twitchings and Convulsions.—These were very uncommon phenomena. Twitchings were recorded in two patients, convulsions in four; one of these four recovered. Neuromuscular irritability was noted in two other patients in whom Chvostek's sign developed. In both, the symptoms followed vigorous alkali therapy.

Hyperpnea.—Dyspnea or hyperpnea was recorded on 12 occasions, with onset ranging from the fourth to the twelfth day. In six instances it appeared approximately coincidentally with the onset of pulmonary edema and may well have been an effect of the latter. In only a few instances was respiration clearly of the Kussmaul type.

Edema.—Evidence of edema was observed in 25 patients. It appeared as early as the third and as late as the eleventh day, largely depending on the extent of intravenous fluid therapy. Clinical evidence of pulmonary edema was recorded in 12 instances. Either pulmonary or peripheral edema might appear first, and each was observed in the absence of the other. Facial edema was noted only 8 times.

Nonfatal Cases

In examining the clinical records of nonfatal cases in this series to see if diagnosis of renal injury could be established beyond reasonable doubt, we were hampered by incompleteness of observation and record. The findings in 44 patients whose records were fairly complete and who manifested 1 or more of the 4 criteria described above are summarized in the accompanying table.

Three patients presented the complete tetrad of characteristic findings. Two showed the triad of pigment excretion, azotemia, and hypertension, but in both there was uncertainty regarding urine output during the first 48 hours after injury. Two presented the combination of pigment excretion, oliguria, and azotemia, but blood pressure determinations at appropriate time intervals were not recorded. In five others with the same triad, hypertension could be definitely excluded.

Among those with a combination of two principal signs, one patient showed oliguria and hypertension, but nonprotein nitrogen was not determined and the urine was not tested with benzidine. In one case hypertension of notable level (170/120) and azotemia were observed, but urine output was not recorded

TABLE 51.—PRINCIPAL FINDINGS IN 44 SURVIVING PATIENTS SUSPECTED OF HAVING RENAL INSUFFICIENCY

Number of Patients	Findings			
	Pigment Excretion	Oliguria	"High Azotemia"	Hypertension (Above 135/90)
3	+	+	+	+
2	+	?	+	+
2	+	+	+	?
1	?	+	?	+
1	?	?	+	+
1	?	+	+	?
5	+	+	+	0
1	+	0	+	0
3	+	+	0	0
6	0	+	0	0
19	+	0	0	0

+ = present.
? = not recorded, or presence uncertain.
0 = absent.

nor was the urine tested with benzidine during the first 5 days. In Case 130, oliguria and unimpressive azotemia of 69 mg. per 100 cc. were demonstrated, but again the urine was not tested and no postoperative blood pressures were recorded. In another patient, azotemia and pigment excretion were present but no elevation of blood pressure occurred, and the urine excretion for the first 24 hours was 750 cc., which was above our arbitrary limit but nevertheless in the lower range of normality.

Three patients presented the remaining pair of findings: pigment excretion and oliguria. Six patients manifested only transitory oliguria without supporting evidence of nephropathy, and 19 pigment excretion with similar lack of confirmatory findings. In the light of the above findings, let us again evaluate our diagnostic criteria.

As in the fatal group, no patient with other evidence of renal insufficiency failed to show *pigment excretion* if the urine was tested with benzidine within the first 48 hours after injury. Nineteen patients out of the 44, however, who at no time showed any other evidence of renal damage, excreted benzidine-positive material.

Oliguria was demonstrated in 15 patients with 1 or more other positive findings. In 3 patients its presence was uncertain and in 6 it was observed in the absence of any other sign. In one questionable case, in which there was pigment excretion and azotemia, oliguria was absent. Oliguria in these patients who survived was, however, sometimes extremely transitory. Among the patients manifesting the complete tetrad, oliguria was of only a day's duration in two cases, and lasted only 2 days in one. The longest duration of oliguria did not exceed 4 days. In none of the cases was output depressed to anuric levels; i.e., below 100 cc. in 24 hours.

Azotemia was observed in 15 of the 44 patients. In no instance was it the sole finding. A plasma nonprotein nitrogen concentration of 88 mg. per 100 cc. accompanied only by pigment excretion occurred in one instance. In 7 patients the maximal level was below 100 mg. per 100 cc., and in 6 the range was between 100 and 150 mg. per 100 cc. of plasma. Two desperately ill patients recovered despite nonprotein nitrogen levels of 247 and 217 mg. per 100 cc. respectively. In 3 patients the azotemia was of such low degree (74, 77, and 69 mg. per 100 cc. respectively) and so transitory (lasting only 1 and 2 days) as to be of doubtful significance. In the other patients it lasted from 3 to 21 days.

Seven patients showed definite *hypertension* which ranged from 128/90 in Case 54 to 180/115 in Case 138. Blood pressure was not recorded for two patients who presented the triad of pigment excretion, oliguria, and azotemia, but did not become elevated in five other patients presenting the same combination. The remaining two patients in this group had, respectively, azotemia of more than 17 days' duration with a maximum nonprotein nitrogen level of 247 mg. per 100 cc., and azotemia of over 7 days' duration with a nonprotein nitrogen level of 140 mg. per 100 cubic centimeters. Hypertension was never observed without other evidence of renal insufficiency. Once hypertension developed it was very persistent, even after the nonprotein nitrogen had dropped to normal levels. The shortest duration of hypertension observed was 12 days, and in one patient it was still present at 22 days.

In summary, pigment excretion appeared to be a constant phenomenon in the shock kidney but was seen also in many patients who never showed evidence of renal failure. Oliguria likewise was frequently seen in the absence of renal failure. In positive cases it might be extremely transitory and the volume not greatly depressed. Azotemia was a constant and, except in the presence of severe complications or in the moribund state, a reliable sign of renal failure. Elevation of blood pressure in the absence of a head injury was inconstant. When present it constituted the most important confirmatory criterion.

On these grounds it is reasonable to conclude that all seven surviving patients manifesting hypertension did, in fact, have "shock kidney." In six of these azotemia was proved, and in the seventh the nonprotein nitrogen level was not recorded. Eight other patients showed azotemia supported by one or more other criteria of renal injury. In three patients azotemia was so slight and transitory as to be of doubtful significance. In the remainder it was of sufficient severity or was bolstered by enough other confirmatory evidence to justify the diagnosis of renal injury.

We conclude, then, that a minimum of 11 and a possible maximum of 14 of our patients developed and survived "shock kidney." In comparison with 38 fatal cases of histologically proved shock kidney, this indicates a case fatality rate of approximately 75 percent.

SUMMARY AND CONCLUSIONS

The clinical records of 60 patients on whom necropsy was performed were analyzed from the standpoint of factors relating to renal function, and the findings in the group of 38 with histologically demonstrated pigment nephropathy were compared with those of the 22 in whom this lesion was not present. It became apparent that the clinical syndrome of renal insufficiency which follows shock is remarkable chiefly for the scarcity and mildness of its symptoms. Little that the patient complained of served to call attention to the condition. Drowsiness slowly deepening into stupor was the most common symptom, but it might be absent almost until death. The only common sign was edema, either pulmonary or peripheral.

Laboratory and blood pressure findings provided more useful criteria. Seven findings were present with great constancy in the nephropathic cases that appeared only sporadically or never in the control group. These were in ascending order of diagnostic importance: proteinuria, persistent acidity of the urine, excretion of benzidine-positive material, oliguria, azotemia, fixation of specific gravity of the urine at a low level, and hypertension. It was found that the diagnosis of nephropathy could only be made by the systematic recording of four factors in every patient who was resuscitated from shock: (1) the total urinary output, (2) the presence of benzidine-positive material in the urine, (3) the nonprotein nitrogen level in the blood plasma, and (4) the systolic blood pressure. The symptom complex of *oliguria, pigment excretion, azotemia,* and *hypertension* established the diagnosis. It is probable that in some cases oliguria was too transient to be recognizable, and certain that in some cases hypertension did not develop. If the patient survived beyond 4 days, fixation of specific gravity and constant acidity of the urine afforded important confirmatory evidence.

These diagnostic criteria of nephropathy were then applied in a review of the records of the nonfatal cases in the series. It was concluded that a minimum of 11 and a possible maximum of 14 had had a pigment nephropathy. Using the former figure, the case fatality rate is approximately 75 percent.

CASES OF SPECIAL INTEREST IN THIS CHAPTER

Nonfatal

13	44	72	109	133
27	54	81	112	138
29	60	87	125	150
37	71	104	130	

Fatal

8	26	52	85	108	122
12	31	55	86	116	123
22	41	65	88	117	129
24	47	66	95	118	131
25	49	74	97	120	136
		80	98	A-30	

Crush Syndrome Fatalities

69 70 78 93 132

CHAPTER V

Clinical, Physiologic, and Biochemic Correlation in Lower Nephron Nephrosis

The importance and frequent occurrence of renal failure in those battle casualties who were severely wounded must be emphasized. In the preceding chapter the diagnosis of posttraumatic renal insufficiency was discussed from a clinicopathologic viewpoint. In this chapter an attempt will be made to present a comprehensive picture of the physiologic and biochemic features of the syndrome and their correlation with the clinical findings.

In studying these patients in whom renal insufficiency developed following trauma we have dealt with a unique group of individuals. They were nearly all young men, and so far as was known, physiologically sound prior to wounding. They had incurred severe wounds which almost immediately began to cause changes in their internal environment. Because of the effectiveness of resuscitation and other early treatment, the wounds and the changes produced were not severe enough to cause early death. These men withstood operation fairly well, largely because they had been adequately treated preoperatively, but beginning with the first day or two after operation (or after trauma, if no surgery was done) they began to show clinical and laboratory evidence of inadequate renal function. The renal failure progressed rapidly and in most instances the patients either died in uremia within 10 days or then began to show signs of improvement of renal function, such as diuresis and clearance of nonprotein nitrogen, and subsequently recovered.

In selecting patients presumed to have diminished renal function, two main criteria were utilized: the nonprotein nitrogen level in the blood plasma, and the degree of urinary suppression. Much of the data presented in this chapter will relate primarily to the patients with high azotemia, since this was a constant and generally reliable indication of renal insufficiency. In many instances the data are also correlated with the degree of urinary suppression because a low urinary output provides a simple and useful clinical means of recognizing many cases of impending renal failure. Our definitions of "high azotemia" and of oliguria and anuria have been given, and the diagnostic features of the syndrome were discussed in Chapter IV.

The incidence of high azotemia, oliguria, and anuria in our series is shown in Table 52. In 5 of the 186 patients no nonprotein nitrogen determinations were made and in 50 the urinary output was unknown. Seventy-three of 181 patients were found to have high azotemia. Thirty-three of 136 patients had anuria for at least 24 hours, 45 oliguria (they did not reach anuric level at any time), and 58 had a normal output of urine. Of the patients with high azotemia, 27 also had anuria and 29 oliguria.

TABLE 52.—PLASMA NONPROTEIN NITROGEN LEVEL AND URINARY OUTPUT IN THE SEVERELY WOUNDED

Nonprotein Nitrogen Level	Urinary Output (Number of Patients)				
	Anuria [1]	Oliguria [2]	Normal Output	Output Unknown	Total
With High Azotemia [3]	27	29	10	7	73
Without High Azotemia	1	16	48	43	108
NPN Unknown	5	....	....	....	5
Total	33	45	58	50	186

[1] Urinary output of less than 100 cc. in 24 hours.
[2] Urinary output of 100–600 cc. in 24 hours.
[3] Plasma nonprotein nitrogen level of 65 mg. per 100 cc. or higher.

Clinical Features

Case Fatality

Sixty-five of the 186 patients in the total series failed to survive. Of the 65 who died, 51, or 78 percent, were among those who had high azotemia or urinary suppression or both. The serious implication of the onset of these conditions is well illustrated by Table 53. Of the 73 patients with high azotemia, 50, or 68 percent, died. Of 33 with anuria, 30, or 91 percent, died. This table likewise shows forcefully the importance of uremia as a primary cause of death in these patients; it was the primary cause of 34 (68 percent) of the deaths among patients with high azotemia and of 22 (73 percent) of the deaths among patients with anuria.

TABLE 53.—CASE FATALITY RATES AND TYPE OF DEATH IN ALL PATIENTS WITH AZOTEMIA AND/OR URINARY SUPPRESSION

Presumptive Renal Damage	Total Cases	Fatal Cases		Role of Uremia in Fatal Cases *Number of cases*				
				Primary Cause of Death		Con-trib-utory	Coinci-dental	None or Un-known
		Number	Percent	Number	Percent			
High Azotemia	73	50	68	* 34	68	3	13	0
Urinary Suppression								
Oliguria	45	21	47	12	57	1	5	3
Anuria	33	30	91	22	73	1	2	5
Total	78	51	65	34	67	2	7	8

* Of the 186 patients studied, 35 were classified as dying primarily of uremia, on 1 of whom (Case 146) no nonprotein nitrogen determination was made. Hence only 34 patients are included in the table.

Degree of Initial Shock

The relationship of the degree of shock on admission to subsequent development of renal failure is shown in Table 54. When the crush cases, a case of true transfusion incompatibility, and a case of sulfathiazole crystalluria in the group without shock are excluded, it becomes evident that a preponderance of patients in whom signs of renal failure appeared were recognized as having had severe or moderate initial shock. With the above-mentioned cases excluded, 86 percent of the azotemia group, 73 percent of the oliguria group, and 76 percent of the anuria group had had moderate or severe shock at the time of hospital admission. Many men may have had transient shock, even of several hours' duration, before hospital entry with no sign of shock on entry. Our figures therefore are doubtless too low. It is not, however, clear that the severity of the renal lesion is entirely determined by the degree of shock. This series includes a few patients (Cases 22, 138, and 120) who, so far as we could determine, at no time had any appreciable degree of shock yet who subsequently manifested renal insufficiency.

TABLE 54.—RELATIONSHIP OF INITIAL SHOCK TO DEVELOPMENT OF RENAL INSUFFICIENCY

Classification of Cases	Total Cases	Degree of Initial Shock				
		None	Slight	Moderate	Severe	Unknown
By NPN Retention						
High Azotemia	73	[1] 6	6	27	33	1
By Output						
Oliguria	45	3	8	13	20	1
Anuria	33	[2] 8	3	6	16	0

[1] Includes 2 crush cases, 1 case of transfusion incompatibility, and 1 case of slight postoperative shock.
[2] Includes 1 case of sulfathiazole crystalluria, 1 case of transfusion incompatibility, and 2 crush cases.

Survival Period after Wounding

The time of death after wounding was considered in 51 patients who had renal insufficiency (Table 55). Of these 51, uremia was the cause of death in 35, a contributory cause in 3, and only coincidental in 13 patients. Of the 35 patients in whom uremia was the primary cause of death, 15, or 43 percent, died in the first 5 days and 17, or 48.5 percent, in the second 5 days—more than 91 percent within 10 days after wounding. Of the entire group of 51 fatalities, 94 percent (48 patients) died within the first 10 days. The significance of this time factor will be illustrated in connection with the biochemic data and in the

TABLE 55.—PERIOD OF SURVIVAL AFTER WOUNDING IN 51 PATIENTS WITH RENAL INSUFFICIENCY

Time from Wounding to Death *Days*	Role of Uremia in Cause of Death		
	Primary *Number of cases*	Contributory *Number of cases*	Coincidental *Number of cases*
1 to 5	15	2	9
6 to 10	17	1	4
11 to 15	3	0	0
Total	35	3	13

following chapter on therapy. Evidence will also be presented that if patients can be carried through this 10-day critical period, they stand a fair chance of recovery. This point will be further discussed later; it emphasizes the importance of avoiding certain therapeutic errors which can result in death, such as overloading the circulatory system by administration of too much fluid.

Type and Location of Wounds

The type and location of major wounds and injuries in patients with renal insufficiency (as indicated by nonprotein nitrogen retention and urinary suppression) is shown in Table 56. In the former classification—the high azotemia group—peripheral wounds with fracture and intra-abdominal wounds are of equal frequency. In the latter, peripheral wounds predominate in the oliguria group whereas in the anuria group intra-abdominal wounds are somewhat more frequent. Thoracic wounds are third in all three groups. Wounds of the liver,

TABLE 56.—TYPE AND LOCATION OF WOUNDS OR INJURIES IN PATIENTS WITH RENAL INSUFFICIENCY

Type and Location of Wound	High Azotemia	Oliguria	Anuria
	Number of cases	*Number of cases*	*Number of cases*
Peripheral, with Fracture	32	18	11
Intra-abdominal	32	14	13
Thoracic	15	10	7
Peripheral, without Fracture	8	5	5
Thoraco-abdominal	6	7	4
Liver	12	7	8
Kidney	[1]10	[2]7	[2]6
Urinary Tract other than Kidney	6	3	4
Crush	4	1	4
Burn	1	1	0
Spinal Cord Injury	2	0	1
Totals			
Multiple Major Wounds	21	10	7
Single Major Wound	52	35	26
Total Cases Included	[3]73	45	[4]33

[1] Six treated by nephrectomy.
[2] Four treated by nephrectomy.
[3] Includes 1 case of incompatible blood transfusion.
[4] Includes 1 case of incompatible blood transfusion and 1 case of sulfathiazole crystalluria.

kidneys, and urinary tract occurred, but not in a high percentage in any group.

Hypertension

Table 57 shows the number of patients having high azotemia who at some time in their course also had a systolic blood pressure of 135 mm. Hg or higher, or a diastolic pressure of 90 mm. Hg or higher. These figures represent the probable upper limits of normal for the age group into which our patients fell. Blood pressures were recorded in 71 of 73 patients with high azotemia, 67 being recorded within the first 7 days after wounding or injury, including crush injury. Hypertension developed in 44 patients, usually during the first week. In the few in whom it was first noted after this period, the probability is that they also had an unobserved hypertension prior to the first determinations recorded. In general the blood pressure rose gradually, reaching a maximum between the third and sixth days after wounding. This agrees essentially with the time of maximum nitrogen retention in the blood.

Of the 27 patients who did not have hypertension, 20 died. Of these 20, thirteen died within the first 4 days after wounding, three within 6 days, and four between 6 and 10 days. Of those who died within a few days after wounding, many had never really recovered from shock. It seems probable that they would

TABLE 57.—INCIDENCE OF HYPERTENSION IN PATIENTS WITH HIGH AZOTEMIA

Patients	Hypertension Present	Hypertension Absent	Total
Survived			
With Minimal Renal Failure	5	7	12
With Recovery Diuresis	10	0	10
Total	15	7	22
Died			
Uremia Primary Cause	27	7	34
Uremia Contributory	1	2	3
Uremia Coincidental	1	11	* 12
Total	29	20	49
TOTAL	44	27	71

* Not including 1 case in which the presence or absence of hypertension was not known.

have developed hypertension if they had lived longer, especially those in whom the primary cause of death was uremia.

Other Clinical Findings

Edema was observed in 23 of the 73 patients with high azotemia. The edema varied in degree, but it was usually generalized, involving all extremities and the face. It was present in 18 patients who died. Three patients had generalized convulsions. Eyegrounds were examined in 7 patients; 2 showed flame-shaped hemorrhages and 1 a small exudate. A pericardial friction rub was heard in 1 patient who died of uremia, and pericarditis was found on necropsy.

Biochemic and Physiologic Features

BLOOD

Biochemic Abnormalities

A large number of blood chemistry studies were made preoperatively and postoperatively on the 73 patients with high azotemia. It was not possible to make daily or even regular determinations on every patient, and the number of cases indicated in the various cells of the tables to follow is conditioned by the available data. The plasma carbon-dioxide combining power, and the concentrations of plasma nonprotein nitrogen, chlorides, phosphate, protein, magnesium, phosphorus, creatinine, and uric acid, and of the serum sodium were determined. Average values are shown in Table 58 A through G and Table 59. When more than 1 determination of any constituent was made on any 1 patient during the postoperative periods specified in the tables, only the most abnormal value was selected for inclusion in the averages.

In both tables the data are presented in two ways: (1) on the basis of survival, and (2) on the basis of the daily output of urine. These findings, together with the changes in the urine (see Tables 75-77) to be discussed later, reflect the typical biochemic and physiologic alterations which occurred in those of the severely wounded patients in whom renal insufficiency developed. The data show the changes taking place during the acute phase either to the time of death or, in those who survived, through the recovery phase as long as we could follow the case. Variations will be mentioned whenever they are important.

Table 58.—Physiologic and Biochemic Findings in Patients with High Azotemia*

A. Plasma Nonprotein Nitrogen**

Classification of Cases	Average Plasma Nonprotein Nitrogen (mg. per 100 cc.)					
	Preoperative Period	Postoperative Period				
		1 Day	2–4 Days	5–7 Days	8–10 Days	11–15 Days
ALL CASES	47.3±4.8 (21 cases)	72.8±4.2 (31 cases)	143.1±9.3 (54 cases)	182.2±17.2 (29 cases)	175.8±29.8 (13 cases)	127.6±23.4 (10 cases)
Patients' Outcome						
Lived	41.5±4.9 (8 cases)	65.3±4.1 (11 cases)	92.8±9.1 (17 cases)	117.3±20.5 (11 cases)	103.4±20.1 (8 cases)	109.9±17.0 (9 cases)
Died—All Causes	50.9±7.2 (13 cases)	77.0±6.0 (20 cases)	166.2±11.0 (37 cases)	221.9±19.9 (18 cases)	291.8±18.8 (5 cases)	287 (1 case)
Died of Uremia	36.0 (3 cases)	80.0±7.9 (11 cases)	190.5±11.3 (27 cases)	258.8±12.6 (14 cases)	291.8±18.8 (5 cases)	287 (1 case)
Died of other Causes	55.4±8.9 (10 cases)	73.2±9.5 (9 cases)	100.6±11.5 (10 cases)	92.8±22.7 (4 cases)	—	—
Urinary Output						
Normal	37.3 (3 cases)	59.4±7.0 (5 cases)	89.6±8.6 (8 cases)	112.4±15.1 (7 cases)	76.0 (3 cases)	29 (1 case)
Anuria	34.5 (2 cases)	75.6 (8 cases)	190.4 (20 cases)	257.1 (12 cases)	258 (4 cases)	155 (2 cases)
Oliguria	43.0 (11 cases)	76.5 (15 cases)	127.9 (24 cases)	141.2 (10 cases)	183.6 (5 cases)	140.4 (5 cases)
Unknown	68.0 (5 cases)	69.0 (3 cases)	66.5 (2 cases)	—	108 (1 case)	117.5 (2 cases)
Anuria and Oliguria	41.7±3.5 (13 cases)	76.2±5.3 (23 cases)	156.3±10.2 (44 cases)	204.4±20.1 (22 cases)	216.7±35.2 (9 cases)	144.6±29.7 (7 cases)
Anuria, Oliguria, and Unknown	49.0±5.5 (18 cases)	75.4±4.7 (26 cases)	152.4±10.2 (46 cases)	204.4±20.1 (22 cases)	205.8±33.4 (10 cases)	138.6±23.1 (9 cases)

* A through G: If more than 1 determination had been made on 1 patient during the specified period, the most abnormal value was used.
** Normal range: 25–40 mg. per 100 cc. "High azotemia": 65 mg. per 100 cc. or higher.

TABLE 58.—PHYSIOLOGIC AND BIOCHEMIC FINDINGS IN PATIENTS WITH HIGH AZOTEMIA

B. Plasma Carbon-Dioxide Combining Power*

Classification of Cases	Average Plasma Carbon-Dioxide Combining Power (mEq./L.)					
	Preoperative Period	Postoperative Period				
		1 Day	2–4 Days	5–7 Days	8–10 Days	11–15 Days
ALL CASES	21.8±1.3 (21 cases)	24.9±1.3 (20 cases)	25.6±0.9 (47 cases)	23.6±1.5 (23 cases)	21.4±2.1 (11 cases)	19.5±1.5 (8 cases)
Patients' Outcome						
Lived	19.3±2.0 (8 cases)	27.4±1.5 (7 cases)	27.7±1.1 (15 cases)	24.8±1.5 (7 cases)	25.2±2.3 (6 cases)	20.3±1.4 (7 cases)
Died—All Causes	23.3±1.7 (13 cases)	23.6±1.8 (13 cases)	24.6±1.1 (32 cases)	23.1±2.1 (16 cases)	16.7±2.3 (5 cases)	13.5 (1 case)
Died of Uremia	24.6 (3 cases)	24.3±2.4 (8 cases)	23.3±1.0 (25 cases)	20.2±1.5 (13 cases)	16.7±2.3 (5 cases)	13.5 (1 case)
Died of other Causes	22.9±2.0 (10 cases)	22.7±3.0 (5 cases)	29.4±3.3 (7 cases)	35.5 (3 cases)	—	—
Urinary Output						
Normal	24.2 (3 cases)	29.7 (3 cases)	31.9±2.5 (8 cases)	34.4±3.6 (4 cases)	36.0 (1 case)	—
Anuria	26.2 (2 cases)	23.0 (6 cases)	23.2 (17 cases)	20.0 (11 cases)	19.1 (4 cases)	22.9 (2 cases)
Oliguria	20.0 (11 cases)	24.7 (11 cases)	25.2 (22 cases)	23.1 (8 cases)	20.4 (5 cases)	18.3 (4 cases)
Unknown	22.4 (5 cases)	—	—	—	20.6 (1 case)	18.6 (2 cases)
Anuria and Oliguria	21.0±1.6 (13 cases)	24.1±1.5 (17 cases)	24.3±0.8 (39 cases)	21.3±1.1 (19 cases)	19.8±1.8 (9 cases)	19.8±1.9 (6 cases)
Anuria, Oliguria, and Unknown	21.4±1.4 (18 cases)	—	—	—	19.9±1.6 (10 cases)	19.5±1.5 (8 cases)

* Normal range: 24–31 mEq./L.

TABLE 58.—PHYSIOLOGIC AND BIOCHEMIC FINDINGS IN PATIENTS WITH HIGH AZOTEMIA

C. Plasma Chlorides*

Classification of Cases	Average Plasma Chlorides (mEq./L.)					
	Preoperative Period	Postoperative Period				
		1 Day	2–4 Days	5–7 Days	8–10 Days	11–15 Days
ALL CASES	98.8±0.8 (21 cases)	96.8±0.9 (31 cases)	93.7±1.6 (54 cases)	93.1±3.0 (28 cases)	91.8±6.3 (13 cases)	103.0±5.3 (10 cases)
Patients' Outcome						
Lived	98.7±1.3 (8 cases)	96.3±1.5 (11 cases)	96.7±2.3 (17 cases)	94.1±3.3 (11 cases)	102.7±7.9 (8 cases)	104.2±5.8 (9 cases)
Died—All Causes	98.9±1.1 (13 cases)	96.9±1.4 (19 cases)	92.7±2.1 (37 cases)	92.2±4.3 (18 cases)	74.4±3.1 (5 cases)	91.4 (1 case)
Died of Uremia	99.1 (3 cases)	93.5±1.7 (10 cases)	90.7±1.9 (27 cases)	89.3±3.2 (14 cases)	74.4±3.1 (5 cases)	91.4 (1 case)
Died of other Causes	98.8±1.4 (10 cases)	100.7±1.3 (9 cases)	98.0±5.9 (10 cases)	102.2 (4 cases)	—	—
Urinary Output						
Normal	102.1 (3 cases)	100.2±2.2 (5 cases)	102.7±6.8 (8 cases)	98.8±10.2 (7 cases)	111.7 (3 cases)	96.4 (1 case)
Anuria	100.0 (2 cases)	94.4 (8 cases)	88.9 (20 cases)	90.7 (11 cases)	76.7 (4 cases)	92.0 (2 cases)
Oliguria	98.9 (11 cases)	96.6 (15 cases)	94.3 (23 cases)	91.7 (10 cases)	83.5 (5 cases)	99.8 (5 cases)
Unknown	96.2 (5 cases)	98.9 (3 cases)	99.4 (2 cases)	—	133.7 (1 case)	125.0 (2 cases)
Anuria and Oliguria	99.1±0.8 (13 cases)	95.8±1.2 (23 cases)	91.8±1.5 (43 cases)	91.2±2.3 (21 cases)	80.5±3.4 (9 cases)	97.6±3.9 (7 cases)
Anuria, Oliguria, and Unknown	98.3±0.8 (18 cases)	96.2±1.1 (26 cases)	92.2±1.5 (45 cases)	91.2±2.0 (21 cases)	85.8±6.1 (10 cases)	103.7±5.9 (9 cases)

* Normal range: 97.5–104 mEq./L.

TABLE 58.—PHYSIOLOGIC AND BIOCHEMIC FINDINGS IN PATIENTS WITH HIGH AZOTEMIA

D. Plasma Phosphate*

Classification of Cases	Average Plasma Phosphate (mEq./L.)					
	Preoperative Period	Postoperative Period				
		1 Day	2–4 Days	5–7 Days	8–10 Days	11–15 Days
ALL CASES	3.9±0.3 (18 cases)	2.6±0.2 (26 cases)	3.7±0.3 (45 cases)	3.7±0.3 (26 cases)	4.7±0.5 (9 cases)	3.3±0.3 (10 cases)
Patients' Outcome						
Lived	4.3±0.3 (7 cases)	2.2±0.2 (9 cases)	2.6±0.3 (12 cases)	2.9±0.4 (10 cases)	3.5±0.3 (4 cases)	3.1±0.3 (9 cases)
Died—All Causes	3.6±0.3 (11 cases)	2.9±0.3 (17 cases)	4.1±0.3 (33 cases)	4.3±0.3 (16 cases)	5.7±0.7 (5 cases)	4.9 (1 case)
Died of Uremia	3.8 (3 cases)	2.7±0.3 (10 cases)	4.3±0.3 (26 cases)	4.6±0.1 (12 cases)	5.7±0.7 (5 cases)	4.9 (1 case)
Died of other Causes	3.6±0.3 (8 cases)	3.1±0.7 (7 cases)	3.6±0.9 (7 cases)	3.5±1.0 (4 cases)	—	—
Urinary Output						
Normal	2.9 (3 cases)	2.1±0.2 (5 cases)	2.1±0.3 (6 cases)	2.9±0.7 (7 cases)	—	2.3 (1 case)
Anuria	3.2 (2 cases)	2.7 (7 cases)	4.3 (18 cases)	4.5 (10 cases)	5.9 (4 cases)	3.9 (2 cases)
Oliguria	4.4 (9 cases)	2.9 (12 cases)	3.7 (20 cases)	3.5 (9 cases)	4.1 (4 cases)	3.1 (5 cases)
Unknown	3.9±0.5 (4 cases)	2.0 (2 cases)	3.0 (1 case)	—	3.1 (1 case)	3.9 (2 cases)
Anuria and Oliguria	4.1±0.3 (11 cases)	2.9±0.3 (19 cases)	4.0±0.3 (38 cases)	4.1±0.3 (19 cases)	4.9±0.6 (8 cases)	3.3±0.3 (7 cases)
Anuria, Oliguria, and Unknown	4.1±0.3 (15 cases)	2.7±0.3 (21 cases)	4.0±0.3 (39 cases)	4.1±0.3 (19 cases)	4.7±0.5 (9 cases)	3.5±0.3 (9 cases)

* Normal range: 1.04–2.0 mEq./L.

956507 O—52——10

Table 58.—Physiologic and Biochemic Findings in Patients with High Azotemia

E. Plasma Protein*

Classification of Cases	Average Plasma Protein (mEq./L.)					
	Preoperative Period	Postoperative Period				
		1 Day	2–4 Days	5–7 Days	8–10 Days	11–15 Days
ALL CASES	14.8±0.1 (21 cases)	15.1±0.1 (32 cases)	15.6±0.1 (53 cases)	15.8±0.2 (31 cases)	15.8±0.3 (13 cases)	15.8±0.3 (10 cases)
Patients' Outcome						
Lived	14.6±0.1 (8 cases)	15.1±0.2 (11 cases)	15.1±0.2 (17 cases)	15.1±0.2 (13 cases)	16.3±0.3 (7 cases)	16.5±0.3 (8 cases)
Died—All Causes	14.8±0.2 (13 cases)	15.1±0.1 (21 cases)	15.6±0.1 (36 cases)	16.5±0.2 (18 cases)	15.6±0.6 (5 cases)	14.1 (1 case)
Died of Uremia	13.9 (3 cases)	15.3±0.2 (11 cases)	15.3±0.1 (27 cases)	15.8±0.2 (14 cases)	15.6±0.6 (5 cases)	14.1 (1 case)
Died of other Causes	15.1±0.1 (10 cases)	14.8±0.2 (10 cases)	16.8±0.4 (9 cases)	18.5±0.3 (4 cases)	—	—
Urinary Output						
Normal	15.6 (3 cases)	15.6±0.2 (6 cases)	16.0±0.3 (8 cases)	17.3±0.3 (8 cases)	17.7 (3 cases)	14.8 (1 case)
Anuria	13.6 (2 cases)	14.8 (8 cases)	15.6 (19 cases)	15.8 (12 cases)	15.8 (4 cases)	18.2 (2 cases)
Oliguria	14.6 (11 cases)	15.3 (16 cases)	15.3 (24 cases)	14.8 (11 cases)	15.1 (4 cases)	15.3 (4 cases)
Unknown	15.1 (5 cases)	12.6 (2 cases)	15.6 (2 cases)	—	15.8 (1 case)	17.0 (2 cases)
Anuria and Oliguria	14.3±0.1 (13 cases)	15.1±0.1 (24 cases)	15.3±0.1 (43 cases)	15.3±0.2 (23 cases)	15.3±0.3 (8 cases)	16.3±0.3 (6 cases)
Anuria, Oliguria, and Unknown	14.6±0.1 (18 cases)	14.8±0.1 (26 cases)	15.3±0.1 (45 cases)	15.3±0.2 (23 cases)	15.3±0.3 (9 cases)	16.3±0.3 (8 cases)

* Converted from Gm. per 100 cc. to mEq./L. for purposes of comparison with electrolytes. Our normal range of plasma protein was 6–7 Gm. per 100 cc.

TABLE 58.—PHYSIOLOGIC AND BIOCHEMIC FINDINGS IN PATIENTS WITH HIGH AZOTEMIA

F. Serum Sodium*

Classification of Cases	Average Serum Sodium (mEq./L.)					
	Preoperative Period	Postoperative Period				
		1 Day	2–4 Days	5–7 Days	8–10 Days	11–15 Days
ALL CASES	146.3±3.7 (5 cases)	147.5±3.7 (6 cases)	141.3±2.5 (21 cases)	137.8±5.1 (8 cases)	140.7±4.4 (6 cases)	151.7±5.7 (7 cases)
Patients' Outcome						
Lived	137.9 (2 cases)	148.0 (2 cases)	139.9 (3 cases)	124.0 (1 case)	147.4 (3 cases)	153.7±6.3 (6 cases)
Died—All Causes	151.9 (3 cases)	147.3±5.1 (4 cases)	141.5±2.8 (18 cases)	139.7±5.5 (7 cases)	134.0 (3 cases)	140.0 (1 case)
Died of Uremia	—	143.3 (2 cases)	139.5±2.5 (16 cases)	139.8±6.5 (6 cases)	134.0 (3 cases)	140.0 (1 case)
Died of other Causes	151.9 (3 cases)	151.3 (2 cases)	157.8 (2 cases)	139.1 (1 case)	—	—
Urinary Output						
Normal	150.8 (2 cases)	160.4 (1 case)	169.6 (1 case)	139.1 (1 case)	—	—
Anuria	—	143.3 (2 cases)	141.2 (14 cases)	142.8 (5 cases)	138.8 (3 cases)	148.1 (2 cases)
Oliguria	137.9 (2 cases)	148.0 (2 cases)	137.6 (7 cases)	124.5 (2 cases)	136.5 (2 cases)	148.0 (3 cases)
Unknown	154.0 (1 case)	—	—	—	154.9 (1 case)	160.9 (2 cases)
Anuria and Oliguria	137.9 (2 cases)	145.6±4.1 (4 cases)	140.0±2.0 (21 cases)	137.6±5.9 (7 cases)	137.9±4.2 (5 cases)	148.0±4.3 (5 cases)
Anuria, Oliguria, and Unknown	143.2 (3 cases)	145.6±4.1 (4 cases)	140.0±2.0 (21 cases)	137.6±5.9 (7 cases)	140.7±4.4 (6 cases)	151.7±5.7 (7 cases)

* Normal range: 139–149 mEq./L.

TABLE 58.—PHYSIOLOGIC AND BIOCHEMIC FINDINGS IN PATIENTS WITH HIGH AZOTEMIA

G. Plasma Magnesium*

Classification of Cases	Average Plasma Magnesium (mEq./L.)					
	Preoperative Period	Postoperative Period				
		1 Day	2–4 Days	5–7 Days	8–10 Days	11–15 Days
ALL CASES	2.0±0.1 (13 cases)	1.4±0.1 (5 cases)	2.4±0.3 (13 cases)	2.8±0.6 (9 cases)	3.3 (3 cases)	2.2±0.3 (5 cases)
Patients' Outcome						
Lived	2.2±0.2 (4 cases)	1.6 (1 case)	2.1±0.2 (4 cases)	1.8 (2 cases)	2.3 (2 cases)	2.1±0.3 (4 cases)
Died—All Causes	2.0±0.2 (9 cases)	1.4±0.2 (4 cases)	2.6±0.4 (9 cases)	3.2±0.7 (7 cases)	5.2 (1 case)	2.6 (1 case)
Died of Uremia	2.1 (3 cases)	1.4 (2 cases)	2.3±0.4 (6 cases)	3.3±1.0 (5 cases)	5.2 (1 case)	2.6 (1 case)
Died of other Causes	1.9±0.3 (6 cases)	1.4 (2 cases)	3.2 (3 cases)	2.8 (2 cases)	—	—
Urinary Output						
Normal	1.6 (3 cases)	1.3 (1 case)	2.5 (2 cases)	2.8 (2 cases)	—	—
Anuria	1.8 (2 cases)	1.7 (1 case)	2.3 (5 cases)	2.4 (4 cases)	1.8 (1 case)	1.8 (1 case)
Oliguria	2.3 (5 cases)	1.4 (3 cases)	2.5 (5 cases)	3.6 (3 cases)	5.2 (1 case)	2.3 (2 cases)
Unknown	2.3 (3 cases)	—	—	—	2.8 (1 case)	2.3 (2 cases)
Anuria and Oliguria	2.2±0.2 (7 cases)	1.5±0.2 (4 cases)	2.4±0.4 (10 cases)	2.9±0.8 (7 cases)	3.5 (2 cases)	2.1 (3 cases)
Anuria, Oliguria, and Unknown	2.2±0.1 (10 cases)	1.5±0.2 (4 cases)	2.4±0.4 (10 cases)	2.9±0.8 (7 cases)	3.3 (3 cases)	2.2±0.3 (5 cases)

* Normal range: 0.8–2.5 mEq./L.

Nitrogenous Waste Products and Phosphorus

Nonprotein Nitrogen.—Averages of nonprotein nitrogen findings are shown in Tables 58A and 59. Although the number is small and the variation great in some periods, giving rise to large standard errors, the data are adequate to give a fairly representative picture. Generally nitrogen retention was already significant by the first postoperative day, increased rapidly during the first 10 days, and then began to decline. This is illustrated in Chart 18, which has been constructed from averages shown in Table 58A, "All Cases."

CHART 18. PLASMA NONPROTEIN NITROGEN IN PATIENTS WITH HIGH AZOTEMIA

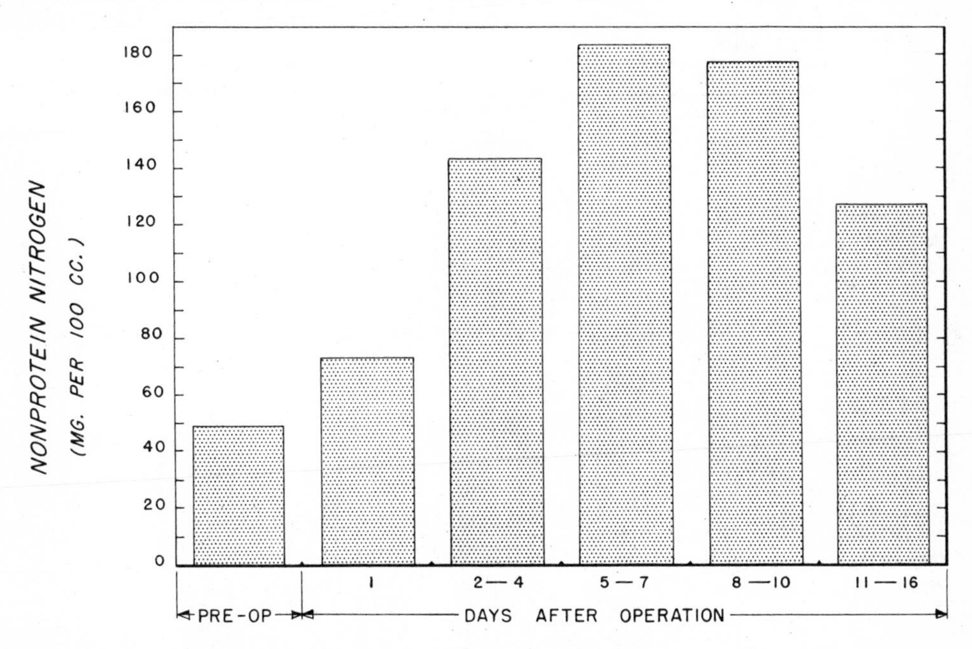

As previously discussed, most of the fatalities occurred in the first 10 days, so the fall in nitrogen retention in the tenth through fifteenth days chiefly represents patients who recovered. In general the nonprotein nitrogen level rose progressively to the day of death in those patients dying primarily of uremia (Chart 19 and Table 60). However, two patients (Cases 66 and 93) who lived longer than 10 days after wounding (14 and 13 days respectively) had begun to show some evidence of returning renal function. The importance of this fact in relation to therapy cannot be too strongly emphasized: it is essential to avoid any measure that might precipitate death before this spontaneous recovery can occur.

CHART 19. PLASMA NITROGENOUS WASTE PRODUCTS AND PHOSPHORUS IN PATIENTS WHO DIED OF UREMIA

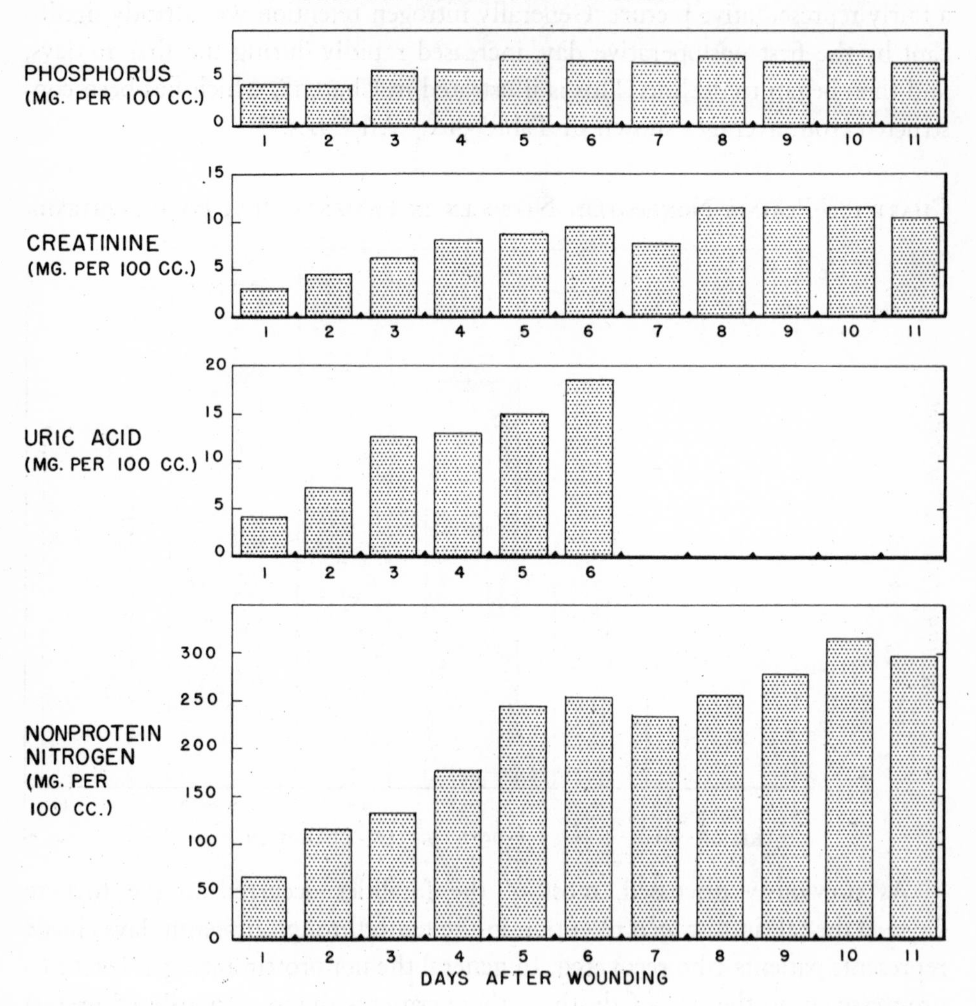

Marked qualitative differences are clear between patients in the different categories shown in Tables 58, 59, and 60. In many instances the standard error of the mean is large, indicating wide variation of values in the cases listed; also the number of cases in many categories is small. Differences in degree of nitrogen retention seem to be evident, however, (1) between those who lived and those who died of uremia, and (2) between those with a normal output of urine and those with oliguria or anuria. The time of greatest retention is essentially in the same periods as shown in Chart 18.

An attempt to determine whether the development of azotemia could be correlated with the degree of initial shock was not successful. As was mentioned previously, of the total number of patients who developed posttraumatic azotemia, oliguria, or anuria, a large proportion had had severe or moderate shock on hospital entry. A few patients who had no shock or only slight initial shock (so far as we could determine) had subsequent renal insufficiency, and the renal failure was as severe as in those with previous moderate or severe shock. Similarly there was no evidence that nonprotein nitrogen retention was initially greater in patients who subsequently died of uremia or who developed oliguria or anuria than it was in those whose renal failure was less severe.

For those interested in further differences between categories of patients and in day-to-day changes in the nonprotein nitrogen and other constituents of the plasma, the detailed analyses in Tables 59 through 62 are included. The essential trends are illustrated in the charts; minor variations are evident in the tables. The lack of effect of ether anesthesia on nonprotein nitrogen levels was discussed in Chapter II.

Creatinine and Urea.—In general, creatinine rose in the plasma at about the same rate as the nonprotein nitrogen (Chart 19). Also, as with other nitrogenous products and the electrolytes, there was no correlation between the degree of initial shock and elevation of creatinine during the period of posttraumatic renal failure. The plasma urea nitrogen level was determined simultaneously with total nonprotein nitrogen and creatinine in 15 cases (Table 63). Like creatinine, it rose approximately as the total nonprotein nitrogen rose. The relationships of these three substances when nonprotein nitrogen was elevated are shown in the table. The averages were obtained by using 38 determinations from a larger series on 15 patients, but including only those in which the nonprotein nitrogen was over 100 milligrams per 100 cubic centimeters. When more than 1 determination was included from the same patient, the samples were drawn at least 24 hours apart.

Although all waste products which make up the total nonprotein nitrogen rose in our patients, they did not accumulate in exactly the same proportions seen in the normal individual, if these figures represent a fair sample. However,

TABLE 59.—AVERAGE PLASMA NITROGENOUS WASTE PRODUCTS AND PHOSPHORUS IN HIGH AZOTEMIA

PREOPERATIVE PERIOD

Classification of Cases	NPN mg. per 100 cc.	Creatinine mg. per 100 cc.	Uric Acid mg. per 100 cc.	Phosphorus mg. per 100 cc.
Patients' Outcome				
Lived	42 (8 cases)	2.0 (8 cases)	5.4 (5 cases)	6.5 (7 cases)
Died—All Causes	51 (13 cases)	2.0 (13 cases)	5.3 (9 cases)	5.4 (11 cases)
Died of Uremia	36 (3 cases)	2.0 (3 cases)	6.8 (3 cases)	5.7 (3 cases)
Died of other Causes	55 (10 cases)	2.0 (10 cases)	4.5 (6 cases)	5.4 (8 cases)
Urinary Output				
Normal	37 (3 cases)	1.2 (3 cases)	5.0 (3 cases)	4.3 (3 cases)
Anuria	35 (2 cases)	1.7 (2 cases)	5.7 (2 cases)	4.8 (2 cases)
Oliguria	43 (11 cases)	2.1 (11 cases)	5.5 (6 cases)	6.6 (9 cases)

FIRST POSTOPERATIVE DAY

Classification of Cases	NPN mg. per 100 cc.	Creatinine mg. per 100 cc.	Uric Acid mg. per 100 cc.	Phosphorus mg. per 100 cc.
Patients' Outcome				
Lived	65 (11 cases)	2.3 (11 cases)	4.4 (3 cases)	3.3 (9 cases)
Died—All Causes	76 (20 cases)	3.2 (20 cases)	6.6 (8 cases)	4.0 (16 cases)
Died of Uremia	77 (11 cases)	3.5 (11 cases)	7.4 (5 cases)	3.8 (9 cases)
Died of other Causes	73 (9 cases)	2.9 (9 cases)	5.4 (3 cases)	4.2 (7 cases)
Urinary Output				
Normal	59 (5 cases)	2.0 (5 cases)	6.1 (2 cases)	3.1 (5 cases)
Anuria	72 (8 cases)	3.5 (8 cases)	7.9 (3 cases)	3.9 (6 cases)
Oliguria	77 (15 cases)	2.9 (15 cases)	5.1 (6 cases)	4.1 (12 cases)

TABLE 59.—AVERAGE PLASMA NITROGENOUS WASTE PRODUCTS AND PHOSPHORUS IN HIGH AZOTEMIA—*Continued*

SECOND POSTOPERATIVE DAY

Classification of Cases	NPN *mg. per 100 cc.*	Creatinine *mg. per 100 cc.*	Uric Acid *mg. per 100 cc.*	Phosphorus *mg. per 100 cc.*
Patients' Outcome				
Lived	75 (11 cases)	2.7 (10 cases)	7.1 (4 cases)	4.5 (6 cases)
Died—All Causes	118 (27 cases)	5.0 (26 cases)	9.0 (8 cases)	5.3 (23 cases)
Died of Uremia	127 (20 cases)	5.5 (20 cases)	9.3 (7 cases)	5.1 (18 cases)
Died of other Causes	91 (7 cases)	3.4 (6 cases)	6.7 (1 case)	5.9 (5 cases)
Urinary Output				
Normal	68 (5 cases)	2.2 (4 cases)	6.7 (1 case)	3.5 (3 cases)
Anuria	125 (15 cases)	5.6 (14 cases)	9.2 (5 cases)	5.0 (12 cases)
Oliguria	104 (16 cases)	4.0 (16 cases)	8.0 (6 cases)	5.7 (13 cases)

THIRD POSTOPERATIVE DAY

Classification of Cases	NPN *mg. per 100 cc.*	Creatinine *mg. per 100 cc.*	Uric Acid *mg. per 100 cc.*	Phosphorus *mg. per 100 cc.*
Patients' Outcome				
Lived	87 (11 cases)	2.9 (10 cases)	8.0 (1 case)	3.3 (7 cases)
Died—All Causes	154 (18 cases)	7.1 (18 cases)	13.3 (7 cases)	5.4 (15 cases)
Died of Uremia	159 (16 cases)	7.4 (16 cases)	14.4 (6 cases)	5.6 (14 cases)
Died of other Causes	115 (2 cases)	4.2 (2 cases)	6.8 (1 case)	2.9 (1 case)
Urinary Output				
Normal	80 (4 cases)	1.8 (4 cases)	6.8 (1 case)	2.3 (3 cases)
Anuria	166 (10 cases)	7.7 (10 cases)	10.3 (3 cases)	5.3 (8 cases)
Oliguria	118 (15 cases)	5.1 (14 cases)	15.8 (4 cases)	5.1 (11 cases)

TABLE 59.—AVERAGE PLASMA NITROGENOUS WASTE PRODUCTS AND PHOSPHORUS IN HIGH AZOTEMIA—*Continued*

FOURTH POSTOPERATIVE DAY

Classification of Cases	NPN *mg. per 100 cc.*	Creatinine *mg. per 100 cc.*	Uric Acid *mg. per 100 cc.*	Phosphorus *mg. per 100 cc.*
Patients' Outcome				
Lived	99 (7 cases)	3.3 (9 cases)	15.9 (2 cases)	4.2 (6 cases)
Died—All Causes	191 (18 cases)	7.4 (18 cases)	9.0 (5 cases)	6.2 (17 cases)
Died of Uremia	224 (14 cases)	8.9 (14 cases)	12.3 (2 cases)	6.9 (13 cases)
Died of other Causes	75 (4 cases)	2.2 (4 cases)	6.9 (3 cases)	3.7 (4 cases)
Urinary Output				
Normal	97 (4 cases)	2.3 (5 cases)	6.9 (3 cases)	3.3 (4 cases)
Anuria	221 (12 cases)	9.0 (12 cases)	14.2 (3 cases)	7.3 (11 cases)
Oliguria	121 (9 cases)	4.3 (10 cases)	13.6 (1 case)	4.6 (8 cases)

FIFTH POSTOPERATIVE DAY

Classification of Cases	NPN *mg. per 100 cc.*	Creatinine *mg. per 100 cc.*	Uric Acid *mg. per 100 cc.*	Phosphorus *mg. per 100 cc.*
Patients' Outcome				
Lived	106 (8 cases)	4.4 (8 cases)	10.5 (3 cases)	4.3 (7 cases)
Died—All Causes	228 (11 cases)	8.2 (11 cases)	15.9 (4 cases)	6.2 (9 cases)
Died of Uremia	243 (10 cases)	8.6 (10 cases)	18.6 (3 cases)	6.3 (8 cases)
Died of other Causes	73 (1 case)	4.1 (1 case)	7.6 (1 case)	5.5 (1 case)
Urinary Output				
Normal	81 (3 cases)	2.7 (3 cases)	7.6 (1 case)	3.5 (3 cases)
Anuria	244 (9 cases)	8.7 (9 cases)	14.6 (2 cases)	5.9 (7 cases)
Oliguria	131 (7 cases)	5.5 (7 cases)	14.6 (4 cases)	5.7 (6 cases)

TABLE 59.—AVERAGE PLASMA NITROGENOUS WASTE PRODUCTS AND PHOSPHORUS IN HIGH AZOTEMIA—*Continued*

SIXTH POSTOPERATIVE DAY

Classification of Cases	NPN *mg. per 100 cc.*	Creatinine *mg. per 100 cc.*	Uric Acid *mg. per 100 cc.*	Phosphorus *mg. per 100 cc.*
Patients' Outcome				
Lived	91 (5 cases)	3.0 (5 cases)	....	3.8 (4 cases)
Died—All Causes	187 (12 cases)	7.6 (13 cases)	16.5 (4 cases)	6.4 (11 cases)
Died of Uremia	235 (8 cases)	9.8 (9 cases)	19.9 (1 case)	7.0 (7 cases)
Died of other Causes	92 (4 cases)	2.7 (4 cases)	15.3 (3 cases)	5.2 (4 cases)
Urinary Output				
Normal	102 (6 cases)	2.9 (6 cases)	15.3 (3 cases)	4.7 (6 cases)
Anuria	245 (5 cases)	11.1 (6 cases)	....	7.1 (4 cases)
Oliguria	144 (6 cases)	5.1 (6 cases)	19.9 (1 case)	5.7 (5 cases)

SEVENTH POSTOPERATIVE DAY

Classification of Cases	NPN *mg. per 100 cc.*	Creatinine *mg. per 100 cc.*	Uric Acid *mg. per 100 cc.*	Phosphorus *mg. per 100 cc.*
Patients' Outcome				
Lived	133 (5 cases)	3.3 (5 cases)	2.2 (1 case)	4.4 (4 cases)
Died—All Causes	212 (5 cases)	8.6 (5 cases)	15.5 (1 case)	6.1 (5 cases)
Died of Uremia	246 (4 cases)	10.3 (4 cases)	....	6.7 (4 cases)
Died of other Causes	76 (1 case)	1.7 (1 case)	15.5 (1 case)	3.9 (1 case)
Urinary Output				
Normal	111 (3 cases)	2.1 (3 cases)	15.5 (1 case)	3.7 (2 cases)
Anuria	239 (4 cases)	9.4 (4 cases)	....	6.5 (4 cases)
Oliguria	145 (3 cases)	5.1 (3 cases)	2.2 (1 case)	4.9 (3 cases)

TABLE 59.—AVERAGE PLASMA NITROGENOUS WASTE PRODUCTS AND PHOSPHORUS IN HIGH AZOTEMIA—*Continued*

EIGHTH THROUGH TENTH POSTOPERATIVE DAYS

Classification of Cases	NPN mg. per 100 cc.	Creatinine mg. per 100 cc.	Uric Acid mg. per 100 cc.	Phosphorus mg. per 100 cc.
Patients' Outcome				
Lived	103 (8 cases)	3.5 (8 cases)	15.0 (2 cases)	5.3 (4 cases)
Died—All Causes	267 (5 cases)	12.1 (5 cases)	....	7.9 (4 cases)
Died of Uremia	267 (5 cases)	12.1 (5 cases)	....	7.9 (4 cases)
Died of other Causes	....	....	....	....
Urinary Output				
Normal	76 (3 cases)	1.4 (3 cases)	....	....
Anuria	235 (4 cases)	12.1 (4 cases)	16.7 (1 case)	8.2 (3 cases)
Oliguria	176 (5 cases)	6.4 (5 cases)	....	5.8 (4 cases)

it would appear that both creatinine and urea make up a greater proportion of the total nonprotein nitrogen in patients with severe renal failure than in the normal individual.

Excretion of Urea and Creatinine.—In two patients who died in the first 6 postoperative days, 24-hour urea nitrogen and creatinine excretion was measured. The relationships of the total amounts of these substances in the urine to plasma nonprotein nitrogen levels, urine specific gravity, and output of urine in these two patients are shown in Table 64.

The relationship of rising plasma levels of nitrogenous waste products to low or decreasing urinary excretion of these same substances is distinctly shown. The fall in output and specific gravity of the urine is directly related to these changes. Twenty-four hour specimens were examined also in two patients who had recovery diuresis and will be discussed under that subject later in this chapter. One of these patients also showed diminished total excretion; the other was examined after his recovery and values were essentially normal.

Phosphorus.—The characteristic retention of phosphorus in renal failure was

TABLE 60.—AVERAGE PLASMA NITROGENOUS WASTE PRODUCTS AND PHOSPHORUS IN PATIENTS WHO DIED OF UREMIA

Days after Wounding	NPN *mg. per 100 cc.*	Creatinine *mg. per 100 cc.*	Uric Acid *mg. per 100 cc.*	Phosphorus *mg. per 100 cc.*
First	69±10.3 (9 cases)	3.0±0.24 (9 cases)	4.1 (3 cases)	4.2±0.47 (8 cases)
Second	118±11.5 (13 cases)	4.8±0.24 (13 cases)	7.3±1.1 (5 cases)	4.1±0.28 (12 cases)
Third	132±6.2 (16 cases)	6.3±0.26 (16 cases)	12.8±2.4 (8 cases)	5.8±0.42 (14 cases)
Fourth	178±5.1 (16 cases)	8.1±0.47 (16 cases)	12.9 (3 cases)	5.9±0.36 (14 cases)
Fifth	245±18.9 (13 cases)	8.9±0.53 (13 cases)	15.0 (3 cases)	7.1±0.96 (12 cases)
Sixth	253±13.0 (8 cases)	9.5±0.70 (9 cases)	18.4 (3 cases)	6.9±0.22 (8 cases)
Seventh	234±26.3 (4 cases)	7.8±1.83 (4 cases)	....	6.6 (3 cases)
Eighth	255 (2 cases)	11.3 (2 cases)	....	7.1 (2 cases)
Ninth	278±16.0 (5 cases)	11.4±0.44 (5 cases)	....	6.8 (3 cases)
Tenth	314 (3 cases)	11.4 (3 cases)	....	7.7 (3 cases)
Eleventh	296 (2 cases)	10.3 (2 cases)	....	6.8 (2 cases)

Note: Data are given on this table for days post-wounding rather than days postoperative as in the preceding table.

also observed in our cases, and in general paralleled the degree of nitrogen retention (see Chart 19 and Tables 58A, 58D, 59, 60, 61, and 62). In these patients with posttraumatic azotemia, phosphorus retention was primarily due to impaired ability to excrete that substance; whereas the hyperphosphatemia seen in patients in shock soon after wounding was possibly due to release of phosphates secondary to muscle damage (Chapter I). Reference to Tables 58 through 62 and to the individual case records shows that the patients with the most severe renal damage had the greatest phosphorus retention.

Relationship of Calcium and Phosphorus.—Calcium and phosphorus determinations were made on 12 patients who had high azotemia. The well-known reciprocal relationship of calcium and phosphorus was present in the majority of these cases (Table 65).

TABLE 61.—AVERAGE NONPROTEIN NITROGEN AND ELECTROLYTES OF PLASMA IN PATIENTS IN WHOM OLIGURIA DEVELOPED

Time of Determination	Plasma					Serum
	Nonprotein Nitrogen *mg. per 100 cc.*	CO_2 Combining Power *mEq./L.*	Chlorides *mEq./L.*	Phosphate *mEq./L.*	Magnesium *mEq./L.*	Sodium *mEq./L.*
Preoperative	39.6±2.6 (21 cases)	22.8±1.4 (19 cases)	100.2±0.8 (20 cases)	3.7±0.3 (16 cases)	2.0±0.2 (10 cases)	138.6 (3 cases)
Postoperative Days						
First	59.9±5.8 (27 cases)	25.7±1.2 (18 cases)	98.1±0.9 (26 cases)	2.5±0.3 (21 cases)	1.4 (3 cases)	146.0 (3 cases)
Second to Fourth	99.6±11.4 (34 cases)	25.3±0.8 (29 cases)	96.4±1.7 (33 cases)	3.2±0.3 (26 cases)	2.4±0.4 (7 cases)	136.8±3.3 (6 cases)
Fifth to Seventh	131.8±29.3 (11 cases)	23.1±1.5 (8 cases)	92.3±2.4 (11 cases)	3.5±0.5 (9 cases)	3.5 (3 cases)	124.5 (2 cases)
Eighth to Tenth	139.1±50.2 (7 cases)	22.2±3.0 (6 cases)	87.4±4.3 (7 cases)	4.1±0.5 (4 cases)	5.2 (1 case)	136.5 (2 cases)
Eleventh to Fifteenth	140.4±42.8 (5 cases)	18.3±2.0 (4 cases)	99.8±5.2 (5 cases)	3.1±0.5 (5 cases)	2.3 (2 cases)	151.0 (2 cases)

TABLE 62.—AVERAGE NONPROTEIN NITROGEN AND ELECTROLYTES OF PLASMA IN PATIENTS IN WHOM ANURIA DEVELOPED

Time of Determination	Plasma					Serum
	Nonprotein Nitrogen *mg. per 100 cc.*	CO_2 Combining Power *mEq./L.*	Chlorides *mEq./L.*	Phosphate *mEq./L.*	Magnesium *mEq./L.*	Sodium *mEq./L.*
Preoperative	34.7 (3 cases)	23.9 (3 cases)	98.7 (3 cases)	2.8 (3 cases)	1.8 (2 cases)	—
Postoperative Days						
First	75.6±4.7 (8 cases)	23.0±3.0 (6 cases)	95.7±2.4 (8 cases)	2.7±0.3 (7 cases)	1.7 (1 case)	143.3 (2 cases)
Second to Fourth	190.4±13.9 (20 cases)	23.2±1.3 (17 cases)	88.9±2.0 (20 cases)	4.3±0.5 (18 cases)	2.3±0.4 (5 cases)	141.2±2.7 (14 cases)
Fifth to Seventh	257.1±14.9 (12 cases)	20.0±1.6 (11 cases)	90.7±3.8 (11 cases)	4.5±0.1 (10 cases)	2.4±0.2 (4 cases)	142.8±6.9 (5 cases)
Eighth to Tenth	258.0±21.8 (4 cases)	19.1±2.3 (4 cases)	76.7±4.2 (4 cases)	5.9±0.9 (4 cases)	1.8 (1 case)	138.8 (3 cases)
Eleventh to Fifteenth	155.0 (2 cases)	22.9 (2 cases)	92.0 (2 cases)	3.9 (2 cases)	1.8 (1 case)	148.1 (2 cases)

TABLE 63.—RELATIONSHIP OF PLASMA TOTAL NONPROTEIN NITROGEN, UREA NITROGEN, AND CREATININE IN 15 PATIENTS

	Plasma Averages *mg. per 100 cc.*			Ratios *Averages*	
	Nonprotein Nitrogen	Urea Nitrogen	Creatinine	Urea / NPN	Creatinine / NPN
Elevated*	193±12	137±9	7.3±0.47	0.71±0.01	0.039±0.001
Normal Value	33	15	1.0	0.51	.028

*Based on 38 determinations made on 15 patients in whom N.P.N. was over 100 mg. per 100 cc.

TABLE 64.—RELATIONSHIP OF URINARY NITROGENOUS WASTE PRODUCTS AND URINARY EXCRETION IN 2 FATAL CASES

Case 108 (Uremia primary cause of death)

Day Specimen was Taken	Urine Output *cc. in 24 hrs.*	Urine Specific Gravity	NPN (Plasma) *mg. in 100 cc.*	Urea Nitrogen (Urine) *Gm. in 24 hrs.*	Creatinine (Plasma) *mg. in 100 cc.*	Creatinine (Urine) *Gm. in 24 hrs.*
Day of Operation . . . . (Postoperative)	*100	*1.032	37	*0.13	1.61	*0.20
Postoperative Day						
First	185	1.014	77	0.54	3.90	0.33
Second	155	1.012	113	....	5.08	0.32
Third (Day of death)	....	....	170	....	6.15	....

Case 107 (Uremia contributory to death)

Day Specimen was Taken	Urine Output *cc. in 24 hrs.*	Urine Specific Gravity	NPN (Plasma) *mg. in 100 cc.*	Urea Nitrogen (Urine) *Gm. in 24 hrs.*	Creatinine (Plasma) *mg. in 100 cc.*	Creatinine (Urine) *Gm. in 24 hrs.*
Day of Operation . . . . (Preoperative)	60	1.028	27	....	1.11	....
Postoperative Day						
First	1,560	1.017	41	7.2	1.61	1.20
Second	1,570	1.019	46	9.4	1.64	1.32
Third	1,540	1.015	....	10.9	....	1.35
Fourth	....	....	91	....	4.44	....
Fifth	800	1.012	73	4.6	4.10	0.50
Sixth (Day of death)	....	....	152	....	5.90	....

*Urine specimen represents 19 hours only.

TABLE 65.—RELATIONSHIP OF CALCIUM AND PHOSPHORUS IN 12 PATIENTS WITH HIGH AZOTEMIA

Case No.	Calcium mg. per 100 cc. (Normal: 9–11)	Phosphorus mg. per 100 cc. (Normal: 1.83.5)	NPN mg. per 100 cc. (Normal: 25–40)	Day of Determination *Postoperative day*	Patient's Outcome
138	10.6	6.4	166	4	Recovery diuresis.
	10.5	6.2	162	14	
133	9.4	4.7	108	10	Do.
	9.5	5.4	101	14	
60	9.9	5.0	98	8	Do.
93	9.0	6.0	155	*5	Death in uremia.
	9.3	7.3	287	*11	
37	9.0	2.1	140	4	Recovery—no oliguria.
112	8.9	4.0	67	2	Recovered with minimal renal failure.
108	8.6	5.1	77	1	Death in uremia.
9	8.4	10.9	224	** 8	Do.
	7.6	12.6	201	** 9	
123	8.0	4.3	120	3	Do.
78	7.8	8.9	178	* 4	Do.
22	7.7	6.5	294	5	Do.
25	7.4	5.3	166	2	Do.
Averages for patients with calcium of 9 or over . . . . (8 determinations)	9.7	5.4	152	....	
Averages for patients with calcium of less than 9 . . . . . . (8 determinations)	8.1	7.2	166	....	

* Days after crush injury.
** Days after transfusion reaction.

Uric Acid.—This substance, like phosphorus and creatinine, rose in patients with high azotemia as the nonprotein nitrogen did, and in roughly the same proportion while retention of both progressed with renal failure (Chart 19 and Tables 59 and 60). Here also the number of determinations was rather small in most categories, but the tendency for greatest retention of uric acid in those patients who had the most severe renal insufficiency will become apparent by inspection of the tables and from the individual case records. The elevated uric acid seen in admission cases has been previously discussed and possible mechanisms for it mentioned in Chapter I.

Summary—Nitrogenous Waste Products

The nitrogenous waste products and phosphorus of the blood plasma all showed progressive retention as renal insufficiency which follows shock or trauma proceeded. In patients with high azotemia the maximum retention was observed between the sixth and tenth postoperative days. The majority of deaths occurred during this period also. Average values for nitrogenous waste products fell from the tenth to the fifteenth days, representing largely patients who recovered. The few patients who died after the tenth day usually showed progressive nitrogen retention up to the day of death, but in a few a falling nonprotein nitrogen level and rising urine output indicated beginning recovery even though they subsequently died of uremia. These time factors emphasize the importance from a therapeutic standpoint of making every effort to carry the patient through the critical first 10 days until the kidneys begin spontaneously to recover.

Acid-Base Balance

Anions

Plasma Carbon-Dioxide Combining Power and Blood pH.—The only group with a sufficient number of determinations of combining power for dependable averages was that of "All Cases" of high azotemia from Table 58B. In these patients, initial low values were followed by a rise toward normal (normal range: 24-31 mEq./L.) during the first 4 postoperative days and a subsequent gradual fall during the next 12 days (Chart 20). A breakdown of these averages according to types of cases does not yield differences which are statistically significant. However, in general, those patients who had the most nitrogen retention, those who died in uremia, and those with oliguria or anuria tended to have the lowest values for carbon-dioxide combining power. Conversely, the patients with the least nitrogen retention, those who survived and who had a normal output of urine, tended to have normal values. There was no correlation of carbon-dioxide combining power with degree of shock after the preoperative day. The acidosis seen in patients who were in shock when they were admitted to the hospital was discussed in Chapter I. Evidence that a low carbon-dioxide combining

CHART 20. PLASMA CARBON-DIOXIDE COMBINING POWER IN HIGH AZOTEMIA

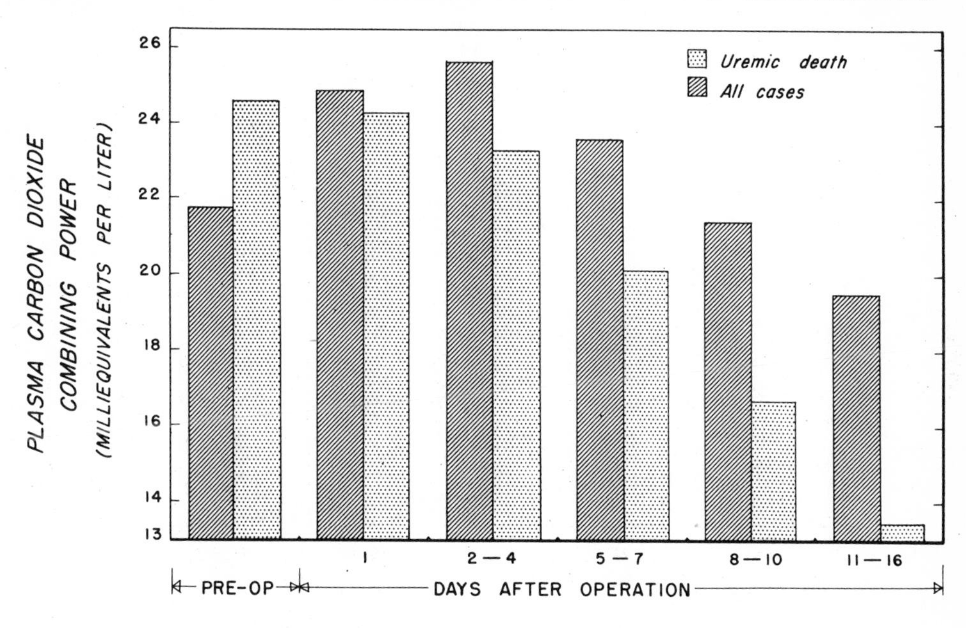

power was a result of diminished alkali reserve in these patients is only indirect.

The pH of the venous blood was measured in five patients who simultaneously had low carbon-dioxide combining power and renal failure. The results were as follows:

Case No.	*Plasma CO_2 Combining Power (mEq./L.)*	*Blood pH (venous)*
69	23	7.39
90	20	7.37
93	16	7.31
112	20	7.04
133	21	7.32

From the limited number of cases in which a blood pH determination was done, and from the indirect evidence to be cited later, it seems likely that there was a metabolic acidosis in the majority of cases. If the low carbon-dioxide combining power had been due to respiratory alkalosis, one would expect to see clinical evidence of hyperventilation and possibly an alkaline urine, depending on the renal function. None of our patients had either. Furthermore, in such cases the blood pH, although probably in the normal range (7.38-7.48), would be in the upper limits of normal. Obviously we do not have enough pH determinations to draw any definite conclusions, and those we do have were made on venous

CHART 21. HYDROGEN-ION CONCENTRATION OF URINE IN HIGH AZOTEMIA

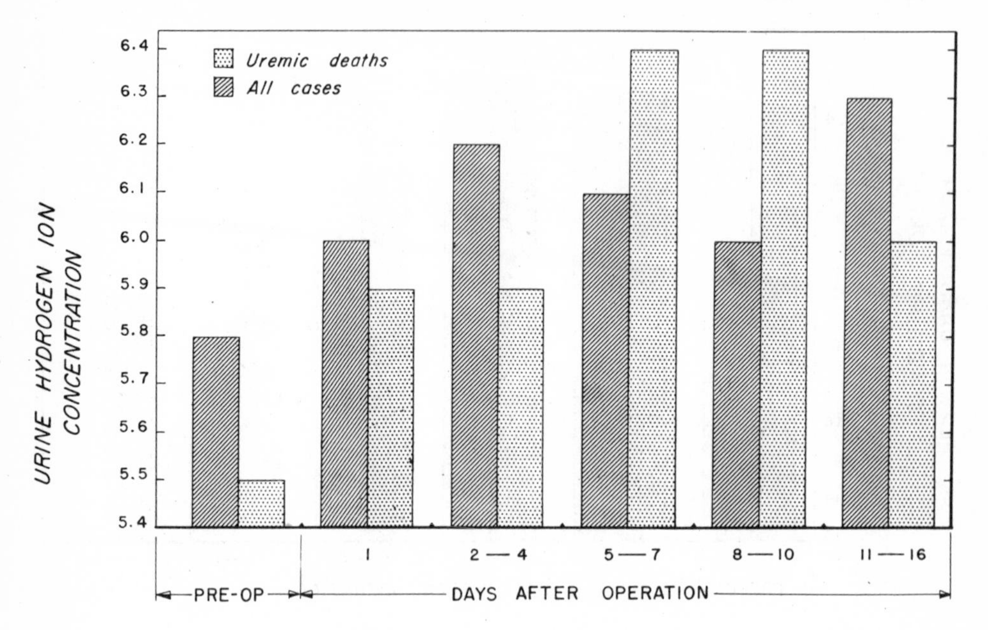

blood, but they support the view that most of these patients were suffering from a metabolic acidosis. This acidosis was not of the hyperchloremic type. For further discussion, see the following sections on chlorides and sodium.

The range of the pH of the urine in patients with high azotemia gave at least a partial explanation for the acidosis; after the first postoperative day none of the patients was able to produce a urine more acid than pH of 6.0 despite an increasingly severe acidosis. In those in whom renal failure was most severe—those who died of uremia—this abnormality was even more evident (Charts 20 and 21). The inference here is that those mechanisms responsible for acidification of the urine, such as tubular transfer of hydrogen ion, were impaired. This subject will be discussed further in the section on Urine; average urine pH is shown in Chart 21 and Table 76. Measurements of urinary ammonia were too few to say whether the deficient formation of this base was also responsible for the acidosis.

Plasma Chlorides.—The relationship of the plasma chloride level to the severity of renal failure is shown in Chart 22 and Table 58C. The averages of all patients with high azotemia show progressive hypochloremia through the first 10 postoperative days and normal values after this time (normal range:

CHART 22. PLASMA CHLORIDES IN HIGH AZOTEMIA

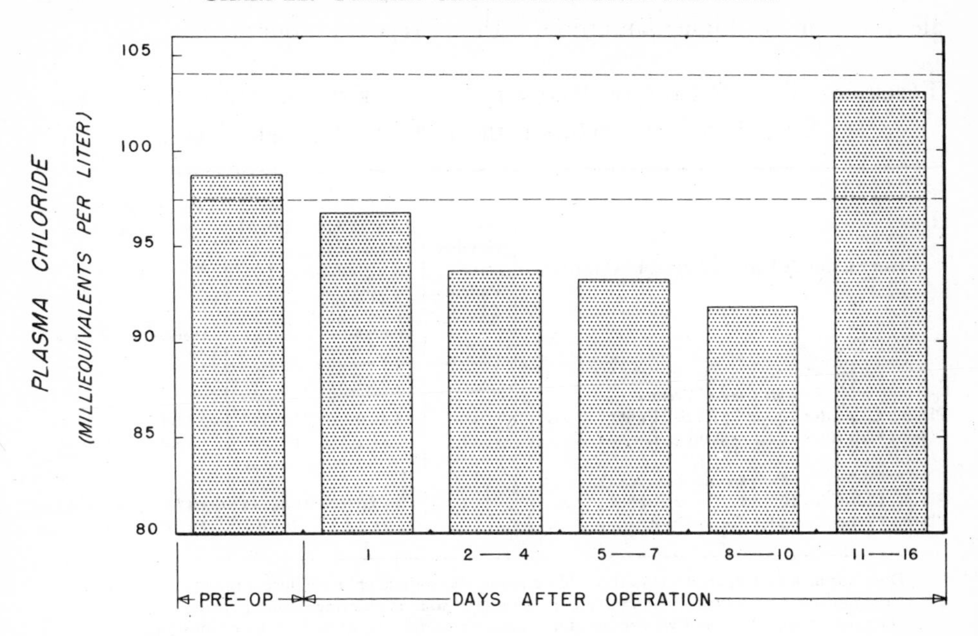

97.5-104). Of the patients who died in uremia, the average values show that an extreme hypochloremia was reached by the tenth day; only one of these patients survived longer than that day. Average values for patients who lived were only slightly low during the period of greatest nitrogen retention. Analysis of individual case records shows that the lowest plasma chloride levels usually occurred in those patients who died before the tenth day, and the rise in the level from the eleventh through the fifteenth day occurred largely in those patients who had a recovery diuresis or only minimal azotemia.

Relationship of Low Plasma Chloride Levels to Intake of Sodium Chloride.— The mechanism of the hypochloremia in these patients is not clear. Most of the patients with a low plasma chloride level were extremely ill and were taking practically no food by mouth; hence their source of salt was almost entirely derived from that administered parenterally. In those patients who presumably had the most severe renal lesions (those who died in uremia), there is a possible correlation between the quantity of parenteral sodium chloride given and the plasma chloride levels (Table 66). The table shows the influence of parenteral sodium chloride intake over a period of 3 days on the subsequent plasma chloride level in 32 patients who died and in 19 who survived. The patients were arbitrarily divided into 2 groups: those with plasma chloride levels of 100 milliequivalents per liter or higher, and those with levels below a hundred.

TABLE 66.—RELATIONSHIP OF PARENTERAL INTAKE OF SODIUM CHLORIDE FOR 3 SUCCESSIVE DAYS TO SUBSEQUENT PLASMA CHLORIDE LEVEL

Plasma Chloride Level and Patients' Outcome	Number of Patients	Plasma Chloride Levels *mEq./L.*		Parenteral NaCl in Previous 3 Days *grams*	
		Average	Range	Average	Range
Patients Died of Uremia					
Plasma Chlorides 100 mEq./L. or Higher	11	104.0	100–111	34.4	8.5–76.5
Plasma Chlorides under 100 mEq./L.	21	84.3	69–94	[1] 23.2	8.5–34.0
Patients Lived					
Plasma Chlorides 100 mEq./L. or Higher	7	119.0	100–144	[2] 42.5	17.0–93.5
Plasma Chlorides under 100 mEq./L.	12	91.2	76–99	[3] 26.9	4.2–51.0

[1] Does not include 10 patients who received no parenteral sodium chloride during the previous 3 days.
[2] Does not include 3 patients who received no parenteral sodium chloride during previous 3 days.
[3] Does not include 9 patients who received no parenteral sodium chloride during previous 3 days.

Of 32 patients who died in uremia, 11 had plasma chlorides of 100 milliequivalents per liter or higher up to the time of death. All of the 11 had received considerable parenteral sodium chloride in the previous 3 days. Twenty-one of the 32 had low plasma chlorides, under 100 milliequivalents per liter; 10 of these patients had received no chlorides parenterally during the previous 3 days, and the remaining 11 had received on an average considerably less salt than those in whom plasma chloride levels were found to be normal or high. It should be emphasized that this analysis of fatalities includes only patients who died in uremia, that is, those in whom the maximum degree of renal impairment could logically be expected.

Among 19 of 23 patients with high azotemia who lived, some relationship of parenteral salt intake to low plasma chloride is also evident in the table. In addition, these patients as a whole were not nearly so ill and it is likely that chloride intake by mouth was considerable, so the total salt intake probably largely exceeded parenteral salt intake. Examination of the individual records of patients who developed severe renal failure and yet lived (see also the section on Recovery Diuresis to follow) indicates that hypochloremia was a part of the chemical picture in most such cases, e.g., Cases 60, 27, 125, but that it was to an appreciable degree associated with the sodium chloride intake. This relationship to intake is also brought out in conjunction with the discussion of sodium to follow.

Several exceptions to these generalizations were evident in individual cases. With apparently adequate salt intake, the chloride level was sometimes low, even in patients in whom there was no loss of chloride through Wangensteen drainage or vomiting. In one patient with high azotemia and with all the other clinical features common to the syndrome of severe renal failure, the plasma chloride levels were abnormally high (Case 133), but in this instance salt intake had been excessive.

It is possible that the hypochloremia might have been due in part to a simple dilution of the chloride ion, since practically all of these patients had an increased plasma volume. This will be discussed further in the section on Plasma Volume. No such connection is apparent, however, in Table 67 which shows plasma volume and plasma chloride determinations done simultaneously in 18 patients who subsequently died of uremia. No correlation between degree of initial shock and plasma chloride level could be demonstrated.

TABLE 67.—PLASMA VOLUME AND PLASMA CHLORIDE DETERMINATIONS IN 18 PATIENTS WHO DIED OF UREMIA

Case No.	Postoperative Days	Plasma Chloride Level *mEq./L.* (normal: 97.5–104)	Plasma Volume (% of calculated normal)	
			Decrease	Increase
9	6	72	....	21.0
22	5	90	....	13.0
26	3	106	....	21.8
47	3	82	....	8.8
52	2	93	....	33.5
55	7	80	....	37.7
69	8	76	....	15.8
80	4	86	5.5	
86	6	76	....	25.5
93	6	82	....	6.1
95	3	92	1.0	
98	5	111	....	32.7
105	7	103	....	39.8
108	3	91	....	3.8
118	5	82	....	6.1
123	3	93	....	18.6
135	4	91	....	63.9
136	3	104	14.5	

Chloride Excretion.—Total chloride excretion was measured in five patients with high azotemia (Cases 104, 105, 107, 112, and 133). Of these, the two patients who died (Cases 105 and 107) had plasma chloride levels which were low or falling. In both of these and in Case 112, chloride excretion was practically nil; chloride intake was probably inadequate in each. Two of them (Cases 107 and 112, to be discussed at greater length in Chapter VII) also had an alkalosis due to administration of excess alkali, chiefly sodium bicarbonate, in an attempt to alkalinize the urine. Two of the three patients who lived had a recovery diuresis. Chloride excretion in one (Case 104) was essentially normal, but determinations were begun after he had actually recovered. The other patient (Case 133) had hyperchloremia, but a high "threshold" for chloride excretion (see Table 78 and Chart 26). This case will be discussed further in the section on Recovery Diuresis.

Chloride concentration in single specimens of urine was measured in 18 patients who died of uremia. In 9 determinations made on 8 patients who had normal plasma chloride levels, the average urine chloride concentration was 72.5±10 milliequivalents per liter. In 21 determinations on 10 patients with low plasma levels, it averaged 54.0±7.0 milliequivalents per liter.

From these data it can, however, be concluded that in cases of renal failure in our series the plasma chlorides in most cases tended to fall as renal failure progressed, the degree of hypochloremia depending to some extent on salt intake. The chloride excreted in the urine was measured in too few cases to state that the hypochloremia was not due to excessive excretion of the chloride ion. No correlation between plasma chloride level and increased plasma volume could be demonstrated, so the low levels, as far as can be determined from our data, were not due to simple dilution. In addition to inadequate salt intake, there must be other factors contributing to hypochloremia.

Plasma Phosphate.—The variations in phosphorus have been discussed in more detail in the preceding section on nitrogenous waste products. The phosphates are mentioned here again only to indicate their relation to total acid-base balance. Reference to Table 58B-E shows that the average plasma phosphates, when converted to milliequivalents, even when elevated to twice normal or over, constitute but a small portion of the total anions; they clearly account for only a portion of the carbon dioxide displaced in those cases in which carbon-dioxide combining power is low.

Plasma Protein.—Plasma proteins have been converted to milliequivalents in

Table 58E. Inspection of these values in all categories shows a remarkable constancy with very small standard errors of the mean. Although the proteins represent a significant proportion of the total anions present, their importance in terms of change in acid-base balance is negligible.

Cations

Serum Sodium.—The number of sodium analyses (Table 58F) was small in comparison with those of anions. However, by grouping all determinations made on patients with high azotemia between the second and tenth postoperative days (or days after trauma) some interesting facts emerge (Table 68).

TABLE 68.—RELATIONSHIP OF SERUM SODIUM, PLASMA CHLORIDE, AND PLASMA CARBON-DIOXIDE COMBINING POWER TO PARENTERAL SODIUM AND CHLORIDE INTAKE IN HIGH AZOTEMIA—32 DETERMINATIONS IN 26 PATIENTS

Classification by Sodium Levels	Average Levels *mEq./L.*			Average Intake in Previous 3 Days * *Total milliequivalents*		
	Sodium (Serum)	Chloride (Plasma)	CO_2 Combining Power (Plasma)	Extra Sodium	Total Sodium	Chloride
Total Determinations	137.6±1.7	87.1±2.1	22.9±1.3	221±39	561±78	339±71
Low Sodium (Below 140—18 determinations)	130.6±1.2	80.7±2.0	22.9±1.8	187±56	369±65	183±54
Normal Sodium (Above 139—14 determinations)	146.5±1.5	95.3±2.7	23.0±2.0	270±48	805±117	541±93

* Calculated from percentage of sodium or chloride present in sodium citrate, sodium bicarbonate, or sodium chloride. Extra sodium therefore represents that given as citrate or bicarbonate.

Thirty-two determinations were made on 26 patients. In 4 instances, 2 determinations for the same patients on different days are included, and in one instance, 3 determinations on different days. Twenty-four of the determinations were among patients dying in uremia, 2 were done on patients in whom uremia was contributory to death, and 1 on a patient in whom uremia was coincident with death. Five determinations were made on patients who survived, 4 of whom had severe renal failure. Nine of the 14 determinations which were above 139 milliequivalents per liter represent patients dying primarily of uremia; 2 determinations, patients in whom uremia was contributory to death; 2 determinations, patients who lived but had severe renal failure, and 1 determination a patient with slight renal failure who survived. Fifteen of the 18 determinations below 140 milliequivalents per liter represent patients dying primarily of uremia, 1 a patient in whom it was coincident with death, and 2 patients who survived but had severe renal failure.

Several facts seem evident from these data: 1. Serum sodium and plasma chloride concentrations were related to intake of these ions, regardless of the severity of the renal insufficiency present. 2. The acidosis, as reflected by the low carbon-dioxide combining power, was equally severe regardless of whether the sodium or chloride levels were normal or low. 3. The outcome was the same in both the normal and low groups; there is no direct evidence that the diminished sodium and chloride concentrations affected the course of the syndrome.

The cause of the acidosis in these cases is not clear. If the acidosis were due to loss of total base, one might expect a lower carbon-dioxide level in the low-sodium group; if due to substitution of chloride for carbon dioxide, the plasma chlorides should be high. As stated before, phosphates were not sufficiently elevated to account for the change entirely in terms of base equivalence. Proteins remained constant and essentially normal. Sulfates and organic acids were not measured; these two components might account for some of the discrepancies evident in our data.

Plasma Magnesium.—There were too few determinations of plasma magnesium to be significant (Table 58G). Because of this, 14 determinations made between the second and tenth postoperative days in 13 cases (two determinations on the same patient on different days are included) were averaged and were 2.3±0.1 milliequivalents per liter. The nonprotein nitrogen determinations done simultaneously on these 13 patients averaged 164±22 mg. per 100 cubic centimeters. If these few determinations are significant, there was no evidence of abnormal magnesium metabolism in this type of renal insufficiency.

Serum Potassium.—Determinations of this substance were made in only seven patients (Cases 78, 80, 107, 112, 133, 135, and 138). In two of these (Cases 78 and 80) the values were 9.1 and 9.8 milliequivalents per liter respectively after several days of anuria or oliguria and just prior to death. In three (Cases 133, 135, and 138) they varied between 6.2 and 7.0 milliequivalents per liter. In the remaining two (Cases 107 and 112) the values were normal (3.9 - 5.3). Analysis of these cases showed that hyperpotassemia occurred only when urine volume was greatly decreased.

Serum Calcium.—This was discussed in the section on Nitrogenous Waste Products and Phosphorus.

Summary—Acid-Base Balance

From the data presented it is apparent that in lower nephron nephrosis resulting from shock or trauma, the most characteristic electrolyte abnormality consists of a progressive, fairly severe acidosis. Hypochloremia was also a frequent but not constant finding, one which we have been unable to explain adequately. Phosphate retention contributes to the acidosis. Serum cation determinations were few. Sodium concentrations followed no constant pattern. Potassium was found to be elevated at the time the patients had oliguria or anuria.

Physiologic Abnormalities

Plasma and Blood Volume

Plasma volume was determined in 23 patients at a time when they had posttraumatic renal insufficiency. The results were striking and of practical importance, for they indicated that increase in plasma volume was a part of the abnormal physiologic picture. Nineteen of these patients died and 4 survived through the mechanism of recovery diuresis. Average plasma volume determinations are shown in Tables 69 and 70, the former for all cases and the latter for fatal cases. Tables 71, 72, and 73 list the individual plasma and blood volume changes and related data on each of the 23 patients.

Relationship of Plasma Volume to Fluid Intake.—Referring first to Tables

TABLE 69.—AVERAGE PLASMA VOLUME CHANGES* IN 23 PATIENTS WITH RENAL INSUFFICIENCY

All Cases (23 Cases)		Increased Plasma Volume (22 Cases)		Decreased Plasma Volume (1 Case)	
Percent Change	Postoperative Days	Percent Change	Postoperative Days	Percent Change	Postoperative Days
43.3±5.7	6.0±0.7	46.2±5.1	6.1±0.7	−19.3	3

* Percent deviation, uncorrected, from the calculated normal plasma volume.

69 and 70, it is evident that the average plasma volume for the entire group was increased significantly above the calculated normal after development of renal insufficiency, the average increase for all 23 cases being 43.3±5.7 percent. In the 19 fatal cases the average increase was 41.6±6.6 percent. The fatal cases were further analyzed as to the quantity of intravenous fluid administered. Average increases for the 15 patients who received an average of 1 liter or more of fluid intravenously daily (Group A, Table 70) were much greater than for the 4 patients who received less than 1 liter daily (Group B, in Table 70). Analysis of Tables 71 and 72, from which the averages in Table 70 were computed, shows that no patient in Group A and only 1 patient in Group B had a normal or subnormal plasma volume after development of renal insufficiency. In this patient (Case 136) there is some reason to question whether deficient circulating blood volume was adequately replaced, and hence whether he ever really recovered from shock during the 3 days he survived after wounding. The four patients who survived all showed increased plasma volume (Table 73).

TABLE 70.—AVERAGE PLASMA VOLUME INCREASE* IN 19 PATIENTS WITH FATAL RENAL INSUFFICIENCY

All Cases (19 Cases)		Group A (15 Cases)		Group B (4 Cases)	
Plasma Volume Increase *percent*	Postoperative Days	Plasma Volume Increase *percent*	Postoperative Days	Plasma Volume Increase *percent*	Postoperative Days
41.6±6.6	4.8±0.4	46.9±6.6	4.8±0.5	21.8	4.8

*Percent increase, uncorrected, over calculated normal plasma volume.

Group A: Patients who received on the average 1 liter or more of fluid (intravenous colloid and crystalloid) per day.

Group B: Patients who received on the average less than 1 liter of fluid (intravenous colloid and crystalloid) per day.

Table 74 represents further analysis of all 23 cases. In 22 of them plasma volume was found to be increased above the calculated normal when renal insufficiency developed. The one exception, a patient (Case 136) who showed a subnormal plasma volume, probably had not been adequately resuscitated, as stated above. Eighteen of the 22 patients with increases had received parenterally an average of 1 liter or more of fluid, crystalloid or colloid, daily. In 10 of the

TABLE 71.—PLASMA AND BLOOD VOLUME CHANGES[1] IN FATAL POSTTRAUMATIC RENAL INSUFFIENCY

Group A: Patients who Received an Average of 1 Liter or More of Intravenous Fluids (Crystalloid or Colloid) Daily

Case No.	Post-operative Days	Plasma Volume Increase	Plasma Proteins	Hematocrit Value	Blood Volume Change	Blood since Wounding	Plasma since Wounding
		percent	*Gm. per 100 cc.*	*percent*	*percent*	*units* [2]	*units* [2]
9	5	....	7.5	36	....	2.2	3.3
	6	43.9	6.8	37	21.0	2.2	3.3
26	3	41.5	6.9	38	21.8	4.5	6
47	1	8.7	5.3	33	....	4.5	2
	3	33.6	4.8	35	8.8	4.5	2
52	2	....	5.7	36	....	8	4
	3	60.1	6.2	38	33.5	8	4
55	6	....	6.4	27	....	6	6
	7	95.1	6.3	25	37.7	7	6
69	[3] 1	....	6.8	70	....	1.5	2
	[3] 2	23.5	6.3	52	13.6	1.5	2
	[3] 5	....	5.4	47	....	1.5	2
	[3] 9	23.5	5.1	42	15.8	1.5	2
80	3	....	6.5	38	....	8	3
	4	10.7	7.1	38	−5.5	8	3
86	2	26.5	6.0	33	−0.1	8	1
	4	....	6.2	39	....	10	1
	6	61.4	6.1	32	25.5	10	1
95	1	....	6.5	48	....	10	1
	3	13.4	6.6	40	−1.0	10	5
98	5	33.9	6.6	47	32.7	8	5
105	7	61.0	7.3	39	39.8	3	6
108	1	6.7	5.1	28	....	11	3
	3	17.7	5.6	40	3.8	13	3
114	6	75.2	5.8	30	31.9	6	1
123	3	52.3	5.8	32	18.6	7	1.3
	6	....	5.8	29	....	7.5	1.3
135	2	17.3	6.5	50	22.9	6	0
	4	80.2	7.3	42	63.9	6	0

[1] Percent deviation from the calculated normal plasma or blood volume. Minus signs indicate decreases.
[2] 1 unit of blood = 500 cc.; 1 unit of plasma = 300 cc. total volume.
[3] Days after release from compression in crush injury.

22 patients multiple determinations were made and 8 of them showed progressive increases in plasma volume as renal failure became more severe. Of the 2 whose plasma volume did not increase further as renal failure progressed, one (Case 69, Table 71) was in Group A in which average fluid intake was high. His plasma volume was increased approximately 23 percent over normal on both

TABLE 72.—PLASMA AND BLOOD VOLUME CHANGES[1] IN FATAL POSTTRAUMATIC RENAL INSUFFICIENCY

Group B: Patients who Received an Average of Less than 1 Liter of Intravenous Fluids (Crystalloid or Colloid) Daily

Case No.	Post-operative Days	Plasma Volume Change	Plasma Proteins	Hematocrit Value	Blood Volume Change	Blood since Wounding	Plasma since Wounding
		percent	*Gm. per 100 cc.*	*percent*	*percent*	*units* [2]	*units* [2]
22	5	67.9	7.1	21	13.0	5	3
93	[3] 1	−31.4	7.3	60	−5.7	0	2
	[3] 3	....	6.2	44	....	0	2
	[3] 6	22.2	6.2	39	6.1	0	2
118	2	34.4	6.7	41	20.7	9	2
	5	16.3	6.6	42	6.1	9	2
136	3	−19.3	8.0	50	−14.5	9	4

[1] Percent deviation from the calculated normal plasma or blood volume. Minus signs indicate decreases.
[2] 1 unit of blood = 500 cc.; 1 unit of plasma = 300 cc. total volume.
[3] Days after release from compression in crush injury. The first determination in this case was made before renal insufficiency developed.

the second and ninth days after crushing injury. The other (Case 118, Table 72) was in Group B, those with restricted fluid intake. His increased plasma volume actually diminished although he subsequently died in uremia.

Among those who had increased plasma volumes were the four patients who had a recovery diuresis and survived. In three of them plasma volume first increased and then decreased as diuresis proceeded and nitrogenous waste products were excreted (Table 73). The progress of the plasma volume changes in relation to the plasma nonprotein nitrogen in these cases is shown in Chart 27. The fourth patient (Case 150) had his first determination after diuresis had begun although he still had severe renal failure and an increased plasma volume.

Relationship of Plasma Volume to Plasma Protein Concentration, Hematocrit Level, and Total Blood Volume.—The relationships of plasma volume to plasma protein concentration, hematocrit value, and total blood volume are evident in Tables 71, 72, and 73. There were considerable individual variations, but in general it can be stated that an expected coincident decrease in plasma protein concentration as the plasma volume rose during renal insufficiency was not usually demonstrated. Thus of the eight patients in whom the already increased plasma volume was known to rise, there were no significant changes in plasma protein concentration in five (three of whom received blood between measurements);

TABLE 73.—PLASMA AND BLOOD VOLUME CHANGES[1] IN 4 PATIENTS WITH POSTTRAUMATIC RENAL INSUFFICIENCY AND SUBSEQUENT RECOVERY DIURESIS

Case No.	Post-operative Days	Plasma Volume Increase *percent*	Plasma Proteins *Gm. per 100 cc.*	Hema-tocrit Value *percent*	Blood Volume Change *percent*	Intra-venous Fluids *cc.*	Oral Fluids *cc.*	Blood since Wounding *units* [2]	Plasma since Wounding *units* [2]
60	0.75	30.3	6.3	25	−8	3,429	....	5.5	10
	2.5	70.1	6.5	25	20	[3] 1,000	[3] 1,435	7.5	10
	6.5	73.5	6.4	24	21	[3] 625	[3] 2,386	8.5	10
	11.5	31.7	6.4	38.4	13	[3] 600	[3] 3,952	13.5	10
133	13	44.3	7.6	40	25	2,518	1,750	23	10.5
	16	49.8	7.4	40	32	[3] 1,583	[3] 1,416	24	12.5
	27	36.1	6.1	32	5	....	....	26	12.5
	35	7.4	5.8	36	−12	....	....	26	12.5
138	4	30.7	6.6	40	16	?	?	2	2
	5	29.7	6.0	40	15	0	[3] 1,525	2	2
	10	55.6	6.6	32	20	1,650	[3] 1,160	2	6
	14	11.1	8.0	40	−1.9	1,000	[3] 2,326	2	6
150	12.5	27.3	6.0	34	1.7	1,000	[4] 3,330	9.2	4

[1] Percent deviation from the calculated normal plasma or blood volume. Minus signs indicate decreases.
[2] 1 unit of blood = 500 cc.; 1 unit of plasma = 300 cc. total volume.
[3] Between determinations.
[4] Approximately.

TABLE 74.—TREND OF PLASMA VOLUME CHANGES DURING POSTTRAUMATIC RENAL INSUFFICIENCY IN 23 PATIENTS

Plasma Volume	Total Patients	1 Liter or more of I.V. Fluid Daily	Plasma Volume Deter-mination Repeated	Results of Repeated Determination		Patients' Outcome	
				Increased Further	Did not Increase	Lived	Died
		Number of patients	*Number of patients*	*Number of patients*	*Number of patients*	*Number of patients*	*Number of patients*
Increased over calculated normal	* 22	18	10	8	2	4	18
Decreased below calculated normal	1	0	0	....	....	0	1

* Four patients with recovery diuresis included. In them the plasma volume was increased until onset of diuresis.

there was an increase in one, and a decrease in only two. Explanation for the absence of a dilution phenomenon is not evident from our data. One can only postulate that in such cases plasma protein was being mobilized from protein sources elsewhere in the body.

The hematocrit level in the eight patients in whom plasma volume increased progressively (as shown by serial determinations) rose in one who received blood between measurements, was unchanged in three, two of whom received blood between measurements, and fell in four, one of whom received blood between measurements. Although the total blood volumes were also increased, the increments clearly were a reflection of the increase in the plasma volume, and because of the low hematocrit level in most cases, they were not as strikingly increased as was the plasma volume.

These data indicate, then, that in posttraumatic renal failure, total circulating plasma volume is increased. This must be due largely to the inability of the kidneys to excrete adequate water. However, because the plasma protein concentration did not usually diminish as plasma volume increased, it is evident that the sole explanation is not simply that hydremia exists. There would seem to be also unexplained extrarenal factors interfering with maintenance of a normal extracellular fluid volume. The practical importance of these observations is self-evident. Administration of excessive quantities of fluids to these patients who already have increased extracellular fluid volume can probably do nothing toward stimulating the kidneys to excrete; it can cause fatal pulmonary edema.

Summary—Plasma and Blood Volume

Plasma volume was determined in 23 patients in whom posttraumatic renal insufficiency developed, 19 of whom died. Averaging all 23 cases, there was an increase over the calculated normal plasma volume of 43.3 percent, and of 41.6 percent in the fatal cases. Considering the patients individually, there was only one in whom plasma volume was less than normal after signs of renal impairment appeared, and there was good reason to believe that this patient had never been adequately resuscitated from shock. Comparison of the plasma volume with simultaneous plasma protein levels indicates that there was an increase in total circulating plasma and not simply an increase in proportion of water in the plasma; i.e., in general, plasma protein did not decrease with increasing plasma volume. In those patients in whom serial determinations were made, including several who had a recovery diuresis, the time of maximum increase in plasma volume coincided with that of maximum azotemia, and in those who recovered, plasma volume and plasma nonprotein nitrogen diminished at parallel rates.

URINE

Specific Gravity

One of the most striking and constant physiologic abnormalities observed in posttraumatic renal insufficiency was impairment of ability of the renal tubules to reabsorb water. Within a day or two postoperatively, those patients who developed renal impairment, almost without exception, lost the power to make a concentrated urine regardless of the amount they were excreting (Chart 23 and Tables 75 and 77). The averages in the tables and chart were calculated from the specific gravities observed in routine specimens, usually the first morning one. They do not, then, represent true concentration tests, but there are several factors which indicate that the values observed, in most cases, were those of practically maximum concentrating ability: (1) Concentration tests were done later on patients who recovered, when it was deemed safe to do them. In these patients, even after the retained nitrogenous products had been cleared and output had returned to normal, specific gravity remained fixed and low. (2) Many of the specimens were taken when the output of urine was very low and hence

CHART 23. URINE SPECIFIC GRAVITY IN PATIENTS WITH HIGH AZOTEMIA

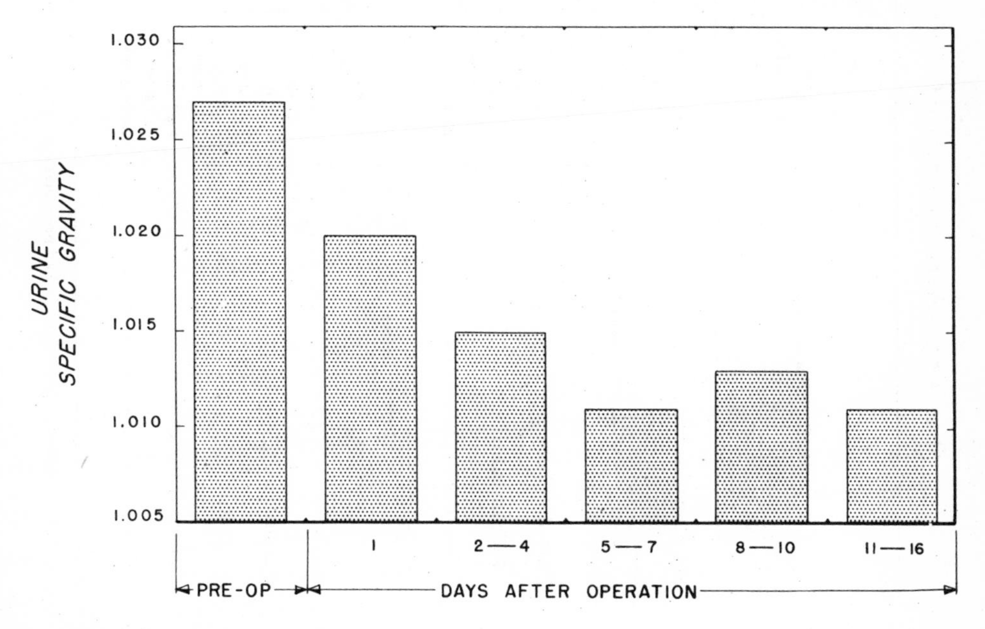

Figures from "Anuria and Oliguria" grouping, Table 75.

956507 O—52——12

TABLE 75.—AVERAGE SPECIFIC GRAVITY OF THE URINE IN PATIENTS WITH HIGH AZOTEMIA*

Classification of Cases	Average Specific Gravity					
	Preoperative Period	Postoperative Period				
		1 Day	2–4 Days	5–7 Days	8–10 Days	11–15 Days
ALL CASES	1.026±.002 (11 cases)	1.020±.001 (21 cases)	1.015±.001 (46 cases)	1.012±.001 (28 cases)	1.014±.001 (13 cases)	1.011±.001 (12 cases)
Patients' Outcome						
Lived	1.026±.001 (4 cases)	1.020±.001 (5 cases)	1.015±.001 (15 cases)	1.012±.001 (13 cases)	1.012±.002 (7 cases)	1.011±.001 (10 cases)
Died—All Causes	1.026±.003 (7 cases)	1.020±.002 (16 cases)	1.015±.001 (31 cases)	1.013±.001 (15 cases)	1.016±.002 (6 cases)	1.011 (2 cases)
Died of Uremia	1.033 (2 cases)	1.021±.002 (9 cases)	1.014±.001 (26 cases)	1.011±.001 (11 cases)	1.013 (4 cases)	1.011 (2 cases)
Died of other Causes	1.023±.003 (5 cases)	1.018±.002 (7 cases)	1.019±.002 (5 cases)	1.018±.003 (4 cases)	1.022 (2 cases)	—
Urinary Output						
Normal	1.028 (1 case)	1.019 (2 cases)	1.016±.001 (7 cases)	1.016±.002 (8 cases)	1.017±.004 (4 cases)	1.007 (1 case)
Anuria	1.032 (1 case)	1.019 (7 cases)	1.014 (18 cases)	1.010 (10 cases)	1.012 (3 cases)	1.013 (3 cases)
Oliguria	1.026 (7 cases)	1.021 (12 cases)	1.016 (21 cases)	1.012 (10 cases)	1.013 (6 cases)	1.011 (6 cases)
Unknown	1.020 (2 cases)	—	—	—	—	1.014 (2 cases)
Anuria and Oliguria	1.027±.002 (8 cases)	1.020±.001 (19 cases)	1.015±.001 (39 cases)	1.011±.001 (20 cases)	1.013±.001 (9 cases)	1.011±.001 (9 cases)
Anuria, Oliguria, and Unknown	1.026±.002 (10 cases)	—	—	—	—	1.012±.001 (11 cases)

* If more than 1 determination had been made on 1 patient during the specified period, the lowest value was used.

when the kidneys were theoretically concentrating urine to the maximum of their ability. (3) In many of the patients, particularly those who died in uremia, fluids were sharply restricted, usually to about 1 liter a day. This could be further reason for assuming that the average urine specimen would be concentrated if the kidneys were capable of making it so; on the other hand, this argument may be rendered untenable by the fact that plasma volume was probably increased in all cases. (4) Twenty-four hour urine specimens were collected from five patients in whom renal failure developed. In these the specific gravity of the total specimens showed the same trend, even though plasma nonprotein nitrogen was rising, and in three cases total output of urine was diminishing.

It will be shown in the section on Recovery Diuresis that in those patients who did recover, the nitrogenous waste products were cleared because of an increasing output of urine but the urine specific gravity remained fixed at a low level. In summary, it appears from our data that in this syndrome one of the earliest functional derangements of the kidney to occur, and probably one of the last to disappear when recovery takes place, is the ability to concentrate the urine.

Hydrogen-Ion Concentration

The tendency of the acidity of the urine to decrease as systemic acidosis and renal failure progress has been previously discussed (see *Plasma Carbon-Dioxide Combining Power* under Acid-Base Balance, Chart 21, and Tables 76 and 77). From our meager data on measurement of titratable acidity and ammonia of the urine (see the section on Recovery Diuresis), it is probable that the mechanism of this failure to make a very acid urine is associated with a decrease in titratable acidity and thus is similar to that seen in most types of renal failure. Inability of the kidneys to produce a urine of maximum alkalinity, if presented with a surplus of base, also seems to be a feature of the syndrome (see Chapter VII) and again is similar to the situation occasionally seen in other types of kidney disease.

There is good evidence[1] that acidification of the urine by active transfer of hydrogen ions, as well as ammonia production is accomplished by the distal

[1] Pitts, R. F.; Lotspeich, W. D.; Schiess, W. A., and Ayer, J. L.: The renal regulation of acid-base balance in man. I. The nature of the mechanism for acidifying the urine. J. Clin. Investigation 27: 48–56, January 1948. Schiess, W. A.; Ayer, J. L.; Lotspeich, W. D., and Pitts, R. F.: The renal regulation of acid-base balance in man. II. Factors affecting the excretion of titratable acid by the normal human subject. Ibid. 57–64.

TABLE 76.—AVERAGE pH OF THE URINE IN PATIENTS WITH HIGH AZOTEMIA*

Classification of Cases	Average pH of Urine					
	Preoperative Period	Postoperative Period				
		1 Day	2–4 Days	5–7 Days	8–10 Days	11–15 Days
ALL CASES	5.8±0.2 (12 cases)	6.0±0.1 (21 cases)	6.2±0.1 (43 cases)	6.1±0.1 (29 cases)	6.0±0.1 (14 cases)	6.3±0.3 (12 cases)
Patients' Outcome						
Lived	5.6±0.2 (4 cases)	6.2±0.3 (5 cases)	6.6±0.2 (15 cases)	5.2±0.3 (13 cases)	5.8±0.2 (7 cases)	6.4±0.3 (10 cases)
Died—All Causes	5.9±0.2 (8 cases)	6.0±0.1 (16 cases)	5.9±0.1 (28 cases)	6.2±0.2 (16 cases)	6.2±0.2 (7 cases)	6.0 (2 cases)
Died of Uremia	5.5 (2 cases)	5.9±0.2 (9 cases)	5.9±0.1 (23 cases)	6.4±0.3 (12 cases)	6.4±0.3 (5 cases)	6.0 (2 cases)
Died of other Causes	6.0±0.3 (6 cases)	6.2±0.2 (7 cases)	6.1±0.3 (5 cases)	5.5±0.2 (4 cases)	5.7 (2 cases)	—
Urinary Output						
Normal	5.7 (2 cases)	6.6 (2 cases)	6.2±0.2 (7 cases)	5.8±0.2 (8 cases)	6.0±0.2 (4 cases)	5.9 (1 case)
Anuria	5.5 (1 case)	5.8 (7 cases)	5.9 (16 cases)	6.2 (11 cases)	6.4 (4 cases)	6.9 (2 cases)
Oliguria	5.8 (7 cases)	6.1 (12 cases)	6.4 (20 cases)	6.1 (10 cases)	5.8 (6 cases)	5.9 (6 cases)
Unknown	6.1 (2 cases)	—	—	—	—	6.9 (2 cases)
Anuria and Oliguria	5.7±0.2 (8 cases)	6.0±0.1 (19 cases)	6.2±0.1 (36 cases)	6.2±0.2 (21 cases)	6.0±0.2 (10 cases)	6.2±0.3 (8 cases)
Anuria, Oliguria, and Unknown	5.8±0.2 (10 cases)	—	—	—	—	6.3±0.3 (10 cases)

* If more than 1 determination had been made on 1 patient during the specified period, the lowest value was used.

tubular cells. This provides further correlation, perhaps, of functional with anatomic findings in patients suffering from lower nephron nephrosis following shock or trauma.

TABLE 77.—AVERAGE SPECIFIC GRAVITY AND pH OF URINE IN PATIENTS WITH OLIGURIA OR ANURIA

Time of Determination	Oliguria		Anuria	
	pH	Specific Gravity	pH	Specific Gravity
Preoperative	5.8±0.1 (10 cases)	1.026±.002 (10 cases)	5.5 (1 case)	1.032 (1 case)
Postoperative Days				
First	6.2±0.1 (22 cases)	1.023±.001 (22 cases)	5.8±0.2 (7 cases)	1.019±.003 (7 cases)
Second to Fourth	6.4±0.2 (31 cases)	1.016±.001 (32 cases)	5.9±0.2 (16 cases)	1.014±.001 (18 cases)
Fifth to Seventh	6.4±0.2 (17 cases)	1.012±.001 (17 cases)	6.2±0.3 (11 cases)	1.010±.001 (10 cases)
Eighth to Tenth	6.0±0.2 (10 cases)	1.015±.001 (11 cases)	6.4±0.2 (4 cases)	1.012 (3 cases)
Eleventh to Fifteenth	6.0±0.2 (6 cases)	1.011±.001 (6 cases)	6.8 (3 cases)	1.013 (3 cases)

Proteinuria and Pigment Excretion

As was pointed out in Chapter IV, all patients with proved renal lesions had proteinuria, and this finding was also a constant one in all patients with posttraumatic renal insufficiency. It was not, however, a specific finding, for it was absent in only 14 of the entire series of casualties studied. The relationship of pigment excretion in the urine to posttraumatic renal insufficiency will be discussed in Chapter VIII.

Summary—Changes in the Urine

The most striking change in the urine was the fixation of specific gravity at low levels within a day or two after the onset of renal failure following shock or trauma. This impairment of maximum reabsorptive capacity of water by the renal tubules persisted after other evidence of kidney damage disappeared in those patients who recovered. Inability to manufacture a highly acid urine in the presence of metabolic acidosis was also a constant feature in the patients studied.

Recovery Diuresis

The arbitrary choice of 65 mg. per 100 cc. or higher concentration of nonprotein nitrogen in the plasma as an index of renal insufficiency in this series of cases has been discussed. Of the 73 patients included in our "high azotemia" group, 23 (32 percent) lived. Those who survived may be further classified according to the degree of renal impairment they exhibited: Twelve had apparently only minimal interference with renal function, with a rapid return to normal after transient nitrogen retention. We were unable to follow one patient with a nonprotein nitrogen level greater than 65 mg. per 100 cc. who lived and so do not know what degree of renal insufficiency he ultimately had. Ten had even greater evidence of renal impairment and their course conformed with the syndrome we have designated as recovery diuresis.

The characteristic features of this syndrome are:

1. A nonprotein nitrogen level greater than 100 milligrams per 100 cubic centimeters.
2. Oliguria or anuria, followed by a substantial diuresis resulting in clearance of nitrogenous waste products and return to normal of the electrolyte pattern.
3. Impaired ability to concentrate the urine.
4. Hypertension (systolic blood pressure above 135 millimeters of mercury; diastolic above 90).

Of the 10 patients exhibiting this syndrome, 9 showed at least three and most of them all four of these characteristics. The tenth patient (Case 44) was observed during a period when the laboratory was not functioning, so his blood and urine could not be examined, but clinically he displayed the characteristics of the syndrome.

This small group of cases is of great interest and practical importance. One would like to know why these patients recovered whereas the majority of those with renal insufficiency died, and whether in their course or treatment there are any clues which might lead to more effective treatment than has been found to the present. Detailed data on a few typical cases (see Charts 25 and 26), together with pertinent clinical and physiologic findings in the group as a whole, are considered of value here. (The 10 cases were Numbers 27, 30, 43, 44, 60, 104, 125, 133, 138, and 150.)

Clinical Features

The degree of initial shock was essentially the same for these 10 patients as for the entire group having renal failure. Three patients had had severe shock, 5 moderate, 1 slight, and 1 no shock. As in other instances, it is entirely possible that there may have been considerable shock in all 10, but so far as we could determine at the time of admission, they must be classified as above.

Five of the 10 patients had multiple major wounds. The major wounds in the entire group were: 6 peripheral with fracture, 4 thoracic, 4 intra-abdominal, and one thoraco-abdominal. One patient had a contusion of the bladder. There were no wounds of the liver or kidney.

The time of onset of oliguria in relation to wounding and operation, and the duration of suppression of urinary output are of interest. Unfortunately the day-to-day records are not as accurate as one would like. Many of these patients were seen in field hospitals during periods of great military activity, when the press of work made it very difficult to make such observations. We have no record of output of urine until the first postoperative day in any of the cases. Eight of the 10 patients are known to have had at least 1 day of oliguria or anuria between the first and sixth postoperative days. Records of output of urine were not kept for the remaining 2 patients at the time they probably had oliguria, but questioning of ward personnel and of the patients suggested very strongly that they too had had oliguria during this period. The duration of oliguria ranged from 1 to 4 days. There followed then a period of gradually increasing output of urine, reaching in some cases 5 or 6 liters a day. The plasma nonprotein nitrogen level did not, as a rule, begin to decrease until several days after diuresis had begun.

Because of the increase in plasma volume during the period of increasing azotemia, it might be expected that total fluid output would exceed intake during the diuresis period. This clearly occurred in two cases (Case 60 (Chart 24) and Case 150). In the remaining eight cases it was impossible to demonstrate this fact from the figures available, for the records kept gave only an approximate estimate of total water balance; they did not account for water lost by perspiration, respiration, or with the stools. Since the plasma volume returned to normal and the edema subsided as diuresis proceeded, it is logical to assume that total fluid output did exceed intake until equilibrium was reestablished.

All these patients had hypertension, by our definition. In general the blood pressure was highest at the time of the most severe nitrogen retention and the

CHART 24. RELATIONSHIP OF FLUID INTAKE AND OUTPUT IN A PATIENT WITH RECOVERY DIURESIS (CASE 60)

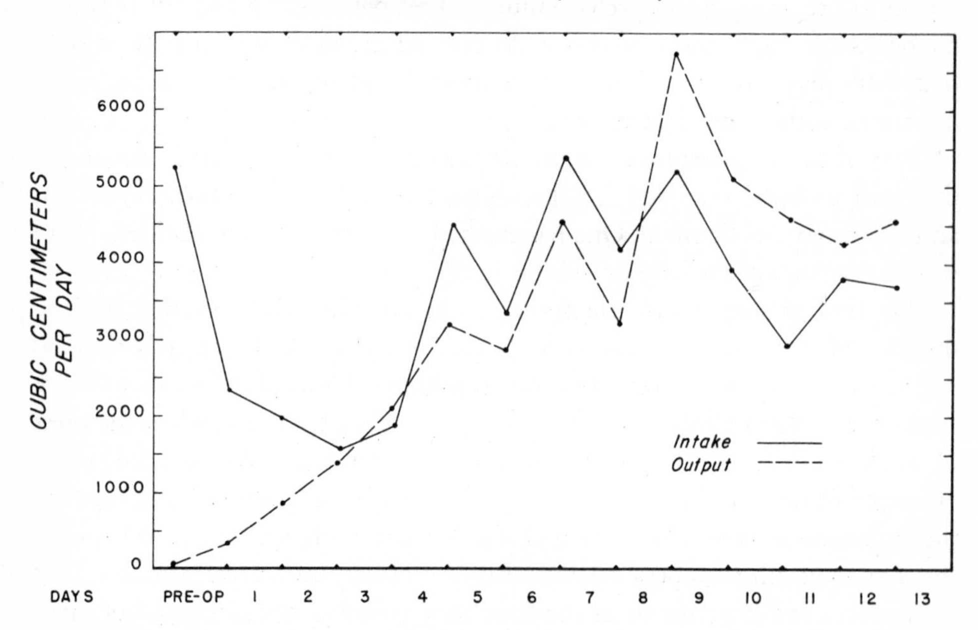

Output exceeded intake from the eighth day. If extrarenal losses were shown, output would have exceeded intake after the fourth day.

Chart 25. Recovery diuresis occurred in this patient following an initial period of renal insufficiency due to severe traumatic shock and great blood loss. Note: (1) Initial period of oliguria and diminished renal function as evidenced by low phenolsulfonphthalein excretion with fixed urine specific gravity which persisted throughout the period of observation. (2) The gradual increase in urinary output during the first week accompanied by rising blood pressure, rising plasma nonprotein nitrogen concentration, falling carbon-dioxide combining power and plasma chlorides. (3) The fall in nonprotein nitrogen occurring only several days after adequate urinary output, accompanied by improvement of phenolsulfonphthalein excretion, rising carbon-dioxide combining power and plasma chloride levels, and return of the blood pressure toward normal. *See page 171.*

CHART 25. COURSE OF A PATIENT WITH RECOVERY DIURESIS (CASE 60)

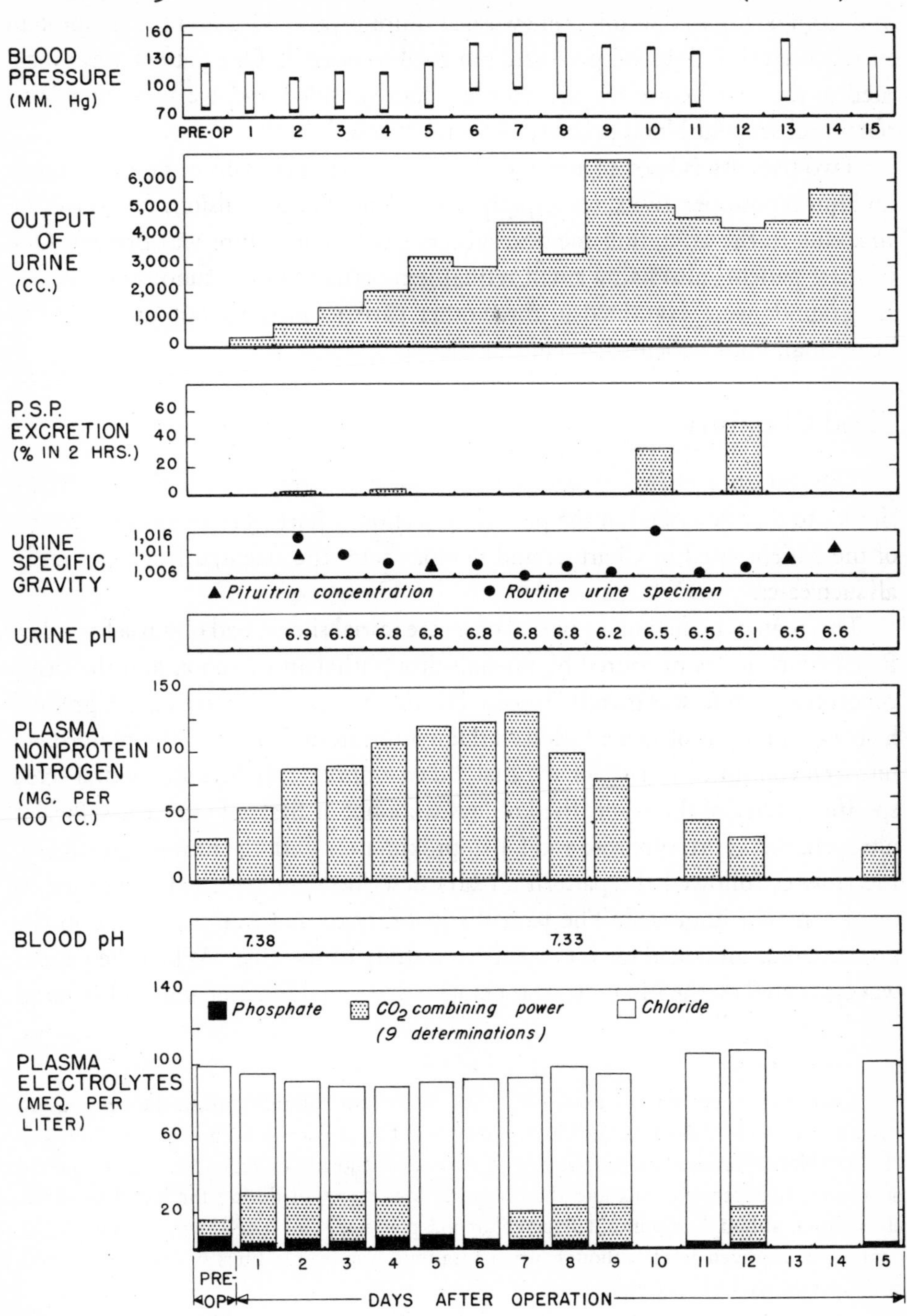

elevation was significant, with levels ranging from 150 to 170 mm. Hg systolic and from 90 to 110 diastolic. Likewise, as diuresis proceeded and the nonprotein nitrogen levels fell, blood pressures returned to normal. One patient was evacuated to the rear before his hypertension had subsided and we were unable to obtain subsequent blood-pressure determinations.

Two patients (Cases 44 and 150) had generalized convulsions on the eighth and ninth postoperative days respectively. In one, the convulsions furnished the first clue to the attending medical officers that renal failure was present. One of these patients also had a small retinal hemorrhage in the fundus of one eye. Eyegrounds were examined in three other patients in the group and found to be normal. Four patients had clinical edema.

Blood Chemistry

The abnormal chemical pattern in this selected group of cases was essentially similar to that described in the preceding section. Chart 25 represents the course of the patient cited in Chart 24 and demonstrates the essential features seen in all such cases.

This man, who had had a period of severe initial shock, had oliguria for 1 day. Renal function, as measured by phenolsulfonphthalein excretion and the urine concentration test, was greatly impaired by the first postoperative day. A gradual increase in output of urine followed. Despite diuresis, however, the nonprotein nitrogen continued to rise for the first 7 days—apparently because, with a fixed specific gravity of the urine, the kidneys were not at first able to clear sufficient nitrogen. Blood pressure rose and fell approximately with the nitrogen retention. Electrolytes followed the pattern already described but returned to normal as renal function improved. The patient's inability to make an acid urine in the presence of a mild acidosis is evident from study of the chart. When the patient was evacuated on the fifteenth postoperative day, renal function was still reduced

Chart 26. There was an excessive intake of sodium chloride during the previous 10 days, which is not shown on the chart. Note: (1) The unusually high serum sodium and plasma chloride levels. (2) A relatively low urinary chloride excretion during the period of maximum hyperchloremia and the extremely low excretion during the last days of the observation, although significant hyperchloremia persisted. (3) The slowly falling plasma nonprotein nitrogen level, although urinary output was over 2 liters a day during most of the period studied. *See page 173.*

CHART 26. COURSE OF A PATIENT WITH RECOVERY DIURESIS (CASE 133)

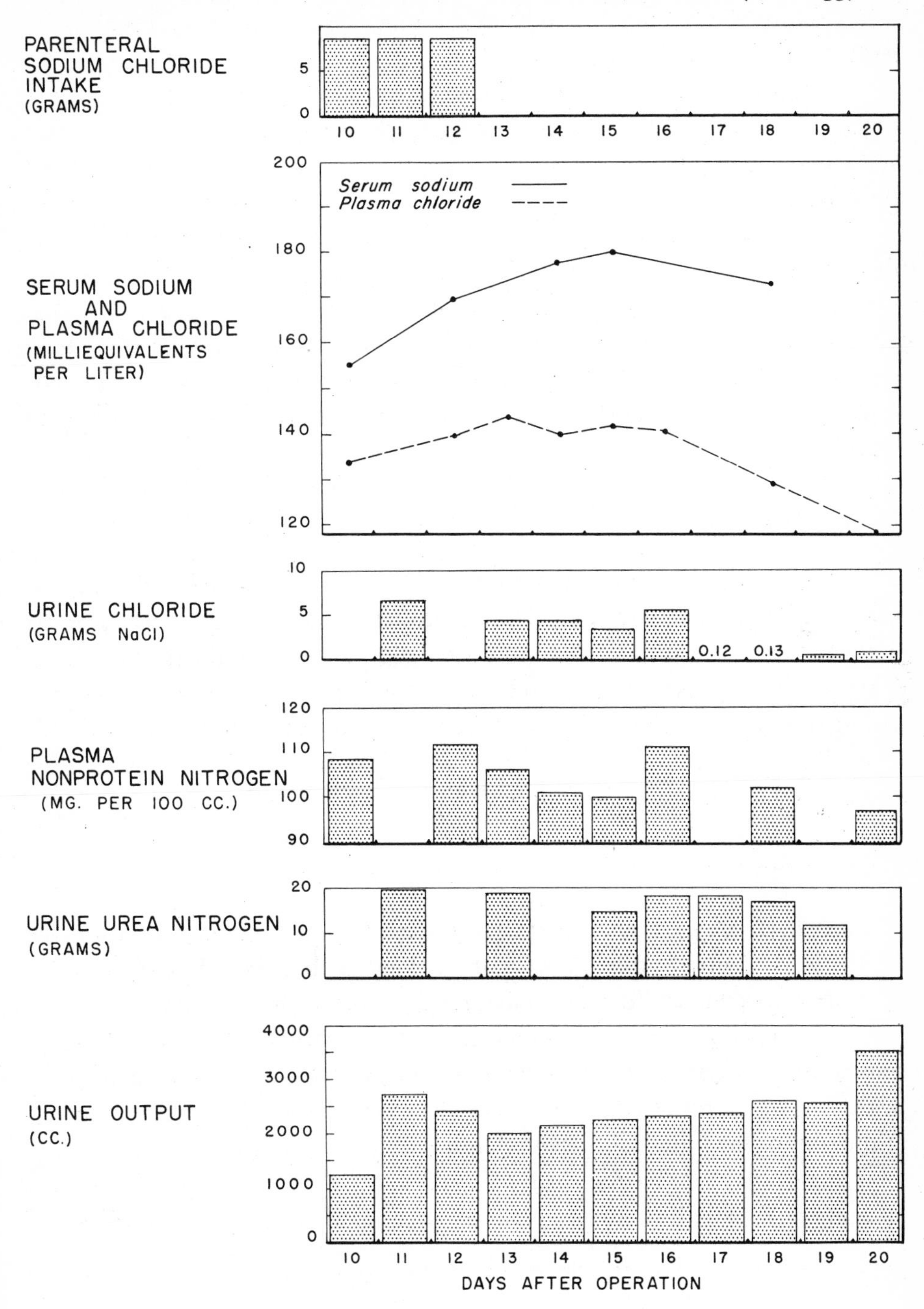

despite normal chemical findings in the blood.[2] Results of blood chemistry and urine examinations, made in eight of the nine other patients, followed essentially the same pattern.

The time of maximum nitrogen retention varied; five patients had their highest nonprotein nitrogen level between the third and ninth days after trauma, and the remaining four between the tenth and thirteenth days. The period of time required for recovery of renal function varied from 6 to 25 days.

As mentioned earlier, hypochloremia was not as prominent a feature in these patients as in those who died in uremia, but it was present to some degree (plasma chlorides under 100 milliequivalents per liter) in five patients. One patient (Case 133), on the other hand, following a high intake of sodium chloride, had a pronounced hyperchloremia (plasma chlorides 144 milliequivalents per liter) about the time of greatest nitrogen retention (Chart 26 and Table 79).

Plasma Volume

Four patients with recovery diuresis in whom the plasma volume was measured showed a significant increase over the calculated normal. It was greatest at the time of maximum nitrogen retention and decreased as diuresis proceeded. Three patients (Cases 60, 133, and 138, Chart 27) were discussed in the preceding section on Plasma and Blood Volume. A fourth patient (Case 150, Table 73) still had a significant elevation in plasma volume when first studied on the twelfth postoperative day after diuresis had begun.

Urinary Findings

Specific Gravity.—Five patients, following administration of pituitrin, were unable to concentrate urine above 1.015 as long as they were followed (up to 49 days postoperatively in one instance). One patient with very transient nitrogen retention could concentrate to 1.020 by the thirteenth day. Concentration tests were not done in the other four patients, but several specimens in three of them were uniformly dilute. In one (Case 30), two routine specimens taken at the time of maximum nitrogen retention were 1.019 and 1.023.

Twenty-four Hour Urine Analyses and Related Findings in Two Patients.—Examinations of 24-hour urine specimens were made in two patients who had

[2] Studies made 10 months later in the United States showed normal kidney function.

CHART 27. PLASMA VOLUME AND PLASMA NONPROTEIN NITROGEN CONCENTRATION IN 3 PATIENTS WITH RECOVERY DIURESIS (CASES 60, 133, AND 138)

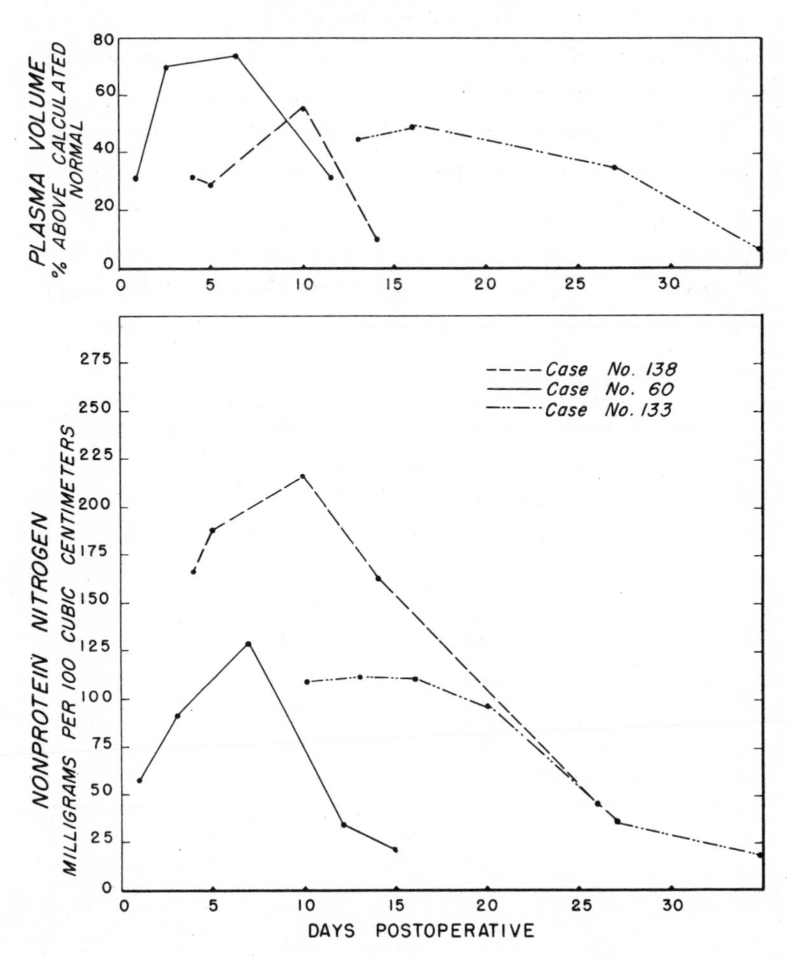

recovery diuresis. In Case 133 the collections were started just at the end of the recovery period. Table 78 lists the findings in one of these patients (Case 104) along with plasma determinations made on the same days. From these data a few conclusions could be drawn regarding this one patient: (1) Titratable acidity values were rather low, considering low plasma carbon-dioxide combining power during the first 3 days of collection. (2) Ammonia production was normal. (3) Chloride excretion and sodium chloride intake were normal. Plasma chloride values were normal. (4) Excretion of urea was high the first day and accompanied a fall in plasma nonprotein nitrogen to normal.

Table 79 and Chart 26 show comparable findings on the other patient (Case 133). Ammonia and titratable acidity determinations of the urine in this case were not numerous enough and varied too widely to draw any conclusions regarding acid-base regulation. Excretion of urea and creatinine was about what would be expected in a normal individual, but not sufficient to clear the retained nitrogen rapidly. Toward the end of the 10-day period during which 24-hour urine collections were made, plasma levels of urea nitrogen and creatinine be-

TABLE 78.—RELATIONSHIP OF 24-HOUR URINALYSES AND PLASMA BIOCHEMIC FINDINGS IN A PATIENT WITH RECOVERY DIURESIS (CASE 104)

Postoperative Days	Fluid Intake cc.	Parenteral NaCl Intake Gm.	Urine Output cc.	Plasma CO_2 Combining Power mEq./L.	Urine pH	Urine Titratable Acidity cc. 0.1 N	Urine Ammonia cc. 0.1 N	Urine Ammonia / Titratable Acidity
Third	1,000	....	900+	....	....	....	....	....
Fourth	3,705	1.6	2,335	25	5.9	257	428	1.7
Fifth	2,100	....	1,590	23	5.6	199	652	3.3
Sixth	3,350	....	1,950	....	5.6	302	688	2.2
Seventh	3,480	....	1,780	23	5.2	444	656	1.4
Eighth	4,850	....	2,480	....	5.4	509	779	1.5
Ninth	3,650	....	2,050	....	6.9	145	414	2.8
Tenth	2,790	....	2,100	26	6.4	69	497	7.1
Eleventh	3,250	....	2,890	....	6.5	93	594	6.4
Twelfth	2,550	....	2,200	....	6.6	154	544	3.4
Thirteenth	2,500	....	2,730	....	6.8	137	475	3.5

Postoperative Days	Urine Chloride Gm. NaCl	Plasma Chloride mEq./L.	Plasma NPN mg. per 100 cc.	Plasma Urea Nitrogen mg. per 100 cc.	Urine Urea Nitrogen Gm.	Plasma Creatinine mg. per 100 cc.	Urine Creatinine Gm.	Urine Specific Gravity
Third	....	....	111	....	....	....	....	....
Fourth	4.7	102	70	....	22.7	1.08	1.42	....
Fifth	3.2	101	44	27	15.4	0.80	1.30	....
Sixth	6.9	....	....	....	19.2	....	1.80	....
Seventh	4.7	102	29	....	12.2	1.39	1.25	1.012
Eighth	9.1	....	....	....	26.1	....	1.72	1.018
Ninth	4.7	....	....	....	13.5	....	1.20	1.016
Tenth	5.9	94	29	....	19.9	0.94	1.48	1.012
Eleventh	8.1	....	....	....	13.5	....	1.33	1.010
Twelfth	8.4	....	....	....	14.5	....	1.25	....
Thirteenth	11.7	....	....	....	15.4	....	0.80	....

gan to fall. Clearance rates of these substances, however, were diminished during the entire period of observation.

The relationship of serum sodium, plasma carbon-dioxide combining power, fluid and sodium chloride intake, urinary output, and urinary excretion of chloride in this same patient are also shown. After a high intake of sodium chloride, sodium and chloride retention developed. Plasma carbon-dioxide combining power fell, in this instance partially as a result of hyperchloremia. Chloride excretion was relatively low considering the high plasma chloride level. As the plasma chloride level fell, chloride excretion decreased to negligible amounts during the last 4 days, even though the plasma chloride level was still unusually high. High serum sodium accompanied the hyperchloremia. There is in this case evidence of a high renal "threshold" for both sodium and chloride excretion.

The course and essential features in this patient were characteristic of recovery diuresis, but he exhibited most unusual electrolyte abnormalities. Although he had an increased plasma volume (Chart 27), there were also marked hypernatremia and hyperchloremia. An elevated serum sodium is most unusual except in the presence of dehydration, which, if the measurements of plasma volume can be accepted, was not present in this patient. Further evidence of inability of the renal tubules to reabsorb maximum amounts of water is seen here in the dilute urines of total specimens in both Cases 104 and 133 during periods of high nitrogen retention.

Renal Clearance Tests and Phenolsulfonphthalein Excretion

The results of renal clearance and phenolsulfonphthalein excretion tests in patients with recovery diuresis were discussed in Chapter III. Briefly, in three such patients in whom clearance measurements were made, all functional components of the kidney were diminished when first observed and gradually returned toward normal over a period of several days or weeks. Similar evidence of functional impairment and subsequent improvement was seen in three additional patients with recovery diuresis on whom phenolsulfonphthalein excretory capacity tests were made.

Summary—Recovery Diuresis

Of the 23 patients with posttraumatic renal insufficiency who lived, 10 exhibited certain features which conform to the syndrome designated as recovery

TABLE 79.—RELATIONSHIP OF 24-HOUR URINALYSES AND PLASMA BIOCHEMIC FINDINGS IN A PATIENT WITH RECOVERY DIURESIS (CASE 133)

Postoperative Days	Fluid Intake cc.	Par-enteral NaCl Intake Gm.	Urine Output cc.	Blood pH (venous)	Plasma CO_2 Combining Power mEq./L.	Urine pH	Urine Titratable Acidity cc. 0.1 N	Urine Ammonia cc. 0.1 N	Urine Ammonia / Titratable Acidity
Fourth	2,500	17	?	...	...	...	...	...	...
Fifth	4,870	25.5	1,600	...	...	...	...	...	...
Sixth	7,000	25.5	1,450	...	...	...	...	...	...
Seventh	4,400	8.5	2,000	...	...	...	...	...	...
Eighth	3,900	8.5	2,950	...	...	...	...	...	...
Ninth	4,395	8.5	3,000	...	...	...	...	...	...
Tenth	3,150	8.5	1,270	7.32	21	...	...	...	...
Eleventh	2,810	8.5	2,650	...	...	5.7	375	377	1.0
Twelfth	3,570	8.5	2,380	...	20	...	...	...	...
Thirteenth	3,110	0	2,030	...	21	5.6	383	244	0.7
Fourteenth	2,540	...	2,150	...	20	...	...	...	...
Fifteenth	3,700	...	2,220	...	20	6.1	461	528	1.1
Sixteenth	3,350	...	2,300	...	21	6.8	242	306	1.3
Seventeenth	4,350	...	2,375	...	...	8.4	...	...	...
Eighteenth	4,400	...	2,610	...	20	8.4	...	...	...
Nineteenth	5,300	...	2,550	...	...	8.4	...	...	...
Twentieth	5,900	...	3,500	...	16	...	...	...	...

TABLE 79.—RELATIONSHIP OF 24-HOUR URINALYSES AND PLASMA BIOCHEMIC FINDINGS IN A PATIENT WITH RECOVERY DIURESIS (CASE 133)—*Continued*

Postoperative Days	Urine Chloride *Gm. NaCl*	Plasma Chloride *mEq./L.*	Serum Sodium *mEq./L.*	Plasma NPN *mg. per 100 cc.*	Plasma Urea Nitrogen *mg. per 100 cc.*	Urine Urea Nitrogen *Gm.*	Plasma Creat-inine *mg. per 100 cc.*	Urine Creat-inine *Gm.*	Urine Specific Gravity
Tenth	....	134	155	108	....	....	4.34	....	....
Eleventh	6.7	....	....	....	....	19.8	....	1.75	1.014
Twelfth	....	140	170	112	92	....	4.87	....	....
Thirteenth	4.6	144	....	106	92	19.2	4.08	1.58	1.015
Fourteenth	4.6	140	178	101	81	....	3.96	1.73	1.015
Fifteenth	3.6	142	180	100	80	14.5	3.96	1.73	1.015
Sixteenth	5.4	141	....	111	86	18.1	3.84	1.32	1.015
Seventeenth	0.12	....	....	....	....	18.3	....	1.32	1.016
Eighteenth	0.13	129	173	102	76	16.5	2.86	1.73	1.017
Nineteenth	0.51	....	....	....	....	11.9	....	1.39	1.018
Twentieth	0.70	119	....	97	....	....	2.37	....	1.016

956507 O—52——13

diuresis; namely, (1) nonprotein nitrogen greater than 100 mg. per 100 cc., (2) oliguria or anuria followed by diuresis and fall in nonprotein nitrogen, (3) low and fixed urinary specific gravity, and (4) hypertension. Their clinical course and physiologic and biochemic changes were entirely similar to those demonstrated in patients who died and were found at necropsy to have had lower nephron nephrosis. This group of patients demonstrates, then, that recovery from this type of renal disease can occur spontaneously if the patient survives the first critical 10 days after onset of renal failure.

SUMMARY

In earlier chapters the changes that began to occur in the internal environment soon after a man had been wounded were described. The effects of these early changes upon the kidney have been reported in this and the preceding chapter. Following severe trauma, accompanied usually by shock, a man could be adequately resuscitated and successfully operated upon. The latent renal incompetency which might develop in this man, who had normal kidneys at the time he was wounded, usually did not become manifest until two or three days later. At this time there appeared signs of failure on the part of the kidneys to withstand the initial insult, the effects of which his body had thus far resisted with fair success.

The first clinical sign of impending renal failure usually was suppression of urinary output. Of 73 patients with "high azotemia" (a plasma nonprotein nitrogen concentration of 65 mg. per 100 cc. or higher at some time during their course), 27 had anuria (urinary output of less than 100 cc. in any 24-hour period) and 29 had oliguria (output of from 100 to 600 cc. in a 24-hour period).

The case fatality rate was high. Fifty patients (69 percent) of the 73 with high azotemia died. Twenty-one (47 percent) of 45 who had oliguria, and 30 (91 percent) of 33 with anuria had a fatal outcome.

Initial shock—if special types of cases such as crush injuries, reaction to incompatible blood transfusion, and sulfathiazole crystalluria are excluded—was observed in a large proportion of the cases. Eighty-two percent of those who had high azotemia, and, in another category, 73 percent of those who had oliguria and 69 percent of those who had anuria had been in moderate or severe initial shock. These figures are undoubtedly too low, for many men probably had been in shock before we saw them.

Death occurred within 10 days after wounding in 48 (94 percent) of 51 patients who died of posttraumatic renal insufficiency. Apparently if the wounded man can withstand this critical 10-day period, recovery of renal function begins and he may survive. In a few patients there was evidence of returning renal function toward the end of their course, even though they died in uremia. The importance of this fact cannot be overemphasized, for a therapeutic error (such as overloading the circulatory system by fluid administration) during this critical period may cause a fatal outcome before natural recovery can take place.

Hypertension (at least 135 mm. Hg systolic and at least 90 mm. Hg diastolic) occurred in 62 percent of the patients with high azotemia, and in 79 percent of those in this group who died in uremia. In many of the fatal cases in which hypertension did not develop, death occurred within 4 days after wounding. Had these patients survived longer, probably they too would have had hypertension.

The important biochemic and physiologic abnormalities in the blood resulting from posttraumatic renal insufficiency were found to be nitrogen and phosphorus retention, acidosis, hypochloremia, and increase in the plasma volume. These blood and plasma changes reflect rapidly diminishing renal function, as indicated by: (1) inability to concentrate the urine; (2) frequent failure to make a highly acid or alkaline urine in the presence of metabolic acidosis or alkalosis; (3) diminished glomerular filtration rate and renal blood flow, and (4) decreased phenolsulfonphthalein and maximum tubular excretory capacity of para-amino hippuric acid.

Nonprotein nitrogen, urea nitrogen, creatinine, uric acid, and phosphorus levels in the plasma rose as renal failure progressed during the first 10 days after wounding. Most observations after this period were on patients who recovered. The level of these waste products fell between the tenth and fifteenth days.

A progressive, fairly severe acidosis was characteristic, manifested by falling plasma carbon-dioxide combining power as renal failure advanced. Loss of ability to make a highly acid urine in most cases suggests that the acidosis was partially to be explained by impairment of the mechanism which produces an acid urine. A few observations also indicated, as expected, an impairment of ammonia production by the renal tubules. There was also good evidence that removal of sodium by excretion as sodium bicarbonate was poorly accomplished in those cases in which alkalosis resulted from administration of large quantities of sodium.

Hypochloremia was severe and progressive, if all fatal cases are averaged. Correlation of the plasma chloride level and sodium chloride intake, however, demonstrated that the low chlorides were to some degree a result of inadequate salt intake. Serum sodium levels showed similar correlation. There was no difference in case fatality between the group with hypochloremia and those with normal plasma chloride levels. One patient with renal failure had severe sodium and chloride retention following a high salt intake. Intake, however, does not entirely explain variations in plasma chloride levels. No correlation with degree of plasma volume increase was apparent, but it is suggested that some interference with water and sodium chloride equilibrium was present in addition to the demonstrated relation to intake.

Phosphates in terms of acid equivalence, contributed toward but did not entirely account for the acidosis. Plasma proteins, if converted to milliequivalents, were normal and constant. Sulfates and organic acids were not measured and possibly account for discrepancies in our anion determinations.

Cation determinations were few. It has already been stated that sodium levels were partially correlated with salt intake. Magnesium was not significantly elevated in most cases. Potassium was determined in only a few cases, but the results suggest that hyperpotassemia was probably a feature of the syndrome. Calcium followed a reciprocal relationship with rising phosphorus levels in the few cases in which such determinations were made.

Total plasma volume was significantly elevated in 22 of 23 patients with posttraumatic renal insufficiency. Nineteen of these 23 died. Three patients with severe renal failure in whom a recovery diuresis developed had plasma volume increases that reached a maximum at the time of greatest nitrogen retention and decreased after diuresis. The degree of increase of the plasma volume was clearly related to fluid intake. The water retention appeared to be largely a result of administration of more fluid than the impaired kidneys could excrete. Comparison of plasma volume with total blood volume indicated that it was the plasma which was increased, rather than all elements of the blood. The expected dilution of plasma proteins was not demonstrated in most cases. The practical importance of this increase in plasma volume has been mentioned.

Ability to concentrate the urine diminished rapidly as the syndrome of posttraumatic renal insufficiency progressed, and specific gravity became fixed in all patients with a severe degree of renal failure. In patients who recovered it was the last of the kidney functions of those measured to return to normal. Since urine concentration is accomplished by the distal tubular cells, whereas mannitol, para-amino hippuric acid, and phenolsulfonphthalein reflect glomerular and proximal tubular function, the lag in recovery of water-reabsorptive capacity may point to greater relative functional impairment of the lower nephron.

Ten patients of the 73 who had high azotemia exhibited all of the features of severe renal failure and subsequently a diuresis developed and they recovered. The course of these patients followed a pattern which has been termed the "syndrome of recovery diuresis." This small group re-emphasizes the importance of avoiding early fatal therapeutic errors (such as overloading the circulatory system with fluid) thereby affording the kidneys an opportunity to recover spontaneously.

CHAPTER VI

Treatment of Lower Nephron Nephrosis

It should be stated at once that treatment of posttraumatic renal insufficiency after the syndrome has become established is disappointing although not hopeless. Evidence has been presented that shock is one factor important in its etiology. As soon as the patient becomes available for treatment, the shock state can usually be corrected fairly rapidly. Primary treatment of the wounded should therefore be directed toward prompt and adequate resuscitation of every man in shock in order to prevent, if possible, development of serious renal insufficiency.

In presenting our experience in the management of patients with posttraumatic renal insufficiency, certain therapeutic errors to be avoided will be stressed and the use of various drugs and procedures to stimulate renal function (most of which are of questionable value) will be discussed.

Fluid Intake

Early in the Italian campaign fatal cases of posttraumatic renal insufficiency began to appear. Therapy almost universally consisted of intravenous administration of large quantities of various crystalloids. Practically every known diuretic was also employed, and attempts were frequently made to alkalinize the urine by administering large quantities of available base by mouth or vein. In the absence of adequate output of urine, the renal insufficiency soon became complicated by cardiac failure as a result of overloading the circulatory system. The majority of patients so treated died rather promptly of pulmonary edema before they had an opportunity either to die in uremia or to regain adequate renal function.

Early in the course of our study it was found that those patients with renal insufficiency almost without exception had increased plasma volumes, as was shown in Chapter V. Here then was an additional explanation for the frequency of pulmonary edema; we were dealing with patients who, as a result of renal failure, already had a circulating plasma volume larger than normal. If additional fluids were added, especially those containing sodium, water retention became more severe. The frequency of pulmonary edema and cardiac failure is therefore not surprising. The therapeutic implications of these physiologic abnormalities are clear. Patients with this type of renal insufficiency already have too much extracellular fluid and too large a plasma volume, apparently primarily as a result of the kidney's being unable to excrete this surplus water. Treatment should therefore include (1) any judicious measures which might possibly encourage the kidneys to excrete more urine, and (2) avoidance of any measures which would further increase plasma volume and secondarily cause cardiac embarrassment.

As was shown in the previous chapter, the critical period in the majority of patients with renal insufficiency appeared to be the first 10 days after wounding, when 94 percent of the total deaths occurred. Evidence has been presented that renal function had begun to improve after this time in a number of patients, even though they subsequently died in uremia. Thus the importance of preventing an early fatal outcome resulting from too enthusiastic fluid administration cannot be overemphasized. Unfortunately most of these patients eventually die in uremia regardless of treatment, but by *judicious* use of fluids they are at least allowed an opportunity to recover renal function spontaneously and their chance of survival is increased.

In cases in which fluids were restricted, the incidence of pulmonary edema was, in our considered judgment, materially lessened, even in those patients who subsequently died primarily of renal failure. A few who recovered (Cases 43, 44, and 138) might have died of heart failure if quantities of fluid comparable to those previously employed had been given.

Our recommendation on fluid intake for the average patient with oliguria or anuria is that ordinarily not more than from 500 to 1,000 cubic centimeters in excess of urinary output be given daily. The patients in this study were seen in the fall, winter, and spring months when the temperature in Northern Italy was such that extrarenal fluid losses were probably minimal. In hot weather or when sweating is excessive this allowance should probably be increased. If urinary output increases to more than 1 liter daily, it is suggested that intake of fluids parallel or slightly exceed output of urine until retained nitrogen is cleared. Oral fluids, whenever their use is feasible, are preferred to parenteral ones in order to avoid sudden augmentation of the already increased plasma volume. Such parenteral fluids as are used should be administered slowly, and the patient should be carefully observed for signs of pulmonary edema during infusion. For reasons to be mentioned later under *Hypertonic Solutions,* the preferred parenteral fluid is an isotonic solution of dextrose.[1]

We have too little data on sodium to compare the level of this cation in the serum with the sodium intake. Hence it cannot be stated whether hyponatremia accompanied the hypochloremia, and therefore whether serious sodium depletion ever occurred. It now appears that as a consequence of the practice of giving almost no salt parenterally, hypochloremia resulted in some patients, although the outcome in those with decreased plasma chlorides apparently was no different from that in patients with normal chlorides. In our opinion, once posttraumatic renal insufficiency has become established, the danger of producing further edema and circulatory failure exceeds the questionable benefit to be derived from continued attempts to replenish deficient sodium by administration of sodium salt. We would therefore now recommend that during the oliguric and anuric phase salt be given only in quantities sufficient to replace extrarenal salt losses and the small quantity lost in the urine. These combined losses can only be estimated; they probably would seldom exceed one or two grams of salt daily.

Procedures and Drugs Used to Stimulate Kidney Function

Our experience revealed no positive and sure measures capable of re-establishing kidney function after renal insufficiency had developed. The aim should always be to avoid measures that might be harmful during the period before

[1] Because of the water-retaining property of the cation in sodium chloride, we suggested that the largest portion of the parenteral fluids given consist of 5- or 10-percent dextrose in distilled water. However, only the 10-percent prepared solution was available during most of the period when these studies were being made. Although 5-percent dextrose can be made up by adding dextrose solution to distilled water, under field conditions and the pressure of work during combat this is troublesome and was not often done.

the kidneys spontaneously begin to clear retained waste products. Well-known methods of stimulating urine flow that were tried will be discussed briefly. It is evident from the results that they were of no value, or at best of questionable value.

Hypertonic Solutions

The advisability of giving hypertonic solutions parenterally in this syndrome is highly debatable. They exert, at least in the presence of normal renal function, a diuretic effect by (1) temporarily increasing plasma volume, and (2) by limiting tubular reabsorption of water due to the osmotic effect of increased concentration of solute in the distal tubules. It is clear that the first of these actions is undesirable, since the circulating plasma volume is already increased; the second is desirable if tubular reabsorption can be altered in the damaged kidney.

Hypertonic saline (10-percent) solution was used in only one patient—the only one in our series with a true transfusion incompatability (Case 9). There was no observed effect on urinary output. It might be argued that early trial of such a solution would be of value in this type of renal insufficiency. If there is no response to 500 cc. of 3-percent saline solution, further attempts at diuresis by this method surely are contra-indicated because of the undesirable increase in plasma volume which must result from excessive salt administration.

Either a hypertonic dextrose solution or 5-percent dextrose in isotonic saline solution was the parenteral fluid most often given to the patients we observed. When solutions rendered hypertonic by sugar are employed, the osmotic effect on the plasma volume must be transient, lasting only until the dextrose is metabolized. The dextrose aids in nourishing patients who, as a rule, are eating poorly or not at all. The concentration of dextrose employed in hypertonic solution varied from 10 to 50 percent, but the 10-percent solution was the one most often used. There was little if any evidence from extensive use of these forms of hypertonic solutions that they influenced the output of urine.

In summary, since hypertonic solutions may dangerously increase plasma volume, and moreover since our data indicate they are ineffective in promoting urinary flow, isotonic solutions would seem to be preferable. If hypertonic solutions are employed, as they occasionally are in oliguria, dextrose is usually the one of choice; limited trial of hypertonic saline solution might be indicated in some cases.

Alcohol

The known diuretic effect of alcohol, and the suggestion that its administration might increase renal blood flow[2] prompted a rather extensive trial of this agent. It was given to 22 patients, 20 of whom subsequently died of renal insufficiency and 2 of whom survived through the mechanism of recovery diuresis. Usually it was given intravenously, slowly, as a 5-percent solution, the total daily dose being from 50 to 100 cc. of 95-percent ethyl alcohol. As an alternative, if the patient could tolerate it, from 120 to 180 cc. of whiskey were given by mouth daily. Of the 20 patients who died, 7 received approximately these doses for 1 day only, 9 for 3 to 4 days, and 4 for 5 to 8 days. Records are not available of the total quantities received by the 2 patients who recovered, but it is known that they received similar daily doses. No symptoms due to the alcohol, other than occasional mild euphoria and drowsiness, were observed in any patient.

In only 2 of the 20 patients who died (Cases 41 and 52) was there a significant increase in urinary output following the use of alcohol. The 2 patients who recovered had marked diuresis. Other patients showed no significant effects, although occasional transitory increases of as much as 300 cc. per day in urinary output were noted. Similar increases, however, occurred in patients with renal insufficiency who had not been given alcohol.

Mercurial Diuretics

Mercupurin, in doses of 1 or 2 cc., was given to three patients who subsequently died of renal failure. No diuretic effect was demonstrable.

Aminophylline

No demonstrable diuresis resulted from intravenous administration of 0.24 to 0.48 Gm. of this drug to four patients who later died of renal failure.

Inorganic Ions

The use of sodium chloride has been mentioned under "Fluid Intake" and *Hypertonic Solutions.*

[2] LAUSON, H. D.; BRADLEY, S. E. and COURNAND, A.: Renal circulation in shock. J. Clin. Investigation 23: 381–402, May 1944.

Sodium sulfate in isotonic (3.2 percent) or hypertonic (4.2 percent) solution was given to two patients in total doses of 800 cc. and 1,000 cc. respectively. Neither any beneficial nor harmful effects were observed. Both patients subsequently died in renal failure.

Magnesium sulfate and potassium chloride were employed on the theory that these solutions might be effective in reducing edema of renal tubular cells and hence perhaps promoting urinary flow. Magnesium sulfate was used in four patients (Cases 69, 78, 93, and 95). From 3 to 8 Gm. were given daily (as 50-percent solution intravenously and intramuscularly) for periods of from 2 to 5 days. Plasma magnesium levels, determined in two of these patients, were 7.0 milliequivalents per liter after 24 Gm. of magnesium sulfate had been administered in 4 days in one (Case 93), and 3.8 milliequivalents per liter after 8 Gm. had been given in 2 days in the other (Case 95). This second patient received in addition 10 Gm. of potassium chloride (as 0.5-percent solution intravenously) at about the same time. No increase in output of urine was demonstrated in these patients and all four died of typical renal failure.

Although no definite symptoms of toxicity due to these cations were demonstrable in these four patients, we believe that the use of magnesium and potassium in such cases is dangerous. In the presence of renal failure, administration of magnesium results in a rapid rise in the plasma concentration of this ion. The danger of reaching toxic levels, it is believed, outweighs any possible beneficial effects. We have no data on potassium levels reached in the one patient who received potassium chloride. However, because this ion likewise exerts toxic effects, in our opinion it should not be used in such cases unless serum potassium levels are known to be normal or low. There is some evidence in the literature to support the contention that retained potassium may play a lethal role in uremia.[3]

Alkalis

The effect of alkalis in wounded patients will be discussed in detail in Chapter VII. Alkalis were given, usually in small doses, to many of the patients after renal insufficiency had developed. Eleven patients who later died of uremia were given between 10 and 20 Gm. of sodium bicarbonate per day for 2 or more days, yet in only two of these patients was an alkaline urine observed. The

[3] Hoff, H. E.; Smith, P. K., and Winkler, A. W.: Cause of death in experimental anuria. J. Clin. Investigation **20**: 607–624, November 1941.

dangers of adding sodium to the extracellular fluid have been discussed. Further, the main reason for giving it in renal insufficiency is to produce an alkaline urine, the therapeutic value of which is debatable. We found no evidence that the use of alkalis has any place in the therapy of established posttraumatic renal insufficiency; in fact it may cause further harm.

Spinal Anesthesia

For many years, whenever anuria developed, it had been customary to suggest that spinal anesthesia be induced in the belief that the kidney failure might perhaps be accounted for, at least in part, by reflex vascular spasm and that this could be interrupted by spinal anesthesia. The results on the whole have been discouraging. Recent information suggests that part of the innervation of the kidney may come from higher origins than was earlier supposed. For this reason, anesthesia to the level of the clavicle was planned. With sensory anesthesia to this level, it is probable that vasomotor anesthesia was higher than this, since it is produced by a lower concentration of procaine hydrochloride than is required for sensory anesthesia. Pertinent data from four cases[4] in this study in which this procedure was tried are summarized briefly as follows.

Case Summaries

1. (*Case 47*)—In 22 hours preceding high spinal anesthesia this patient had voided 30 cc. of urine. The bladder was empty at the time anesthesia was induced.

0800 hours—Blood pressure 128/90.
0820 " —175 mg. procaine hydrochloride in 4 cc. spinal fluid were injected into the third lumbar interspace. Height achieved by barbotage.
0830 " —Blood pressure 135/88.
0835 " —Blood pressure 118/80.
0843 " —Blood pressure 120/80.
0830 " —Sensory anesthesia (pinprick) was present to the top of the second rib at the sternum.
0850 " —Blood pressure 112/80.
0915 " —Blood pressure 118/80. Sensory anesthesia persisted at the same level as at 0830.
0925 " —Blood pressure 118/80.
0945 " —Sensory anesthesia was beginning to wear off. There was no respiratory impairment at any time.

[4] Capt. Gerald Shortz of the 2d Auxiliary Surgical Group carried out the spinal anesthesias on three of these patients.

The patient was catheterized 5½ hours after the spinal anesthesia had been induced. The bladder was still empty. *Conclusion:* The anesthesia had no diuretic effect.

2. (*Case 95*)—The details concerning this case are similar to those of Case 47, except that in this one anesthesia was obtained to about the nipple line, where it persisted for 70 minutes. The blood pressure did not fall during the period of anesthesia. Sixty-five cc. of urine were present in the bladder just before induction of anesthesia. In the 24 hours following induction of anesthesia there was no formation of urine; this was checked by catheter.

3. (*Case 135*)—In 8 hours preceding spinal anesthesia 65 cc. of urine had formed and were obtained by catheter just before anesthetization.

1410 hours—180 mg. procaine hydrochloride in 10 cc. of spinal fluid were injected into the third lumbar interspace.
1415 " —Anesthesia was present to the eighth cervical vertebra.
1430 " —Anesthesia was present to the fourth thoracic vertebra.
1500 " —Anesthesia was present to the seventh thoracic vertebra.
1515 " —Anesthesia was present to the ninth thoracic vertebra.
1535 " —Anesthesia was present to the second lumbar vertebra.
1600 " —Anesthesia of the saddle area and legs only.
1630 " —Full recovery.
2015 " —85 cc. of urine were obtained by catheterization.

There was no fall of blood pressure during this test. Since 65 cc. of urine had been formed in 8 hours preceding anesthesia, and 85 cc. in 6 hours following, no definite effect could be attributed to the anesthesia.

4. (*Case 138*)—In 11 hours preceding spinal anesthesia, 40 cc. of urine had been formed. The bladder was emptied of this just before anesthesia was induced. The blood pressure remained at 120/72 throughout the test.

1500 hours—200 mg. procaine hydrochloride were dissolved in 12 cc. of spinal fluid and injected into the third lumbar interspace.
1505 " —Anesthesia was present to the eighth cervical vertebra.
1515 " —Anesthesia was present to the fifth thoracic vertebra.
1535 " —Anesthesia was present to the second lumbar vertebra.
1600 " —Saddle and leg anesthesia only.
1650 " —Complete recovery.
2100 " —60 cc. of urine were obtained by catheterization.

Sixty cc. of urine were excreted in 6 hours following induction of anesthesia and 40 cc. had been formed in 11 hours preceding anesthesia; hence no definite effect of the spinal anesthesia was evident. The patient's low point in output was 2 days preceding the anesthesia; in other words, a steady increase in urinary output had already begun. This patient was the only one of this group who recovered. One cannot say that the spinal anesthesia either did or did not play a part in his recovery.

No definite evidence was obtained from the four patients studied that spinal anesthesia influenced the output of urine. We had planned to try this procedure earlier, that is, soon after the onset of progressive oliguria. These plans were interrupted by the end of the war in Italy.

Kidney Decapsulation, Sympathectomy

This was carried out in one patient (Case 129) 54 hours after initial operation, during which time the patient had voided 150 cc. of urine. The right kidney was decapsulated and a periarterial sympathectomy performed. There was no effect on urinary output, and the patient died in uremia 48 hours later, having excreted 180 cc. of urine since the second operation.

Correction of Anemia

In instances in which whole blood transfusions were indicated for the correction of severe anemia, these were given. Relatively fresh bank blood was used to avoid possible pigment insult secondary to intravascular hemolysis of aged cells. No benefit or detriment to the already failing kidney was observed.

Nutrition

Ideally, nutritive requirements during the acute phase of the syndrome should be met by an adequate caloric intake, but with such foods that there will be minimal destruction of body protein and production of urea nitrogen from exogenous proteins. These demands would best be served by a carbohydrate and fat intake sufficient to furnish from 1,500 to 2,000 calories per day. If the patient is unable to take food by mouth, it is practically impossible to administer enough dextrose intravenously to furnish such a caloric intake and still adhere to the more important rules of restricting fluids and prohibiting hypertonic solutions. During the acute phase of renal insufficiency one must be content with merely furnishing the small requirement of sodium chloride as isotonic saline solution, and with an attempt to meet caloric requirements by supplying dextrose in a 5-percent solution in water in the additional small fluid allowance remaining—that is, a total daily intake of 500 to 1,000 cc. in excess of total urinary output.

SUMMARY

Various procedures were tried in the treatment of lower nephron nephrosis which occurred as a complication in severely wounded men. Among these were control of fluid intake, the use of relatively fresh blood for transfusions to combat anemia, attempts to make the urine alkaline, spinal anesthesia, kidney decapsulation, and the administration of a number of drugs commonly believed to stimulate the excretion of urine. Except for evidence that avoiding excess fluid administration reduced the incidence of early death from pulmonary edema, all were essentially disappointing, leading to the conclusion that "the best treatment of posttraumatic renal insufficiency is its prevention." Since shock is known to be a major factor in its development, prompt and adequate resuscitation of every man in shock is most important.

Once renal insufficiency has developed, avoidance of the therapeutic error of administering too much fluid and hence accentuating an already increased plasma volume becomes of first importance. Types and quantities of fluids to be administered during the period when renal failure is most severe (usually the first 10 days after trauma) have been recommended. Although we employed various drugs or procedures directed toward promoting urine flow or improving kidney function, we met with little success in their use. These measures included the use of hypertonic solutions, alcohol, mercurial and xanthine diuretics, and solutions of various inorganic ions, the induction of spinal anesthesia, and decapsulation of a kidney. The essential requirement appears to be that of tiding the patient over the critical period until natural recovery of renal function begins. Dialysis procedures, which attempt to remove waste products by routes other than the kidneys until the kidneys resume their function, offer possibilities that were not tried in this study.

CASES OF SPECIAL INTEREST IN THIS CHAPTER

9	43	47	69	93	129	138
41	44	52	78	95	135	

CHAPTER VII

Effect of Alkalis in Treatment of Traumatic Shock

The use of alkalis has been recommended by some as an adjunct in the treatment of the severely wounded for two reasons. First, it was proposed as a means of combatting the acidosis known to exist in shock; second, it was suggested that production of an alkaline urine might make more soluble any blood or muscle pigments or sulfonamide crystals in the urine. Evidence will be presented here that with judicious use of alkalis it is possible to relieve metabolic acidosis, but that in the presence of shock and the accompanying decrease in renal function, it may be very difficult and even dangerous to attempt to produce an alkaline urine.

Any patient who receives whole blood or blood substitutes of necessity also gets sodium citrate which is employed as an anticoagulant when the blood is collected from the donor. Although the quantity varies slightly, we have assumed that each unit* of blood or plasma contained 2 Gm. of U.S.P. sodium citrate. The quantity of alkali received by a patient transfused with several liters of blood or plasma was therefore considerable. In the patients we observed, any additional alkali given was usually in the form of a 2-percent solution of sodium bicarbonate. This was prepared by adding sodium bicarbonate to distilled water shortly after the water was removed from the autoclave. Although some sodium carbonate undoubtedly resulted from this procedure, no untoward reactions were encountered in a large series of patients to whom this solution was given intravenously. Sodium citrate, 4 or 2.5 percent, in sterile ampules, was also employed in a few instances. The sodium administered in excess of that given as sodium chloride was calculated from the quantity present in sodium citrate or sodium bicarbonate. This figure furnished a convenient index of the total alkali

* 1 unit of blood = 500 cc.; 1 unit of plasma = 300 cc. total volume.

received, since both sodium citrate and sodium bicarbonate were frequently administered.

In Table 80 the effect of increasing quantities of alkali in relation to the degree of initial shock is shown. Those patients who received between 1 and 5 Gm. of sodium (approximately from 5 to 20 Gm. of sodium bicarbonate or sodium citrate) still had an acid urine after 20 to 30 hours, and they showed no remarkable rise in plasma carbon-dioxide combining power. In those who received between 5.1 and 10 Gm. of sodium the urine became alkaline only if they had had little or no initial shock. There was a significant change in preoperative and postoperative plasma carbon-dioxide combining power only in those who had had moderate or severe shock, but their urines remained acid.

Inspection of the data on individual patients (Table 80) who received between 10.1 and 20 Gm. of sodium shows that of six who had been in moderate or severe shock, only one was producing an alkaline urine 24 hours later and the remaining five still had acid urines 26 to 34 hours after wounding. The two patients with no shock and slight initial shock respectively both had highly alkaline urines. The plasma carbon-dioxide combining power rose significantly in five of seven patients on whom postoperative determinations were made.

These observations show rather clearly that in patients who have had severe or moderate shock, an alkaline urine is not usually produced even after administration of large quantities of alkali, although the metabolic acidosis may be relieved. The dangers of producing severe alkalosis in such patients, and a partial explanation of their inability to form an alkaline urine become apparent in Tables 81, 82, and 83, and Chart 28 which show the sequence of events in three patients with moderate or severe initial shock who received large quantities of alkali. The cases are summarized as follows:

Cases of Alkalosis

Case 108 (*Table 81*).—This patient, who had severe shock on hospital entry, received 34 Gm. of sodium bicarbonate and 24 Gm. of sodium citrate within the first 24 hours after admission. The plasma carbon-dioxide combining power responded to this excess alkali by rapidly rising to 34 milliequivalents per liter, but despite this relative alkalosis the urine did not become alkaline until the third postoperative day. The plasma chloride level fell although scarcely any chloride was excreted in the urine. Coincident with these changes in acid-base metabolism, the output of urine was very small, the specific gravity of the urine fell, the plasma nonprotein level rose, and the urea nitrogen excretion was minimal. The patient died in uremia on the third postoperative day.

956507 O—52——14

TABLE 80.—RELATIONSHIP OF SODIUM INTAKE AND DEGREE OF INITIAL SHOCK TO PLASMA CARBON-DIOXIDE COMBINING POWER AND pH OF URINE

Excess Sodium Intake Gm.	Degree of Shock on Admission	Preoperative Specimen		Postoperative Specimen			
		Plasma CO_2 *mEq./L.*	Urine pH	Plasma CO_2 *mEq./L.*	Hours after Wounding	Urine pH	Hours after Wounding
1.0 to 5.0 (Average of cases)	None or slight	24.0±1.3 (6 cases)	5.9 (4 cases)	31.0 (2 cases)	21.5 (2 cases)	6.8±0.24 (7 cases)	26.4±4.4 (7 cases)
	Moderate or severe	24.2±1.4 (9 cases)	5.7 (2 cases)	26.0±2.1 (7 cases)	32±3.8 (7 cases)	6.2±0.13 (10 cases)	31.7±4.0 (10 cases)
5.1 to 10.0 (Average of cases)	None or slight	24.0±1.7 (6 cases)	5.6 (3 cases)	24.0±1.8 (6 cases)	27.5±3.5 (6 cases)	7.2±0.22 (9 cases)	25.8±3.1 (9 cases)
	Moderate or severe	21.3±1.7 (12 cases)	5.9 (4 cases)	25.5±1.8 (8 cases)	25.1±1.6 (8 cases)	6.1±0.12 (14 cases)	24.1±1.6 (14 cases)
10.1 to 15.0 (Individual cases)	None or slight	25	....	26	29	7.4	29
		26	5.8	33	17	8.0	15
	Moderate or severe	19	5.9	25	34	6.7	34
		11	....	25	39	5.6	33
		23	5.6	....	....	6.7	33
		22	5.5	34	35	5.4	28
15.1 to 20.0 (Individual cases)	Moderate or severe	15	6.1	33	26	5.5	26
		26	....	26	24	8.1	24

The preoperative specimens were taken when no alkali, or very small quantities, had been given; the postoperative specimens after the patients had received the amount of alkali indicated under "Excess Sodium Intake." The time between wounding and collection of the postoperative specimens is also indicated. Enough patients received between 1 and 10 Gm. of sodium to permit statistical analysis; determinations are listed individually for those who received between 10.1 and 20 grams. The excess sodium intake in grams was calculated from the percentage of sodium in sodium citrate or sodium bicarbonate. Sodium administered in isotonic saline solution is not included in the data.

TABLE 81.—CHANGES IN ACID-BASE METABOLISM AND COINCIDENT FINDINGS IN A PATIENT WHO RECEIVED EXCESS ALKALI

Severe Initial Shock and Subsequent Death from Posttraumatic Renal Insufficiency

Case 108

Period	Parenteral Intake		Plasma CO_2	Plasma Cl	Urine pH	Urine NaCl
	Na *mEq.*	Cl *mEq.*	*mEq./L.*	*mEq./L.*		*Gm.*
Preoperative . . . . . . (18-hr. period)	811	300	22	100	5.5	0.04
Postoperative Day						
First	417	300	34	97	5.4	0.26
Second	115	75	30	96	5.4	——
Third	. . . . .	. . . . .	23	91	7.6	——

Period	Parenteral Intake		Plasma NPN	Urine Urea Nitrogen	Urine Specific Gravity	Urine Output
	Na *mEq.*	Cl *mEq.*	*mg. per 100 cc.*	*Gm.*		*cc.*
Preoperative . . . . . . (18-hr. period)	811	300	37	0.13	1.032	100
Postoperative Day						
First	417	300	77	0.54	1.014	185
Second	115	75	113	. . . . .	1.012	155
Third	. . . . .	. . . . .	170	. . . . .	. . . . .	——

Case 112 (*Table 82*).—Twenty Gm. of sodium bicarbonate and 16 Gm. of sodium citrate were administered within 6 hours after this patient entered the hospital in severe shock. The pH of the venous blood and the plasma carbon-dioxide combining power promptly rose to levels indicative of moderate alkalosis, but the urine did not become alkaline until nearly 24 hours after the alkali had been administered. Although urinary output was normal after the first day, the plasma nonprotein nitrogen level had risen to 67 mg. per 100 cc. by the second postoperative day, when the patient was evacuated. Plasma chloride levels fell and chloride excretion was low. Subsequent follow-up revealed that nitrogen retention persisted for 6 days; the status of the acid-base metabolism could not be followed.

Case 107 (*Table 83 and Chart 28*).—This patient, admitted in moderate shock, received 35 Gm. of sodium bicarbonate and 28 Gm. of sodium citrate on the day of operation, and 15 additional grams of sodium bicarbonate early on the first postoperative day. The resulting severe and prolonged alkalosis is evident in the high plasma carbon-dioxide combining

TABLE 82.—CHANGES IN ACID-BASE METABOLISM AND COINCIDENT FINDINGS IN A PATIENT WHO RECEIVED EXCESS ALKALI

Severe Initial Shock, Subsequent Nitrogen Retention, and Recovery

Case 112

Period	Parenteral Intake		Blood pH (venous)	Plasma CO_2	Plasma Cl	Urine pH	Urine NaCl	Plasma NPN	Urine Specific Gravity	Urine Output
	Na *mEq.*	Cl *mEq.*		*mEq./L.*	*mEq./L.*		*Gm.*	*mg. per 100 cc.*		*cc.*
Preoperative . . . (21.5-hr. period)	400	0	7.04 to 7.45	20 to 30	99	5.4 to 6.5	....	40	1.025	530
Postoperative Day										
First	0	0	7.45	32	86	7.1	0.43	53	1.010	2,180
Second	0	0	....	36	87	7.2	1.4	67	1.010	1,945
Sixth	....	....	....	....	....	....	....	57	....	....
Twelfth	....	....	....	....	....	....	....	34	....	....

TABLE 83.—CHANGES IN ACID-BASE METABOLISM AND COINCIDENT FINDINGS IN A PATIENT WHO RECEIVED EXCESS ALKALI

Postoperative Alkalosis and Azotemia, Resulting in Death

Case 107

Period	Parenteral Intake		Blood pH (venous)	Serum Na	Plasma CO_2	Plasma Cl	Urine pH	Urine NaCl	Plasma NPN	Urine Output
	Na *mEq.*	Cl *mEq.*		*mEq./L.* (n:142)	*mEq./L.* (n:27)	*mEq./L.* (n:103)	(n:7.38-7.48)	*Gm.*	*mg. per 100 cc.*	*cc.*
Preoperative. . . (18-hr. period)	681	0	....	....	15	103	6.1	....	27	60
Postoperative Day										
First.	324	146	....	160	30.2	100	5.5 to 7.3	0.3	41	1,560
Second	0	0	7.44	170	41	91	8.2	0.23	46	1,570
Third	146	146	....	....	....	....	7.7	0.80	....	1,540
Fourth.	332	482	7.48	160	47	73	6.8	....	91	875
Fifth	0	245	7.52	140	43	65	5.8	0.0	73	800
Sixth	60	0	....	....	37	56	7.3	....	152	200(?)

power and blood pH. Considerable ammonium chloride was given on the fourth and fifth postoperative days in an unsuccessful attempt to relieve the alkalosis. In this case also there was a marked lag in the production of an alkaline urine after metabolic alkalosis appeared. By the fourth postoperative day, although severe alkalosis persisted, the patient was no longer able to excrete an alkaline urine. Plasma chlorides fell to phenomenally low levels

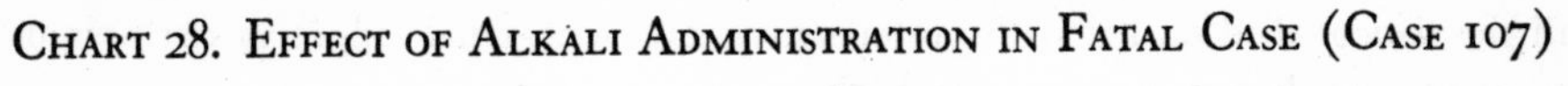

Chart 28. Effect of Alkali Administration in Fatal Case (Case 107)

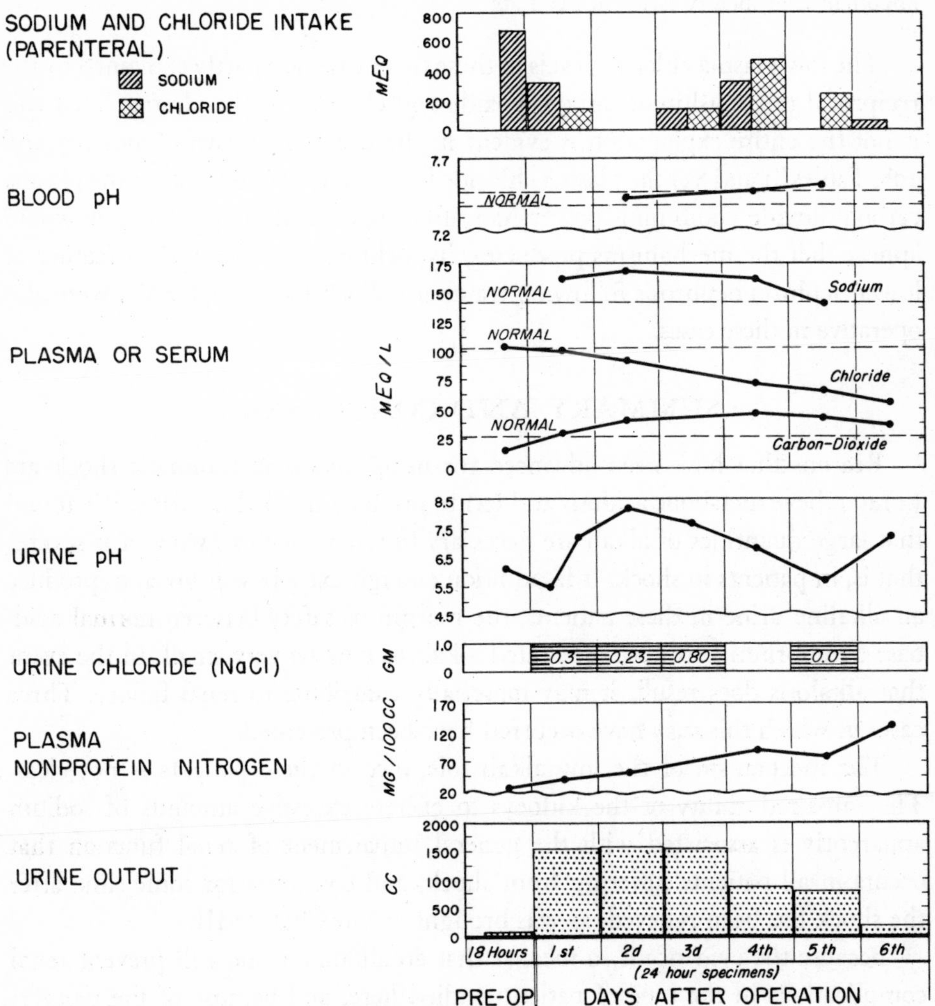

NOTE: (1) The lag in development of an alkaline urine in the presence of alkalosis and sodium retention, and presumptive evidence of inability to excrete excess sodium, as indicated by a fall in the pH of the urine after the second postoperative day; (2) the low plasma chloride levels and negligible urinary chloride excretion; (3) a rising plasma nonprotein nitrogen level and decreasing urinary output, and (4) the fixed specific gravity of the urine.

in this patient (56 milliequivalents per liter the day before death); urinary chloride excretion was practically nil throughout his course. The plasma nonprotein nitrogen level rose, and the patient died on the sixth postoperative day, with renal failure in our opinion an important contributory factor in his death.

The low plasma chloride levels in these three cases are partly explained by the reciprocal relationship of carbon dioxide and chloride in the plasma. That this is not the entire explanation is evident in the fact that in two (Cases 107 and 108, Tables 81 and 83) the plasma chloride level continued to fall after the plasma carbon-dioxide combining power had also begun to decline. Hence it would appear that the mechanisms producing hypochloremia, frequently a feature of lower nephron nephrosis following traumatic shock (see Chapter V), were also operative in these cases.

SUMMARY AND CONCLUSIONS

Reasons that have been advanced for using alkalis in traumatic shock are (1) to relieve metabolic acidosis and (2) to produce an alkaline urine. We found that large quantities of alkali are necessary to relieve acidosis when it is severe; that is, in patients in shock. If in addition enough extra base is given to produce an alkaline urine in these patients, the margin of safety between normal acid-base equilibrium and uncompensated alkalosis may be very small. In the event that alkalosis does result, it may materially contribute to renal failure. Three cases in which this may have occurred have been presented.

The mechanism of the low alkali tolerance in these patients is not clear. The impaired ability of the kidneys to excrete excessive amounts of sodium apparently is associated with the general impairment of renal function that occurs in all patients suffering from shock, and continues for some time after the shock has been relieved, as was brought out in Chapter III.

Because the evidence is so meager that an alkaline urine will prevent renal complications in the type of patient studied here, and because of the dangers inherent in trying to produce such a urine, the use of alkalis for this purpose is not recommended. Small quantities of alkali sufficient to relieve metabolic acidosis, if judiciously employed, probably are advisable. The amount routinely given with citrated whole blood or blood substitutes will in most instances be adequate for this purpose.

CHAPTER VIII

Pigment Mobilization in Severely Wounded Men

It was shown in Chapter IV that severely wounded men commonly excrete heme-containing pigments, either hemoglobin or myoglobin, in the urine and that such excretion was constantly observed in patients destined to develop the syndrome of posttraumatic renal insufficiency. In Chapter IX the significance of pigment excretion will be further emphasized by demonstrating that pigment precipitation in the lower segments of the nephrons was a constant feature of the renal lesion observed in fatal cases. The importance of pigment mobilization, its transport via the plasma to the kidneys, and its excretion in the urine was therefore obvious early in our investigations, and the present chapter will be devoted to presentation of the available data and discussion of their significance.

Materials and Methods

We were severely handicapped by the lack of a spectroscope of sufficient sensitivity to distinguish between the closely similar spectrums of hemoglobin and myoglobin, and even if a suitable instrument had been available it is doubtful if it could have been utilized under field conditions. We resorted therefore to use of the benzidine method, which gave a color reaction strong enough to read in a Coleman Junior spectrophotometer in a dilution of 1 milligram of benzidine-positive material per 100 cubic centimeters. The method did not, however, permit distinction between myoglobin and hemoglobin in plasma, so throughout this chapter the term "plasma hemoglobin" is used to indicate the total amount of benzidine-reacting material, though in many instances a significant proportion was undoubtedly myoglobin. A further small fraction of the total was probably contributed by nonspecific oxydases, but it is improbable that this was large enough to affect comparative results. Under these conditions, results of the test were always positive for "hemoglobin," ranging from 6 to 12 mg. per 100 cc. in the majority of initial samples and also in samples procured during convalescence. We therefore considered values up to 12 mg. per 100 cc. as being within normal range.

In the urine it did prove possible to distinguish between the two pigments within certain limits by taking advantage of the greater stability of myoglobin in alkaline solutions. By cautiously alkalinizing the urine, hemoglobin could be converted to alkaline hematin and precipitated while the greater portion of the myoglobin remained in solution. Tests with known mixtures of the two pigments showed that the separation was approximately 80-percent effective, and analyses of normal and decolorized muscles from patients who died of the crush syndrome provided further confirmation of the validity of the method. When enough pigment for quantitative determination was present in a urine specimen, this method was applied. Values of "myoglobin" that were less than 20 percent of the hemoglobin present were considered negative; findings of 20 percent or more were recorded as myoglobin. Details of the methods used will be found in Appendix C.

Determinations of plasma "hemoglobin" and of urine hemoglobin and myoglobin were made routinely upon all patients in the series from whom suitable specimens could be obtained. In some instances high plasma values were undoubtedly due to hemolysis incurred in taking samples of blood. Great care was used in cleaning and drying needles and syringes and in the technique of venepuncture, but needles and syringes were not paraffinized. In certain patients injury to the kidney or other portion of the urinary tract resulted in gross hematuria, and urine hemoglobin levels in these cases were considered valueless; however, if myoglobin was discovered in such specimens, it was recorded.

Bank Blood

Since hemolysis is inevitable in stored blood, many samples of bank blood, taken at the time the blood was given out for transfusion to our patients, were analyzed. The plasma hemoglobin and the blood sugar levels were determined, the latter in order to check upon the effectiveness of added dextrose as a preservative. Confirmation of the serologic blood group of the bank blood was not attempted because the triple check used in the theater blood bank was as accurate as any method we could have tried. We did, however, take the precaution of checking the blood group of the recipient whenever possible since the "dog tags" were known to be approximately 8-percent erroneous, and since the grouping was often too difficult for hospital technicians because of the large quantities of group O blood that some patients had already received before the first test-specimen was obtained.

Few Rh factor determinations were made because very little typing serum was available. All patients, however, who were conscious at the time of observation were carefully questioned regarding previous transfusion and answers were uniformly negative. Previous sensitization was therefore improbable, and the short duration of the period of transfusion therapy—from 1 to 3 days—made active sensitization of no importance in our problem.

Specifications of Bank Blood.—Blood given to patients in this study was derived from the theater blood bank in all but two instances.[1] All bank blood was group O and the plasma agglutinins against A and B cells had been determined. If these were below 1:64, the blood was labeled *Universal Donor;* if above this level, *O-Blood, for Use in O-Recipients Only*. The blood had been drawn into sodium citrate, and dextrose had been added to give a concentration approximating 0.3 percent. Blood was stored at all times, including periods of transportation, in refrigerators at approximately 8° Centigrade. It was never used after the tenth day.

Analyses of Bank Blood.—Since all blood samples contain cells of varying maturity, progressive hemolysis is inevitable in all stored specimens. This is apparent in Chart 29 and Table 84 which show average plasma hemoglobin levels at the time of transfusion in 213 samples of blood from 2 to 10 days old. The rate compares favorably with Gibson's[2] figures based on storage in A-C-D solution. In occasional samples, usually those from 6 to 8 days old, considerable hemolysis was evidenced by plasma hemoglobin levels from 100 to 300 mg. per

[1] Case 9 was an example of a transfusion accident—A blood to an O recipient. The patient was seen in consultation at a neighboring hospital and was studied for comparison only. The second patient (Case 22) belonged to group A. He received three transfusions of bank blood in a forward hospital and subsequently was given 2 units of group A blood at a general hospital. He had already given evidence of renal insufficiency before the type-specific blood was administered.

[2] Gibson, J. G., 2nd; Evans, R. D.; Aub, J. C.; Sack, T., and Peacock, W. C.: The post-transfusion survival of preserved human erythrocytes stored as whole blood or in resuspension, after removal of plasma, by means of two isotopes of radioactive iron. J. Clin. Investigation **26**: 715–738, July 1947.

CHART 29. RELATIONSHIP BETWEEN FREE PLASMA HEMOGLOBIN AND AGE OF STORED BLOOD—213 SAMPLES

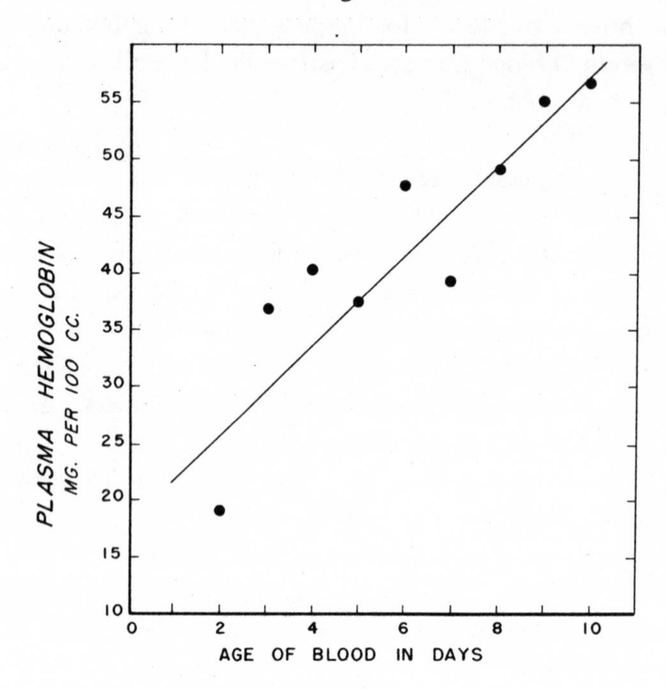

100 cc. (see Charts 30, 31, and 32). The average levels in samples from 5 to 8 days old, the age period of most of the blood used, were in the range from 38 to 50 milligrams per 100 cubic centimeters.

The possible effect of blood transfusions on the level of free hemoglobin in the blood plasma of the recipients is made readily apparent by a few simple calculations. Since the average amount of free hemoglobin in the bank blood at the time of transfusion was approximately 40 mg. per 100 cc., and 500 cc. of blood was the amount per unit, each patient receiving a unit of blood received at the time 200 mg. of free hemoglobin. Our patients received an average of 4.2 units of blood, or 840 mg. of hemoglobin, and in the fatal cases an average of 7.3 units, or 1,460 mg. of hemoglobin was given. Seven patients received from 10 to 14 units, or 2,000 to 2,800 mg. of free hemoglobin. Assuming an average blood volume to be 5,000 cc., such quantities of infused hemoglobin could have resulted in plasma levels of free hemoglobin in the patients of 16 to 58 mg.

per 100 cubic centimeters. It must not be forgotten, however, that these approximations are based on the assumption that all infused free hemoglobin would remain in the circulating plasma. This would certainly not be true, since in many patients significant quantities would be excreted in the urine and in all instances some would escape with the plasma into traumatized tissues.

TABLE 84.—RELATIONSHIP OF AVERAGE PLASMA HEMOGLOBIN LEVEL TO AGE OF STORED BLOOD—213 ANALYSES

Age of Stored Blood *days*	Number of Analyses	Mean Plasma Hemoglobin *mg. per 100 cc.*	Age of Stored Blood *days*	Number of Analyses	Mean Plasma Hemoglobin *mg. per 100 cc.*
2	2	19	7	56	39.6±5.8
3	15	36.7±6.6	8	39	49.5±10
4	10	40±6.5	9	6	55
5	30	38±8	10	3	57
6	52	47.4±8	Total	213	Av.: 43.4

Charts 30 through 33 show the relationship between hemolysis and sugar levels in the stored blood. It is evident that most instances of extreme hemolysis occurred in blood samples with low sugar levels. Table 85 and Chart 33 show average sugar levels in relationship to age of the blood. The chart shows that the sugar level was well maintained until the seventh day and dropped sharply thereafter.

TABLE 85.—RELATIONSHIP OF AVERAGE BLOOD SUGAR TO AGE OF STORED BLOOD—223 SAMPLES

Age of Stored Blood *days*	Number of Analyses	Mean Blood Sugar *mg. per 100 cc.*	Age of Stored Blood *days*	Number of Analyses	Mean Blood Sugar *mg. per 100 cc.*
2	2	256	7	60	289±17
3	15	295±33	8	40	266±25
4	11	276±59	9	6	211
5	31	326±34	10	3	160
6	55	290±21	Total	223	Av.: 286

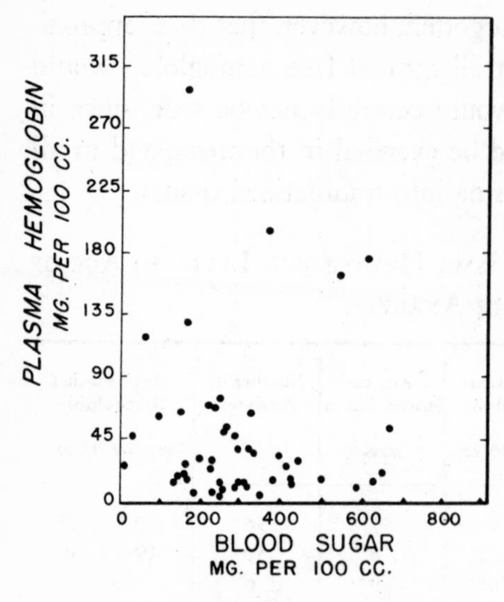

CHART 30. Relationship between Plasma Hemoglobin and Blood Sugar in Blood Stored 6 Days—52 Samples

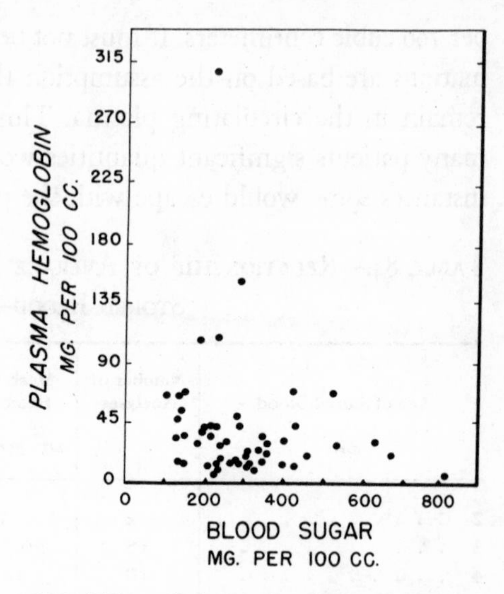

CHART 31. Relationship between Plasma Hemoglobin and Blood Sugar in Blood Stored 7 Days

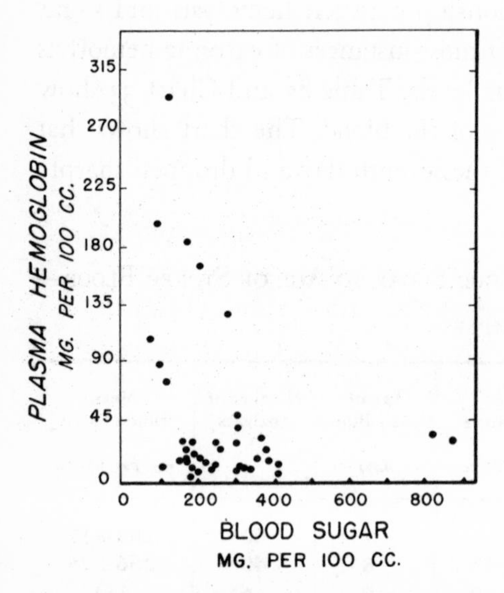

CHART 32. Relationship between Plasma Hemoglobin and Blood Sugar in Blood Stored 8 Days

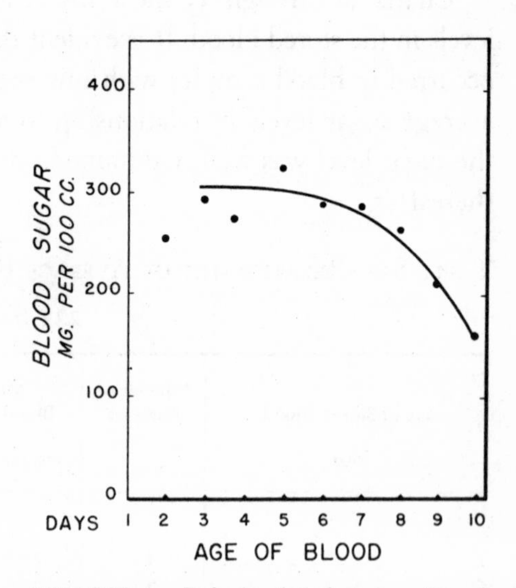

CHART 33. Relationship between Blood Sugar and Age of Stored Blood—223 Samples

Plasma "Hemoglobin" Levels in Wounded Men

The pattern of plasma "hemoglobin" (benzidine-reacting material) levels in severely traumatized men is shown in Charts 34 through 37. In Chart 34, based upon findings in 133 patients, the mean plasma hemoglobin level for each day after injury is plotted. From an initial figure of 10 mg. per 100 cc., it climbs in 72 hours to 17.3 mg., then slowly falls in the course of the next 13 days to a level of 3 mg. per 100 cc. of plasma. Chart 35 shows daily mean levels of 64 patients who had high azotemia, over half of whom died. The curve is essentially similar, though the peak is higher and is delayed 24 hours. In Chart 36 only the fatal cases with histologically proved pigment nephropathy are shown, exclusive of crush cases. In this group the peak is sharp and high, occurring at 24 hours and attaining a maximum of 36.8 mg. per 100 cubic centimeters. This figure is still far below the generally accepted threshold level of 135 mg. per 100 cc. at which a normal kidney begins to excrete hemoglobin.[3 4 5]

The plasma bilirubin level as determined by the van den Bergh diazo test has also been plotted on these charts, omitting cases of direct liver trauma. As would be expected, the bilirubin curve roughly paralleled that of hemoglobin but its peak occurred from 3 to 4 days later. Strict parallelism could not be expected since the bilirubin level is also affected by efficiency of liver function; evidence of liver injury in these patients is presented in Chapters II and XII.

In considering the significance of the plasma hemoglobin levels, two possible relationships at once come to mind: does the level depend upon the severity of shock? or upon the quantity of blood the patient was given? The answer is not obvious since the patients with the most severe shock usually received the most blood. Available evidence compiled from the first specimen of blood obtained for analysis is presented in Table 86. The following cases have been excluded: all crush cases, in which benzidine-reacting pigment in the plasma

[3] GILLIGAN, D. R., and BLUMGART, H. L.: March hemoglobinuria; studies of clinical characteristics, blood metabolism and mechanism, with observations on three new cases, and review of the literature. Medicine **20**: 341–395, September 1941.

[4] GILLIGAN, D. R.; ALTSCHULE, M. D., and KATERSKY, E. M.: Studies of hemoglobinemia and hemoglobinuria produced in man by intravenous injection of hemoglobin solutions. J. Clin. Investigation **20**: 177–187, March 1941.

[5] OTTENBERG, R., and FOX, C. L., JR.: Rate of removal of hemoglobin from circulation and its renal threshold in human beings. Am. J. Physiol. **123**: 516–525, August 1938.

TABLE 86.—MEAN PLASMA "HEMOGLOBIN" LEVELS IN RELATION TO SHOCK AND QUANTITY OF TRANSFUSED BLOOD—76 CASES

Quantity of Blood Received (units)	Plasma Hemoglobin Levels [1]					
	Blood Specimen Drawn Less than 24 Hours after Injury [2]			Blood Specimen Drawn 24–96 Hours after Injury [2]		
	Shock		Total Cases	Shock		Total Cases
	Minimal	Moderate-Severe		Minimal	Moderate-Severe	
None	12.4 (7 cases)	9.8 (7 cases)	11.1 (14 cases)	....	9.2 (5 cases)	9.2 (5 cases)
1 to 3	14.0 (2 cases)	8.7 (20 cases)	9.2 (22 cases)	16.0 (10 cases)	12.4 (3 cases)	15.1 (13 cases)
4 to 14	6.8 (2 cases)	7.9 (3 cases)	7.5 (5 cases)	....	20.5 (17 cases)	20.5 (17 cases)
Average	11.7 (11 cases)	8.8 (30 cases)	9.6 (41 cases)	16.0 (10 cases)	17.3 (25 cases)	16.9 (35 cases)

[1] Mg. of benzidine-reacting material per 100 cc. of plasma.
[2] Determinations based on first blood specimen obtained for this analysis.

CHART 34. AVERAGE LEVELS OF PLASMA "HEMOGLOBIN" AND BILIRUBIN RELATED TO TIME FROM WOUNDING IN 133 SEVERELY WOUNDED PATIENTS

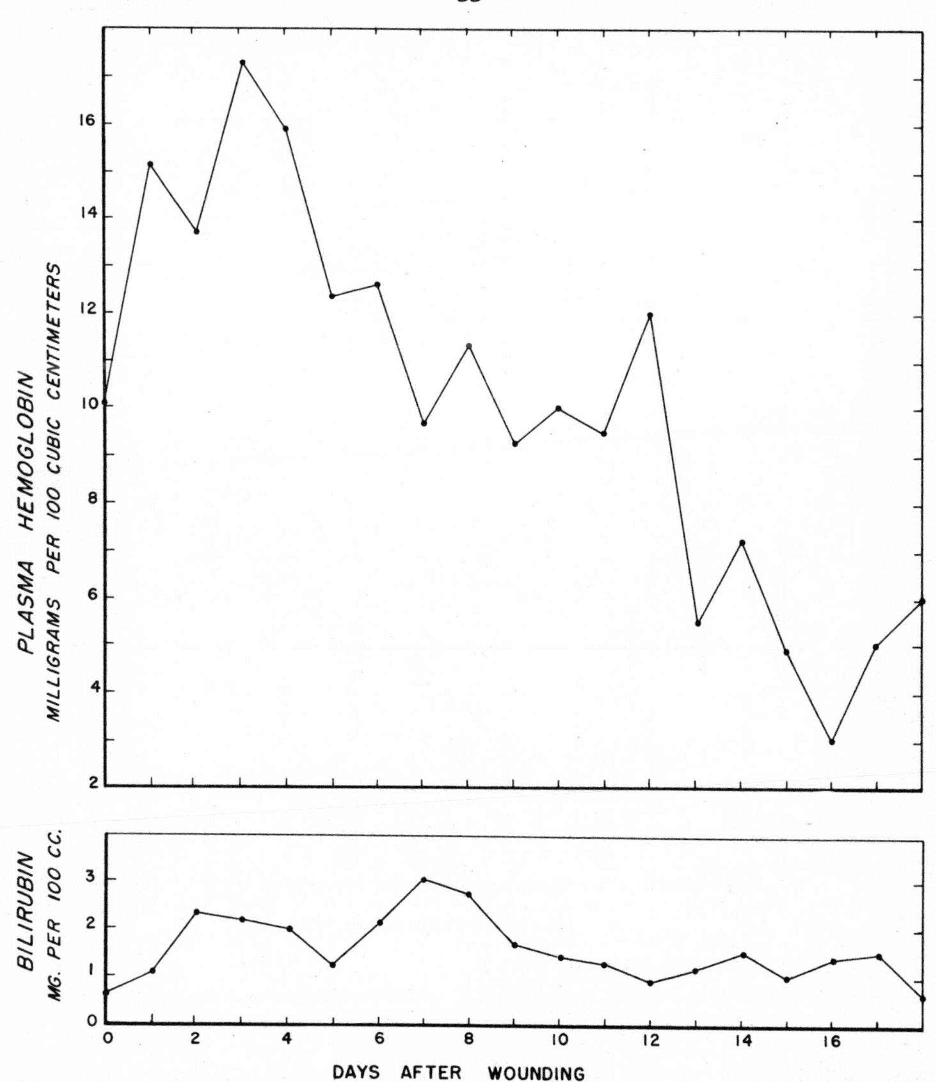

Plasma "hemoglobin": Benzidine-positive material.

may be assumed to have been predominantly myoglobin, all cases in which the initial specimen was not obtained within 3 days of injury, and Case 37 with several plasma hemoglobin levels above two hundred. This figure was so completely out of line with all other cases that a unique and unexplained mecha-

CHART 35. AVERAGE LEVELS OF PLASMA "HEMOGLOBIN" AND BILIRUBIN RELATED TO TIME FROM WOUNDING IN 64 PATIENTS WITH HIGH AZOTEMIA

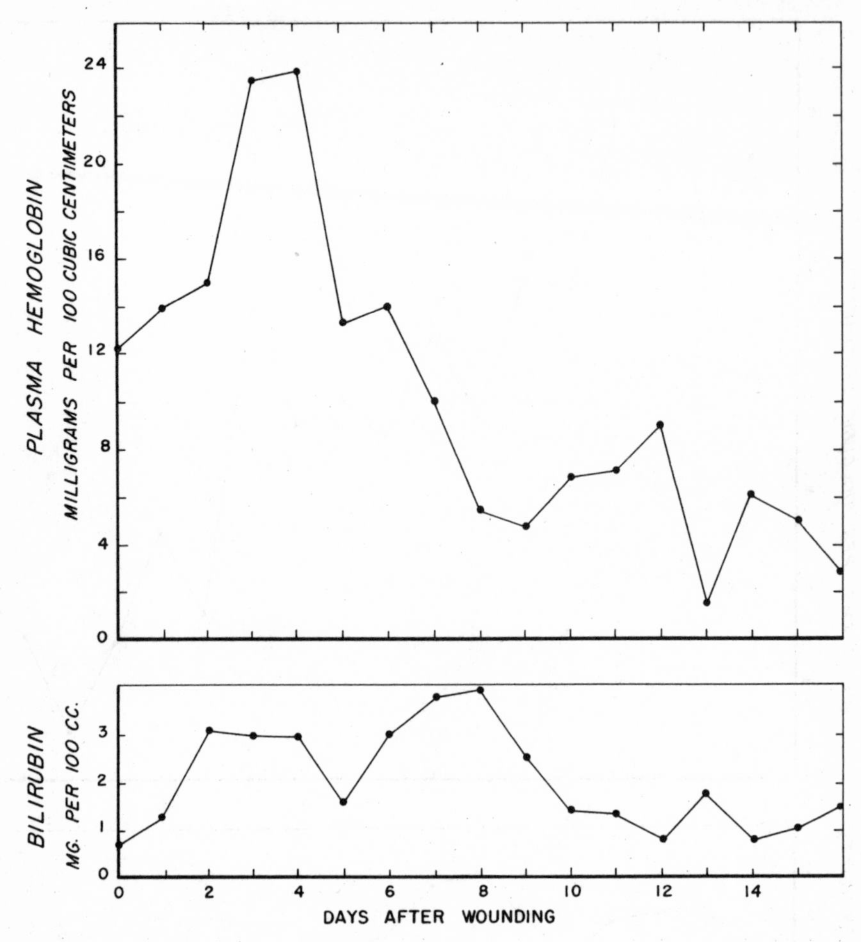

Plasma "hemoglobin": Benzidine-positive material.
High azotemia: Plasma N.P.N. level of 65 mg. per 100 cc. or higher. Over half of these patients died.

nism of hemolysis must be assumed. Seventy-six cases were available for analysis after these exclusions.

In compiling the table, the patients were divided into three groups: (1) those who had received no blood transfusion prior to drawing of the first blood specimen for analysis; (2) those who had received small to moderate amounts of blood—from 1 to 3 units or 500 to 1,500 cc.—and (3) recipients of large quan-

CHART 36. AVERAGE LEVELS OF PLASMA "HEMOGLOBIN" AND BILIRUBIN RELATED TO TIME FROM WOUNDING IN 33 PATIENTS WITH PIGMENT NEPHROPATHY AT NECROPSY

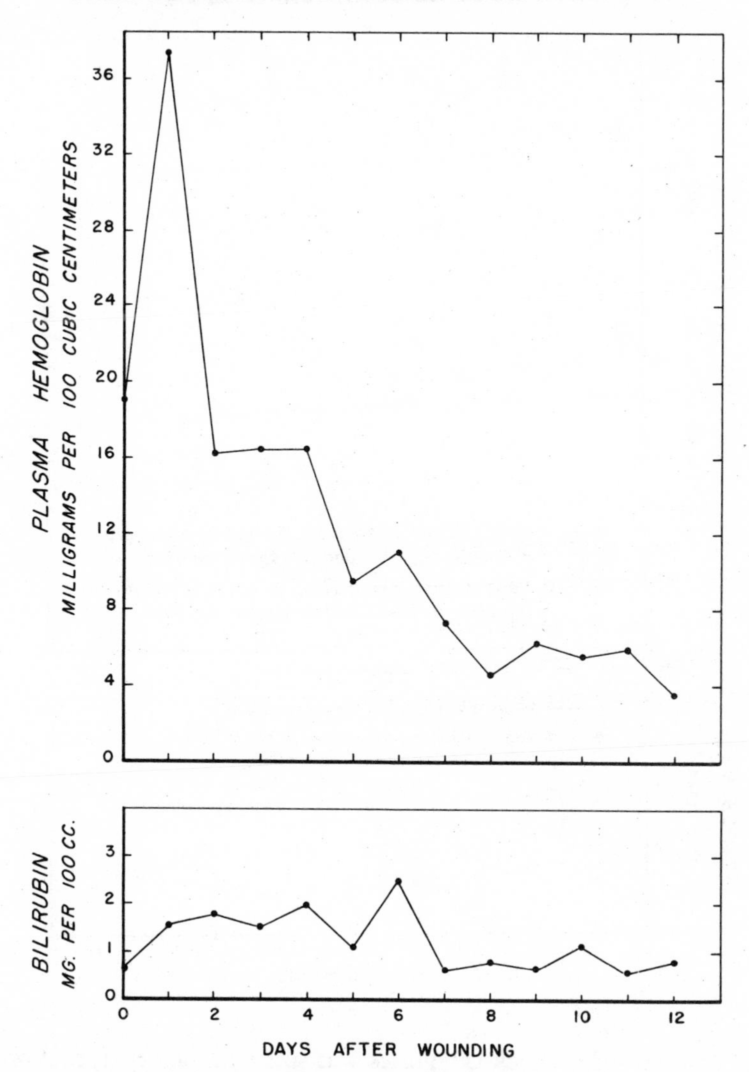

Plasma "hemoglobin": Benzidine-positive material. Cases 9, 41, 85, 115, 116, 132, and A-30 are omitted.

tities of blood—from 4 to 14 units or 2 to 7 liters. Shock had been estimated in three grades of severity, and there were a few patients without shock. The

956507 O—52——15

CHART 37. AVERAGE LEVELS OF PLASMA "HEMOGLOBIN" AND BILIRUBIN RELATED TO TIME FROM WOUNDING IN 107 PATIENTS OF BLOOD GROUPS A OR O

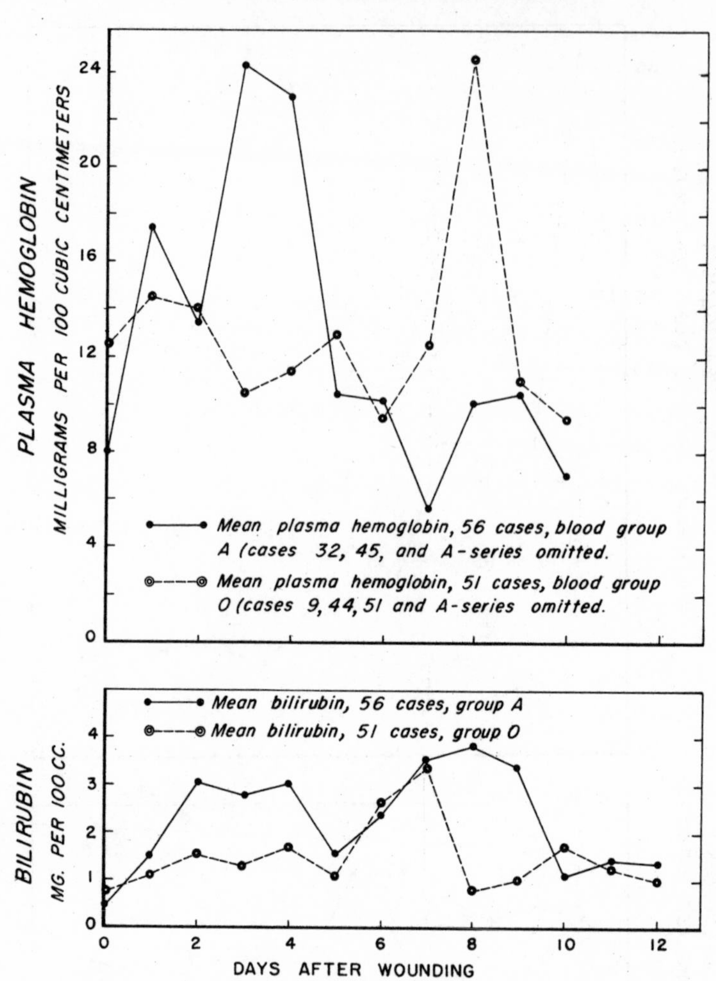

number of cases in some shock categories was so small, however, that only two categories were utilized: (1) patients with no shock or only slight shock (the "minimal-shock" group), and (2) patients with moderate or severe degrees of shock. Data are shown separately for blood samples drawn within 24 hours of injury and those taken from 24 to 96 hours after injury.

It is apparent from inspection of the table that plasma hemoglobin levels during the first 24 hours after injury showed no elevation which could be attributed either to shock or to infusion of bank blood. The mean plasma hemoglobin level for the entire group examined within 24 hours of injury was 9.6 mg. per 100 cc. of plasma, a normal figure for the technique used (See Materials and Methods). The mean for the moderate-and-severe shock group (8.8) was actually lower than the mean (11.7) of the minimal-shock group. More surprising are comparisons based on the quantity of transfused blood. The plasma hemoglobin levels actually appear to decline from a mean of 11.1 mg. per 100 cc. in the 14 patients who had received no blood to 9.2 in 22 patients who had had from 1 to 3 transfusions, and a minimum level of 7.5 in the 5 patients who had received the largest quantities of blood—from 4 to 14 units. These apparently paradoxical differences are not statistically significant, but it is clear that in this study no evidence emerged to indicate that during the first 24 hours after injury infused hemoglobin from stored blood produced any rise in plasma hemoglobin concentration.

In the succeeding 3 days, from 24 to 96 hours after injury, some rise in plasma hemoglobin was usually apparent. The average for the 35 cases in this category was 16.9 mg. per 100 cc. of plasma. Once again no evidence was obtained that shock per se produced any mobilization of hemoglobin. The mean of 17.3 mg. per 100 cc. for the moderate-and-severe shock group is not appreciably greater than the 16 mg.-figure for the minimal-shock category. In contrast to the findings in the first 24 hours, however, there does appear to be evidence that the plasma hemoglobin level rose in proportion to the quantity of transfused blood. It rose from a mean of 9.2 mg. per 100 cc. in the patients who had received no blood, to 15.1 in those who had received from 1 to 3 units, and to 20.5 in the patients treated with 4 or more transfusions. The difference between the first and third of these means, 11.3, is more than three times the standard error of 3.08.

In summary, the initial plasma free-hemoglobin levels of 76 wounded men who had had various degrees of shock, and who had received from none to 14 units of bank blood before the first sample of plasma was obtained for analysis, showed no rise in plasma hemoglobin concentration within 4 days after injury that could be attributed to the state of shock. During the first 24 hours after injury, the plasma hemoglobin concentration was surprisingly constant regardless of the amount of blood the patients had received. Hemoglobin in solution in the plasma of the infused bank blood was therefore not sufficient to raise the plasma hemoglobin level of the recipient. After the first 24 hours, plasma hemoglobin levels did rise in the majority of patients. This rise could not be correlated with the degree of shock but did show an apparently significant correlation with the amount of transfused blood. Such a delayed hemolytic action could be due either to nonspecific, accelerated hemolysis of the infused group O red cells or to hemolysis of the recipients' red cells from accumulation of infused iso-agglutinins. Evidence bearing upon this possibility will be presented in the following section.

Iso-Agglutinins

Relationship to Pigment Nephropathy

In Chart 37, the mean plasma hemoglobin level of 56 patients belonging to blood-group A is compared with that of 51 patients belonging to blood-group O. A distinct peak in the former curve on the third and fourth days after injury is apparent. On the third day the mean level in the A group was 24 mg. of hemoglobin per 100 cc. of plasma as compared with 10 mg. per 100 cc. for the O group at the same period. The difference is large enough to indicate some degree of hemolysis due to *a*-agglutinins. No reason is apparent for the rather surprising delayed rise in plasma hemoglobin concentration in the O group, which appears on the eighth day. The precipitate character of this peak, with its sudden rise and drop and the lack of equivalent rise in the plasma bilirubin, suggests that this may reasonably be ascribed to inadequate sampling or technical error.

Relationship to Lower Nephron Nephrosis

If hemolysis due to iso-agglutinins in plasma or bank blood were of importance in the pathogenesis of lower nephron nephrosis, the lesion should have appeared with greater frequency in our patients of blood-groups A, B, and AB than in those of group O, since all transfusions, with the two exceptions previously noted, were of O blood. No evidence was obtained of any relationship of blood group to case fatality or to development of renal insufficiency.

Blood grouping in the 186 patients in the study was checked in our laboratory in 137 instances. The distribution of blood groups among these 137 patients is shown in Table 87, both for all cases and for fatalities. It is evident that in both categories the distribution approximates closely the usual figures for a sample of the American population. Equally negative evidence of any effect of blood group is shown when the fatal cases of lower nephron nephrosis are considered. Blood group was known in 37 such cases which are shown on the table. It is evident that the distribution again approximates that of an average population.

TABLE 87.—DISTRIBUTION OF BLOOD GROUPS (CHECKED) AMONG ALL PATIENTS,[1] THOSE DYING FROM ALL CAUSES, AND THOSE DYING FROM RENAL FAILURE

Blood Group	All Cases in which Blood Group was Checked (137 Cases)		All Fatal Cases in which Blood Group was Checked (57 Cases)		Fatal Cases with Pigment Nephropathy in which Blood Group was Checked [2] (37 Cases)	
	Number of Patients	Percent	Number of Patients	Percent	Number of Patients	Percent
O	55	40.1	23	40.3	17	46.0
A	59	43.1	27	47.4	16	43.2
B	13	9.5	4	7.0	2	5.4
AB	10	7.3	3	5.3	2	5.4

[1] Total patients on whom blood grouping was rechecked in our laboratory.
[2] Blood group was not checked in 1 of the 38 cases of proved pigment nephropathy.

Hemoglobinuria and Myoglobinuria in Wounded Men

Relationship of Plasma Hemoglobin Levels to Excretion of Hemoglobin in the Urine

Excretion of hemoglobin in the urine is dependent upon two factors: the concentration of hemoglobin in the blood plasma and the permeability of the glomerular filter. As has already been pointed out, only one patient, Case 37, (crush cases excluded) showed a plasma hemoglobin concentration above 135 mg. per 100 cc., the usually-accepted threshold level for hemoglobinuria. An altered permeability of the glomeruli must therefore be assumed in all other patients manifesting hemoglobinuria. If the increase in permeability was more or less constant, it might be expected that the degree of hemoglobinuria would be influenced by the level of plasma hemoglobin. If the alteration in permeability was variable, no such relationship would be demonstrable.

The concentrations of hemoglobin in plasma and urine are compared in Table 88 for 21 cases in which the two determinations were made upon samples collected at approximately the same time. The possibility that the urine might have been retained within the bladder for many hours before voiding could not always be excluded. No evidence of correlation is present, and the Spearman rank order coefficient of correlation (rho) is 0.03, indicating only chance relationship between the two series of figures.

TABLE 88.—COMPARISON OF HEMOGLOBIN CONCENTRATION IN PLASMA AND URINE IN 21 CASES

Case No.	Plasma "Hemoglobin"	Urine Hemoglobin	Case No.	Plasma "Hemoglobin"	Urine Hemoglobin
8	22.3	110.0	62	4.0	12.2
13	6.0	8.0	64	2.7	1.9
18	18.5	12.4	71	68.0	80.8
19	20.5	4.0	86	13.4	8.7
22	9.2	193.0	89	4.0	3.8
34	2.8	13.8	95	44.6	10.5
38	4.3	92.0	108	11.7	6.0
41	34.6	5.9	112	6.5	8.5
49	13.5	11.0	123	25.0	3.0
54	5.3	18.7	125	8.7	15.0
57	6.1	25.8			

Excretion of Myoglobin in the Urine

Analyses for hemoglobin and myoglobin in the urine were carried out in 42 cases in which measurable amounts of benzidine-positive material were present. Myoglobin was positively identified in 19 cases and was the dominant pigment in nine. (Comparison was impossible in 5 of these because wounds of the urinary tract made urine hemoglobin figures unreliable.) In 8 additional cases the test for myoglobin was positive but the proportion found was so small (from 10 to 20 percent of the benzidine-reacting material) that the results were classed as doubtful and were disregarded. The analyses in the remaining 15 cases were recorded as definitely negative (myoglobin from 0 to 10 percent).

The 19 positive cases are listed in Table 89 together with the degree of shock, the concentration of myoglobin and hemoglobin in the urine, the level of benzidine-positive material in the blood plasma, and the major clinical diagnoses.

TABLE 89.—OCCURRENCE OF MYOGLOBINURIA AND CORRELATIVE FINDINGS IN 19 SEVERELY WOUNDED PATIENTS

Case No.	Degree of Shock	Urine		Plasma	Major Diagnosis
		Myoglobin	Hemoglobin *	Benzidine-Positive Material	
		mg. per 100 cc.	mg. per 100 cc.	mg. per 100 cc.	
4	Severe	16.0	....	10.3	Gas gangrene; peritonitis.
7	None	16.0	2.5	5.5	Lacerated femoral artery; anastomosis.
9	. . . do . . .	4.0	11.4	3.1	Thoracic wounds; transfusion reaction.
19	Moderate . .	4.0	3.5	20.5	Traumatic amputation; gas gangrene.
25	Severe	72.0	....	24.5	Abdominal wound; peritonitis.
37	Moderate . .	1.0	2.5	266.0	Thoracic and liver wounds.
38	Severe	420.0	92.0	4.3	Volvulus.
49	. . . do . . .	3.0	11.0	13.5	Abdominal wound.
69	None	588.0	0.0	37.6	Crush syndrome.
70	. . . do . . .	288.0	142.0	8.2	Do.
74	Slight	147.0	61.0	38.2	Burn.
78	. . . do . . .	2.5	2.1	920.0	Crush syndrome.
88	Severe	36.6	....	7.4	Abdominal and extremity wounds; peritonitis.
89	. . . do . . .	1.5	3.8	4.0	Traumatic amputation.
93	. . . do . . .	67.0	80.0	30.0	Crush syndrome.
97	. . . do . . .	205.0	25.0	....	Abdominal wound; peritonitis.
98	Moderate . .	30.0	....	....	Abdominal and cerebral wounds.
126	. . . do . . .	7.0	....	9.3	Thoraco-abdominal wound; peritonitis.
137	None	203.0	41.0	38.4	Lacerated femoral artery.

* Blanks in this column indicate that a wound of the urinary tract rendered the determination useless for purposes of comparison.

Inspection of this table reveals several points of interest. As in the case of hemoglobinuria, it is obvious that there is no correlation between the level of benzidine-positive material in the plasma and the amount of myoglobin excreted in the urine. For example, in Case 38 only 4.3 mg. per 100 cc. were found in the plasma, while the urine contained the enormous concentration of 420 mg. per 100 cubic centimeters. In Case 78, a patient with crush syndrome, the situation was reversed. The plasma concentration was 920 mg. per 100 cc., the maximal figure of the entire series, whereas the urine contained barely enough to measure—only 2.5 milligrams.

If the myoglobinuric cases are considered as a whole, the degree of myoglobinuria shows no relationship to the severity of shock. In the "minimal-shock" group (as previously defined), the concentrations of myoglobin in the urine ranged from 2.5 to 588.0 mg. per 100 cubic centimeters. In the moderate-and-severe shock group, the range was from 1 to 420 mg. per 100 cubic centimeters. The average of seven cases in the minimal-shock group was 321 mg. in comparison with 63.7 mg. for the more severe-shock group, but with such wide variation in the data the averages are meaningless.

TABLE 90.—RELATIONSHIP OF MUSCLE NECROSIS TO SHOCK IN 19 PATIENTS WITH MYOGLOBINURIA

With Muscle Necrosis		Without Muscle Necrosis	
Case No.	Degree of Shock	Case No.	Degree of Shock
69	None.	74	Slight.
70	Do.	37	Moderate.
7	Do.	98	Do.
137	Do.	126	Do.
78	Slight.	25	Severe.
19	Moderate.	38	Do.
93	Severe.	49	Do.
89	Do.	88	Do.
4	Do.	97	Do.
9	None.		

When the nature of the major injury or lesion in these myoglobinuric cases is taken into consideration, however, an interesting correlation does become apparent. The cases fall readily into two groups: those with extensive necrosis of skeletal muscle (either ischemic or infectious) and those without such muscle necrosis. They are so listed, with the estimated degrees of shock, in Table 90.

Five of nine patients with extensive necrosis of skeletal muscles showed minimal or no clinical evidence of shock; in those without extensive muscle necrosis, in contrast, eight were in the moderate-and-severe shock group and only two in the minimal-shock group. One of the latter, Case 74, with extensive burns showed sufficient hemoconcentration to suggest a more severe grade of shock than was clinically apparent. These findings strongly suggest, on the one hand, that myoglobin is rarely liberated in the absence of shock unless there has been extensive necrosis of skeletal muscle, and on the other, that in the presence of severe shock, there is some mechanism for its mobilization other than muscle necrosis.

Relationship of Hemoglobinuria to Myoglobinuria

Attempts to correlate the variety of pigment excreted in the urine with the type of injury or lesion provided extremely puzzling results, as may be seen from the tabulation to follow in which cases have been classified by the predominant pigment, though many of them showed simultaneous excretion of both pigments. Because of the frequency of multiple injuries, the same case has often been included under more than one heading. Cases of trauma to the urinary tract have been excluded from the hemoglobinuric but not from the myoglobinuric category.

Type of injury or complication	*Number predominantly hemoglobin*	*Number predominantly myoglobin*
Crush syndrome	2	3
Wounds of extremity	19	5
Major vascular interruption	11	3
Clostridial myositis	1	2
Urinary tract injury	—	2
Liver injury	4	1
Abdominal wound	11	3
Peritonitis	4	3
Burn	0	1
Volvulus	0	1

It is at once evident that any type of injury may be associated with either hemoglobinuria or myoglobinuria and that in most types, except the crush syndrome and in clostridial myositis, the former is by far the more common. It is noteworthy that in two typical crush cases no evidence of myoglobin excretion was obtained (see Chapter XI). Neither massive trauma to the extremities nor interruption of a major vessel, with consequent ischemic necrosis of muscle, usually resulted in predominant myoglobinuria, and in two of the three patients in whom it did appear, a successful arterial anastomosis had re-established circulation of the leg before myoglobinuria was observed. In three patients (Case 70, extensive but superficial burns; Case 38, volvulus, and Case 9, mismatched transfusion) injury of voluntary muscle can be absolutely excluded. In considering the findings, however, it must be remembered first that our test for myoglobinuria was crude and results were recorded as positive only when considerable quantities of myoglobin were present, and second that myoglobin is rapidly excreted in the absence of renal insufficiency and the loss of a single urine specimen might cause a falsely negative result.

TABLE 91.—GREATEST CONCENTRATIONS[1] OF HEMOGLOBIN AND MYOGLOBIN OBSERVED IN THE URINE

Case No.	Hemoglobinuria *mg. per 100 cc.*	Case No.	Myoglobinuria *mg. per 100 cc.*
22	193	69	588
70[2]	142	38[2]	420
109	123	70[2]	288
8	110	97	205
56	110	137	203
38[2]	92	74[2]	147
71	81	25	72
93[2]	80	93[2]	67
74[2]	61	88	37
72	58	98	30
118	38	7	16
128	34	4	16

[1] Highest of a number of determinations in each case.
[2] Cases that appear in both columns.

One final comparison is of interest. In Table 91 the 12 patients showing the highest concentrations of hemoglobin and the 12 with the highest myoglobin concentrations are listed. As before, cases of trauma to the urinary tract have been eliminated from the hemoglobinuric category. It is apparent from these figures that myoglobinuria was frequently massive whereas hemoglobinuria was rarely so when cases of direct trauma to the urinary tract are eliminated. It is also noteworthy that four cases (Cases 38, 70, 74, and 93) appear in both lists, suggesting that the conditions for the liberation of myoglobin and of hemoglobin may not be unrelated.

SUMMARY

The concentration of benzidine-reacting heme pigment in the blood plasma (recorded as plasma hemoglobin) and the individual concentrations of hemoglobin and myoglobin in the urine were measured in our patients to determine the extent of pigment mobilization. These data, together with determinations of plasma hemoglobin in the bank blood administered to the patients, were analyzed in an attempt to determine the mechanism of pigment mobilization in the body and of pigment excretion by the kidney.

It was found that the bank blood used in therapy was in a satisfactory state of preservation, with an average of only 43 mg. of free hemoglobin per 100 cc. of plasma at the moment of utilization. Even in patients who received as many as 10 to 14 transfusions, the plasma "hemoglobin" levels of the recipients showed in the first 24 hours no elevation which could be attributed to free hemoglobin in the transfused blood. Comparison of the plasma hemoglobin concentrations with the degree of shock in 76 patients showed no evidence that shock itself induced any immediate increase in plasma hemoglobin concentration.

Twenty-four hours after injury, however, a progressive rise in plasma hemoglobin began to be apparent which reached a peak between 48 and 72 hours and then slowly dropped to normal over a period of 2 weeks. This peak was approximately twice as high (36.8 mg. per 100 cc.) in 33 cases of fatal nephropathy as in the series as a whole (17.3 mg. per 100 cc.) and occurred only 24 hours after wounding. No evidence was obtained that it was higher in patients with severe shock than in those without shock or with only minimal shock. It was, however, significantly higher in patients who had received multiple transfusions than in those who had received no blood.

Evidence that this delayed rise in plasma hemoglobin was largely due to iso-agglutinins was afforded by comparison of group A and group O recipients. In 56 of the former, the mean plasma hemoglobin on the third day was 24 mg. per 100 cc., whereas in a sample of 51 group O recipients the corresponding level was only 10.2 milligrams. This difference was of no significance, however, in the development of pigment nephropathy as shown by the percentage distribution of blood groups among the nephropathies, which was essentially identical with the distribution of blood groups in the entire series of cases studied by the Board and with an average sampling of the American population.

In 21 cases in which plasma hemoglobin levels were obtained at approximately the same time that the first urine specimen was voided, the concentrations of pigment in the two fluids were compared. No evidence of correlation was found. It was concluded that the threshold of hemoglobin excretion in wounded men must vary over a wide range.

Myoglobin was positively identified in the urine of 19 patients in the series and these cases were subjected to special scrutiny. As in the case of hemoglobin, no correlation was found between the concentrations of benzidine-reacting pigment in the plasma and of myoglobin in the urine.

With the exception of clear-cut cases of the crush syndrome, excretion of myoglobin could not be predicted from the nature of the patient's injury or its complications. It was rarely seen in wounds of the extremities, even those associated with extensive necrosis of muscle, unless they were complicated by clostridial myositis, or, as in two cases, circulation was re-established after a period of ischemia by a successful arterial anastomosis. It was sometimes very severe in patients with little or no muscle damage. When muscle damage was extensive, the mobilization and excretion of myoglobin appeared to be independent of the development of shock. When there was insignificant or no muscle injury, myoglobinuria was rarely found in the absence of moderate or severe shock.

Two further observations are noteworthy though their significance is not apparent. Myoglobinuria was frequently massive, hemoglobinuria rarely so in the absence of injury to the urinary tract. Myoglobinuria and hemoglobinuria of significant degree frequently occurred in the same patient, suggesting a common but undiscovered mechanism.

CONCLUSIONS

1. Neither the development of shock nor the therapeutic use of multiple transfusions of group O bank blood produced immediate elevation of the plasma "hemoglobin" levels in severely wounded men.

2. The delayed rise in mean plasma "hemoglobin" for the series as a whole in the period from 24 to 96 hours was largely attributable to iso-agglutinins in the O bank blood, since it was absent in a sample of 51 O recipients.

3. Mean plasma "hemoglobin" concentrations were higher in the patients in whom pigment nephrosis developed than in other wounded men but were still far below the threshold level at which the normal kidney excretes hemoglobin.

A depression of the threshold for hemoglobin excretion must be assumed.

4. The lack of correlation between concentrations of benzidine-reacting pigment in the plasma and of hemoglobin or myoglobin in the urine suggests that this alteration of threshold was variable.

5. The irregularity with which extensive muscle injury was followed by myoglobinuria indicates that some factor other than necrosis of muscle cells is involved. This factor is not shock and appears to be the maintenance or re-establishment of the circulation in the involved muscles.

6. In a small number of cases severe myoglobinuria developed in the absence of demonstrable muscle injury. The almost constant presence of moderate or severe shock in such cases suggests the possibility of diffuse ischemic injury of muscle which is not morphologically recognizable.

7. The fact that severe myoglobinuria and severe hemoglobinuria were often observed in the same patient suggests the possibility of a common mechanism.

CHAPTER IX

Pathology of the Kidney in Traumatic Shock

The kidney lesion associated with the clinical syndrome of renal insufficiency following resuscitation from shock is constant but not pathognomonic. Lucké,[1] in a study of material from the Army Institute of Pathology, has shown that a similar lesion, which he has called "lower nephron·nephrosis," develops in a variety of conditions such as mismatched blood transfusion, infusion of human hemoglobin, the crush syndrome, heat stroke, blackwater fever, thermal burns, carbon tetrachloride poisoning, mushroom poisoning (*Amanita phalloides*) and sulfonamide sensitivity. The author, from his own experience, can add to the list of etiologic agents chemical burns, anaphylactic shock following therapeutic use of antipneumococcus rabbit serum, and hemolytic reactions following transurethral resections in which the operative field is irrigated with tap water. Many years ago F. B. Mallory[2] noted the lesion in an occasional patient with hemolytic streptococcus infection. There can be little doubt that with increasing breadth of experience many other causal agents will be brought to light.

Descriptions of the lesion in various stages may be found in innumerable case reports under such titles as transfusion kidney,[3] hemoglobinuric nephrosis,[4] interstitial nephritis,[5] hepatorenal syndrome,[6] and other terms, but surveys of

[1] LUCKÉ, B.: Lower nephron nephrosis (renal lesions of crush syndrome, of burns, transfusions, and other conditions affecting lower segments of nephrons). Mil. Surgeon 99: 371–396, November 1946.

[2] MALLORY, F. B.: Personal communication.

[3] DENAVASQUEZ, S.: Excretion of haemoglobin, with special reference to "transfusion" kidney. J. Path. & Bact. 51: 413–425, November 1940.

[4] MALLORY, T. B.: Hemoglobinuric nephrosis in traumatic shock. Am. J. Clin. Path. 17: 427–443, June 1947.

[5] KIMMELSTIEL, P.: Acute hematogenous interstitial nephritis. Am. J. Path. 14: 737–761, November 1938.

[6] HELWIG, F. C., and ORR, T. G.: Traumatic necrosis of liver with extensive retention of creatinine and high grade nephrosis. Arch. Surg. 24: 136–144, January 1932.

any considerable mass of material are few. The most notable contributions are those of Lucké[7] and of Bywaters and Dible[8] in their studies of the crush syndrome. The present study is based primarily on a review of material from 60 out of 63 necropsies on patients studied by the Board, but is fortified by experience gained from review of more than 150 similar nephropathies at the 15th Medical General Laboratory. The records and material from the 60 cases, correlated with the clinical and biochemic data, provided the means for surveying the lesion in all stages of development as manifested in wounded soldiers resuscitated from shock by human plasma or whole blood transfusions.

Microscopic Pathology

The characteristic features of the lesion emphasized to a greater or lesser degree by different authors are seven: pigment casts; internal hydronephrosis; degeneration of epithelial elements, particularly in the lower segments of the nephrons; rupture of tubules with extrusion of their content into the stroma; interstitial inflammation; granulomatous inflammation, and thrombophlebitis of small intrarenal veins. Let us examine them successively.

Pigment Casts

Pigment casts, as in other forms of lower nephron nephrosis, are the most conspicuous feature of the "shock kidney." They were present in all cases of proved renal insufficiency in the present series in which the survival period was 3 days or longer. Their absence in many of the more acute cases is an interesting feature which will be considered later.

The pigment casts were found in the distal convoluted and collecting tubules and in the ducts of Bellini, their relative frequency in these respective locations varying considerably from case to case. The number of nephrons involved was difficult to estimate in routine sections, since only portions of each nephron were visualized. In most cases with clinically demonstrated renal insufficiency, the proportion was obviously high but the range was wide, probably from 20 to 80 percent.

[7] See footnote 1.

[8] BYWATERS, E. G. L., and DIBLE, J. H.: Renal lesion in traumatic anuria. J. Path. & Bact. 54: 111–120, January 1942.

The pigment, when viewed in unstained sections or sections only lightly stained with hematoxylin, shaded from orange through orange-green to a muddy greenish-brown. It might precipitate as separate coarse globules 4 to 8 microns in diameter (which are frequently mistaken on casual examination for red blood cells); as ropes of globules, rather like strings of sausages; or as granular debris usually embedded in a cast-like matrix. The staining reactions of the pigment were not consistent. A portion of it almost always showed the usual staining reactions of hemoglobin; namely, an affinity for eosin and for the fuchsin in the Masson trichrome, a dense blue color with phosphotungstic acid hematoxylin, and a positive benzidine reaction. Another portion of the pigment, indistinguishable in the unstained or eosin-stained preparations, failed to accept the fuchsin in the Masson or the hematoxylin in the phosphotungstic stain, and was benzidine-negative. Characteristic staining reactions with hematoxylin and eosin, phosphotungstic acid hematoxylin, and Masson trichrome are illustrated in Figures 1, 2, and 3.

Although there were some exceptions, two generalizations could be made regarding the staining reactions of the pigment: First, the shorter the time interval between injury and death, the greater was the proportion of pigment which gave the staining reactions of hemoglobin. Second, the farther down the nephron the pigment was located, the less was this tendency. Figures 4 and 5 illustrate this difference in the pigment casts of the cortex and medulla. The obvious conclusion is that with the passage of time and with the chemical changes in the glomerular filtrate as it passed along the tubule, the original hemoglobin-like material was altered, presumably by a process of degradation in the direction of acid hematin. This degradation never reached the point where iron could be demonstrated with the ferrocyanide reaction. One other differential point has been noted: The hemoglobin-like pigment rarely excited a significant inflammatory reaction, whereas the altered pigment sometimes attracted leukocytes in considerable number (Fig. 6).

Internal Hydronephrosis

Many authors have described marked dilatation of portions of the nephron above the obstructing pigment casts. Their illustrations often show great dilatation of proximal tubules and of Bowman's capsule. Our experience suggests that this apparent dilatation is largely a shrinkage artefact. If formalin-fixed kidney tissue is rapidly dehydrated and embedded in paraffin, shrinkage is difficult to avoid. The glomeruli appear as tiny spheres occupying less than half of the capsular space, and the diameter of the lumen of the proximal tubules is from 50 to 70 percent of the external diameter of the tubule. If the tissue is Zenkerized before embedding, the shrinkage is reduced and primary embedding in Zenker-formol or in Zenker with acetic acid lessens it still further. In such sections Bowman's capsule is rarely dilated, although some dilatation of tubules may be apparent. A still better check upon this debatable issue is provided by the examination of frozen sections in which the factor of dehydration is excluded.

The following statements are based primarily upon the examination of frozen sections which were prepared from almost every case in this series. No dilatation of Bowman's capsule was observed, but tubular dilatation of moderate but unmistakable degree was usual, with the proximal convoluted tubule the segment most commonly involved. Dilatation was not observed before the third day after injury, was almost constant between the third and fifth days, and became less frequent in the cases with longer periods of survival. Dilatation of distal convoluted tubules and upper collecting tubules, usually those situated in the cortical rays, was less common and was ordinarily seen in the more chronic stages from the sixth day onward. In some cases, however, dilatation was marked in these segments and minimal or absent in the proximal tubules (Figs. 7 and 8).

Dilatation of proximal tubules, to judge from frozen sections, correlated well with two characteristic phenomena noted on gross examination: enlargement of the kidney, particularly widening of the cortex, and a wet surface wherever freshly cut.

Degeneration and Regeneration of Tubular Epithelium

Degenerative changes in the epithelial cells were rare in the proximal tubules, absent in the descending limb of Henle's loop, usual in the ascending limb and the distal convoluted tubule, and inconstant in the collecting tubules. The proximal tubule was usually normal except for slight to moderate dilatation. The brush border was well maintained, the cells were not swollen, and the cytoplasmic granules were normal in size and distribution. The tubular lumens frequently contained granular nonpigmented precipitate, but this is not surprising in view of the constant albuminuria demonstrable in patients with severe trauma and constitutes no proof of tubular injury.

In only five cases were the proximal tubules clearly abnormal. In two there

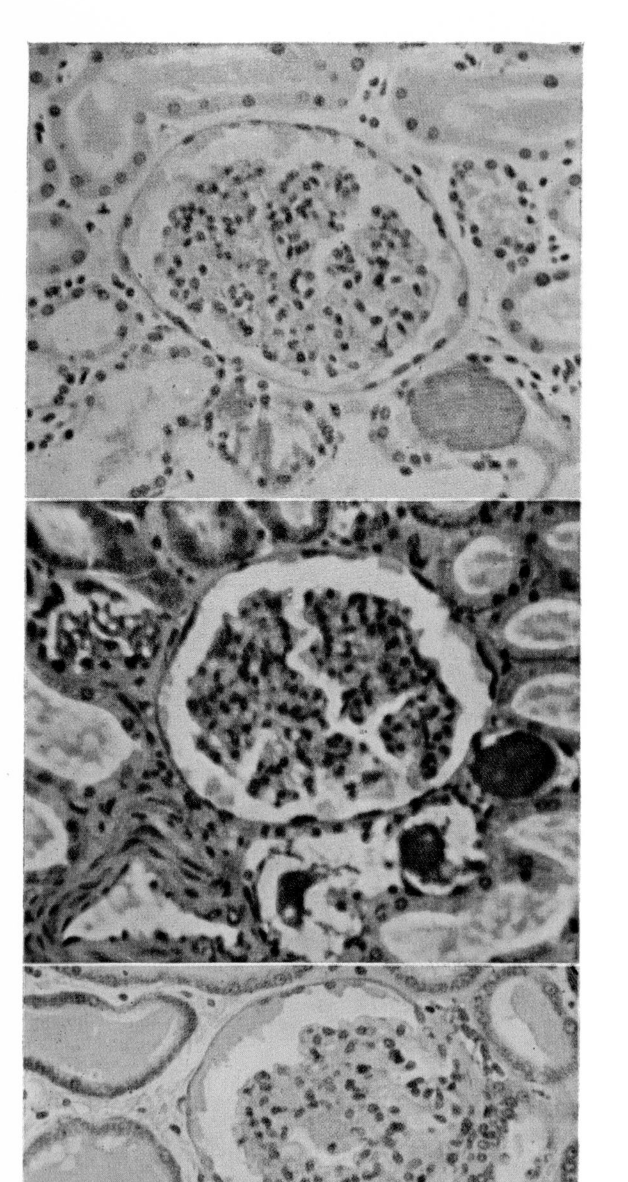

FIGURE 1. *Stain:* Hematoxylin and eosin. The glomerulus is normal. The distal convoluted tubules contain orange colored casts of precipitated hemoglobin. X 330

FIGURE 2. *Stain:* Masson trichrome. The casts stain deep red as do red cells with this stain. X 330

FIGURE 3. *Stain:* Phosphotungstic acid hematoxylin. The deep blue staining of the pigment casts is characteristic of the reactions of hemoglobin with this stain. The proximal convoluted tubules are dilated and contain precipitated albumin, but the epithelial cells show no degenerative changes. X 330

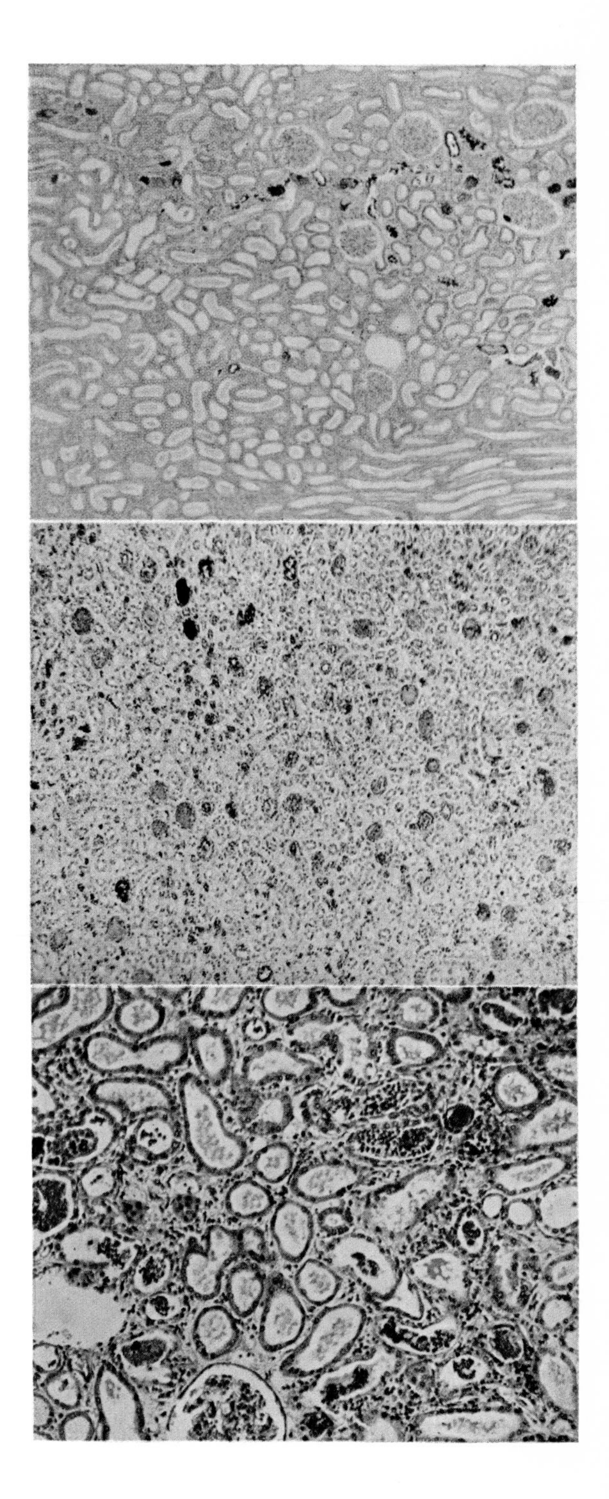

FIGURE 4. *Stain:* Phosphotungstic acid hematoxylin. Renal cortex, low magnification, showing blue-staining casts in the distal convoluted tubules. The proximal tubules are uniformly slightly dilated and contain precipitated albumin but they are otherwise normal. X 80

FIGURE 5. *Stain:* Phosphotungstic acid hematoxylin. Section from the kidney pyramid of the case shown in Figure 4. This patient died 3 days after injury. A considerable proportion of the pigment casts have lost their ability to stain blue with the phosphotungstic acid stain. X 80

FIGURE 6. *Stain:* Masson trichrome. Note the acute exudation into the distal tubules about the masses of pigment which have begun to lose their hemoglobin-like staining reactions. X 200

was extensive fat vacuolation; in the two others the cells were swollen, the brush border was obscured, and the cytoplasm filled with hyaline, presumably albuminous droplets. Nothing in the clinical picture served to distinguish these cases from others of the series. The infrequency of albuminous droplets in the cells of the proximal tubules under conditions of marked albuminuria might be interpreted as evidence of failure of resorptive function in this segment of the nephron. Such functional paralysis would also explain the surprising fact that only once in 200 hemoglobinuric cases was absorption of hemoglobin by the proximal tubules observed. In one instance (Case 86) there were numerous foci of complete coagulative necrosis of proximal tubular epithelium. The possibility of direct traumatic injury of the kidneys could not be excluded here.

The descending limbs of Henle's loops frequently contained considerable amounts of orange pigment, which was not iron-positive with ferrocyanide but accepted the fuchsin counterstain as does so-called hemofuchsin. It was sometimes weakly sudanophilic, and because of its orange-yellow color was difficult to distinguish from fat in Sudan preparations. Since this pigment was also frequently found in cases of sudden death used as controls, we believe it to be a normal phenomenon.

The earliest and most frequent evidence of tubular degeneration appeared in the form of fat vacuolation in the ascending limbs of Henle's loops. The vacuoles were extremely small, mostly from 1 to 2 microns; were hard to identify in paraffin sections; were intensely red in frozen sections stained with Sudan IV; and were not doubly refractile under polarized light. In some cases they were found only in a limited segment of the ascending limb, always the portion closest to the corticomedullary junction; in others the process extended almost to the apex of the pyramid, involving the entire ascending limb (Figs. 9 and 10). A rough quantitation of the severity of this change was attempted by visual estimation, using a 1- to 4-plus scale.

Well-marked (2- to 4-plus) fat vacuolation was present in 6 of 8 cases in this study in which death followed injury by less than 48 hours, including Case 77 with a survival period of only 20 hours. It was present, usually in 3- or 4-plus grade, in 14 of the 15 cases in which death occurred between the second and fourth days. From the fifth day onward it decreased in frequency and intensity; it was found in only 14 of the 27 cases and in only 1 was it above 2-plus grade. A more extensive discussion of this process will be found in Chapter XII in connection with similar observations on other organs.

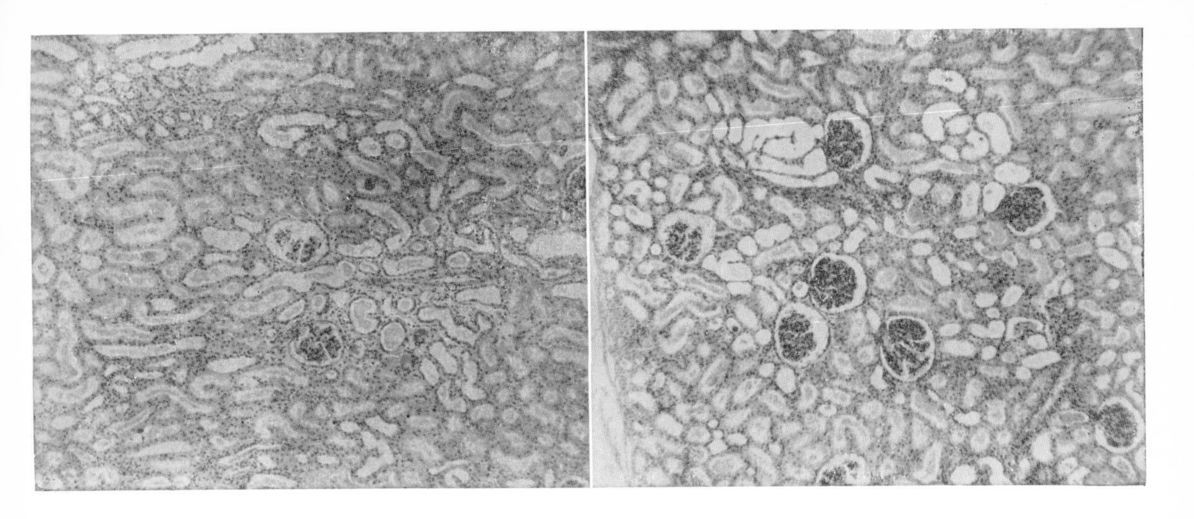

INTERNAL HYDRONEPHROSIS

FIGURE 7. (*Left*) Moderate dilatation of both proximal and distal convoluted tubules is shown in a case of 6 days' duration. A rare sulfonamide crystal is present. *Stain:* Hematoxylin and eosin. X 150

FIGURE 8. (*Right*) Marked dilatation of the distal convoluted tubules with comparatively slight widening of the proximal ones is apparent. *Stain:* Hematoxylin and eosin. X 180

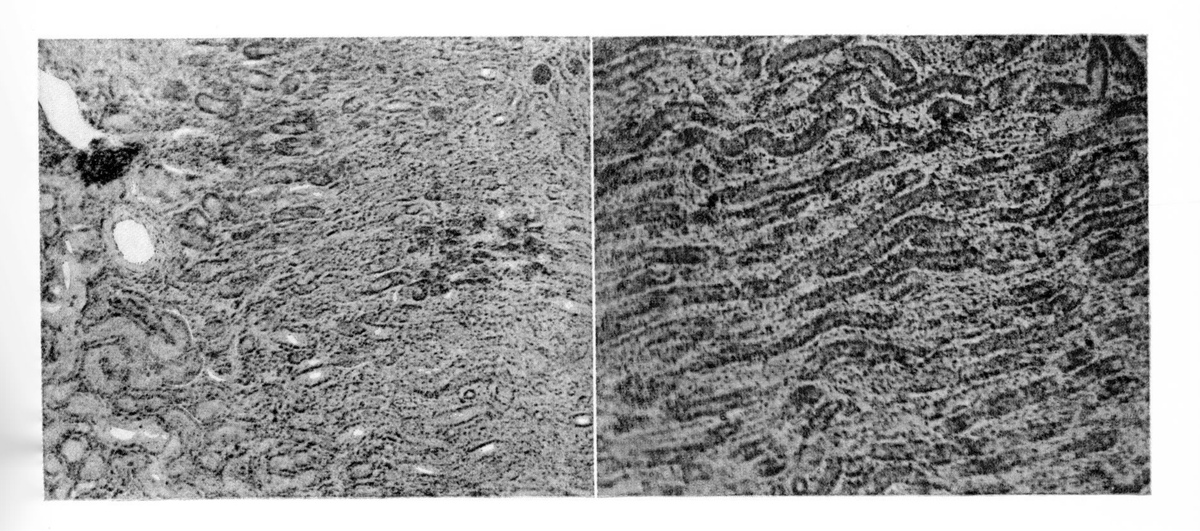

STAINING REACTIONS OF FAT

FIGURE 9. (*Left*) *Stain:* Sudan IV. Fat vacuolation limited to a segment of the ascending limb adjacent to the corticomedullary junction. X 180

FIGURE 10. (*Right*) *Stain:* Sudan IV. Diffuse fat vacuolation of entire ascending limb of Henle's loop. X 180

Occasionally on the third or fourth day, but always by the fifth, other forms of epithelial reaction were obvious. The cells became shrunken, their nuclei pyknotic, and they frequently lost their attachment to the basement membrane and desquamated. At almost the same period, mitoses became apparent and sometimes so numerous that two or three were seen in a single cross-section of a tubule. These degenerative and regenerative changes were frequently limited to, and always most severe in a comparatively limited zone close to the corticomedullary junction.

Distal Convoluted Tubules.—The distal convoluted tubules in apparently normal individuals frequently contain small granules of lipid. In some cases of shock it was evident that the sudanophilic material was increased in amount, but variation in the normal range makes the significance of this observation very difficult to assess. By the fourth or fifth day after injury, degenerative and regenerative changes sometimes became apparent in the distal tubule. They were never as marked or as widespread as in the ascending limbs, but the difference was quantitative, not qualitative.

Collecting Tubules.—Alterations in the character of the epithelium of the collecting tubules are difficult to recognize with certainty, since these tubules are particularly susceptible to postmortem degeneration, including desquamation. Fat stains do not help, since lipoid degeneration rarely occurs. In well-fixed material, however, it was often evident that the cells were hyperchromatic. Frank necrosis was rarely seen, yet mitoses were not infrequent. In other cases reduplication of the epithelial layer was evident and sometimes, where no desquamation was apparent, sheets of epithelial cells filled the lumina of the tubules and encircled or even invaded the pigment casts. Sometimes mitoses were numerous in these detached or semidetached cells. In the collecting tubules, in contrast to other segments of the nephron, the epithelial changes closely paralelled the presence of pigment casts in the affected segments.

Interstitial Inflammation

Interstitial inflammation was not noted before the third day; from the third to the fourth day it was found in half the cases, and from the fifth day onward it was a constant phenomenon. It was first manifested as focal infiltration limited to a fairly narrow zone at the corticomedullary junction. The component cells were predominantly lymphocytes and plasma cells, but variable proportions of neutrophils and eosinophils were usually mingled with them (Fig. 11). The

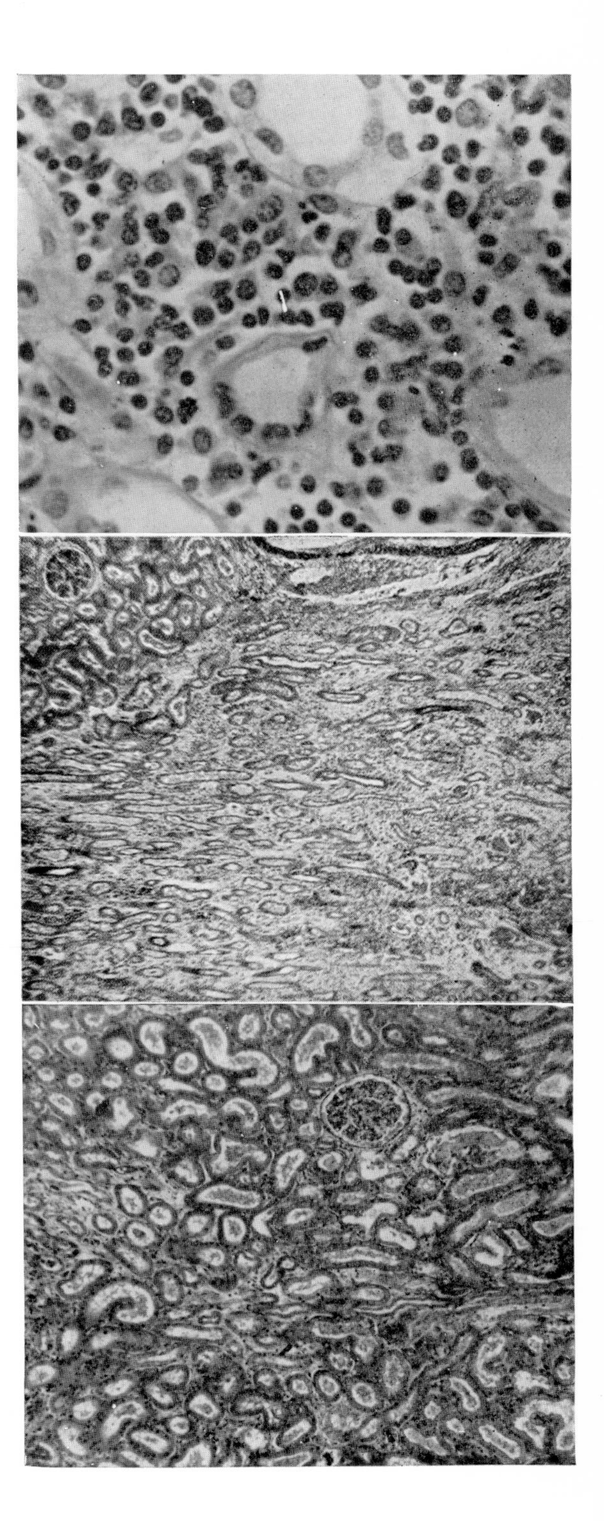

FIGURE 11. Interstitial inflammatory infiltrate between tubules near the corticomedullary junction in case of 8 days' duration. Lymphocytes and plasma cells predominate. *Stain:* Hematoxylin and eosin. X 300

FIGURE 12. *Stain:* Masson trichrome. Low-power view of corticomedullary junction, showing interstitial edema of moderate grade and both diffuse and granulomatous inflammatory reaction. Some extruded casts are visible. Case of 8 days' duration. X 80

FIGURE 13. Case of 12 days' duration. The formation of a second zone of interstitial inflammatory reaction beneath the capsule is shown. *Stain:* Masson trichrome. X 150

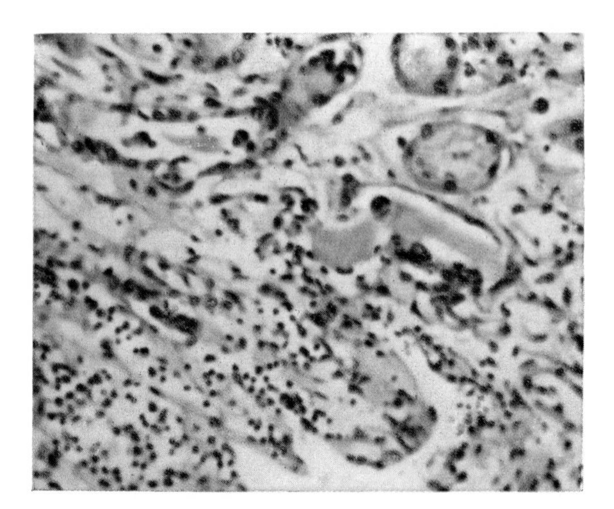

TUBULAR RUPTURE

FIGURE 14. *Stain:* Masson trichrome. A nonpigmented cast found in the process of extrusion from a ruptured tubule. The cells of the tubule show pyknosis and reduplication of nuclei. X 250

infiltrate tended to be most marked in the neighborhood of the blood vessels and also to run in strands between the straight tubules. Edema, though usually present, was rarely a conspicuous feature (Fig. 12). As days passed, the zone of inflammatory infiltration widened and new foci appeared both in the cortex and the medulla. In the former, they tended to be concentrated about the distal convoluted tubules. In a few of the most severe lesions, a clearly-defined second zone of inflammatory infiltration was noted in the outer millimeter of the cortex beneath the capsule (Fig. 13).

Tubular Rupture

The distinctive phenomenon of tubular rupture was generally apparent in any well-developed lesion from the fifth day onward. It was usually associated with the presence of hyaline, non-pigmented casts in the affected segment, which was most commonly the ascending limb but sometimes the distal convoluted tubule. These casts were chromophobic with hematoxylin and eosin or phosphotungstic acid hematoxylin, but stained a fairly bright green in the Masson trichrome. In the affected segments containing the casts, portions of the epithelial lining and of the underlying basement membrane disappeared without trace as if by solution. The casts at this point were frequently seen half within the tubular remnant and half extruded into the stroma (Fig. 14).

Interstitial Granulomas

In the process of tubular rupture and cast extrusion, the advancing margin of the cast abutting on the stromal cells was quickly surrounded by histiocytes. With further extrusion or with complete destruction of the tubular segment, the cast became completely surrounded by histiocytes which occasionally but rarely fused to form giant cells (Figs. 15 and 16). The histiocytes soon invaded the cast and appeared to break it up into comparatively small fragments. It was possible to observe all stages from the original encapsulation to complete disintegration, leaving a focal aggregate of histiocytes with no trace of the original cast material (Fig. 17).

Although this process unquestionably accounts for many, perhaps for most, of the granulomatous lesions found in these kidneys, the evidence is inadequate to prove that it was the only mechanism for their formation. Granulomas were frequently found in the walls of veins and occasionally in the capsule of the kidney, separated from the nearest tubule by apparently intact fibrous tissue of considerable density. Some of these lesions were quite similar in appearance to the Aschoff bodies of rheumatic fever.

Hyaline masses, indistinguishable from the intratubular casts by any staining method tried, were also occasionally found in the walls of veins, even jutting into the lumen to become the basis for thrombus formation (Fig. 18). The question whether these represent extruded casts which have wandered surprisingly from their original location or which have developed in situ in some entirely different manner cannot be answered at present. It is of interest that on only one occasion in over 200 cases studied did the author note extrusion of a pigment cast and consequent granuloma formation.

Thrombophlebitis

In a considerable proportion of cases of 5 or more days' duration, thrombi were readily found in the large but thin-walled veins of the corticomedullary junction. These thrombi were attached to a portion of the vein wall and they jutted into and narrowed but almost never occluded the lumen. Beneath some points of attachment a mass of hyaline material as described in the preceding

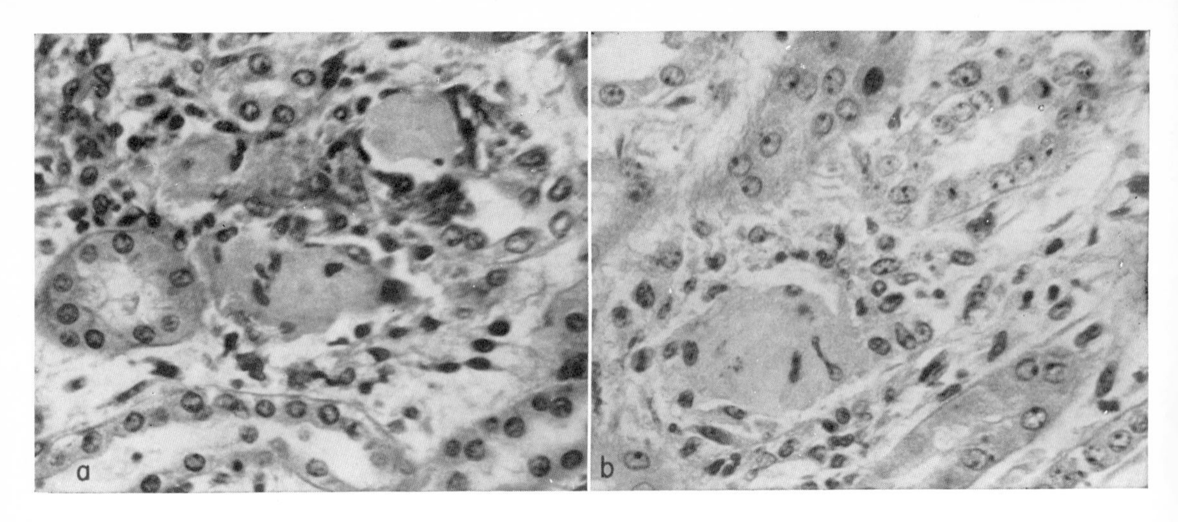

Interstitial Granulomas

FIGURE 15. (*Left*) A granulomatous reaction is developing around several extruded casts. *Stain:* Masson trichrome. X 250

FIGURE 16.—(*Right*) Beginning collection of histiocytes about an extruded hyaline cast and invasion of the cast by the same cells. The adjacent tubule shows a mitotic figure. *Stain:* Phosphotungstic acid hematoxylin. X 250

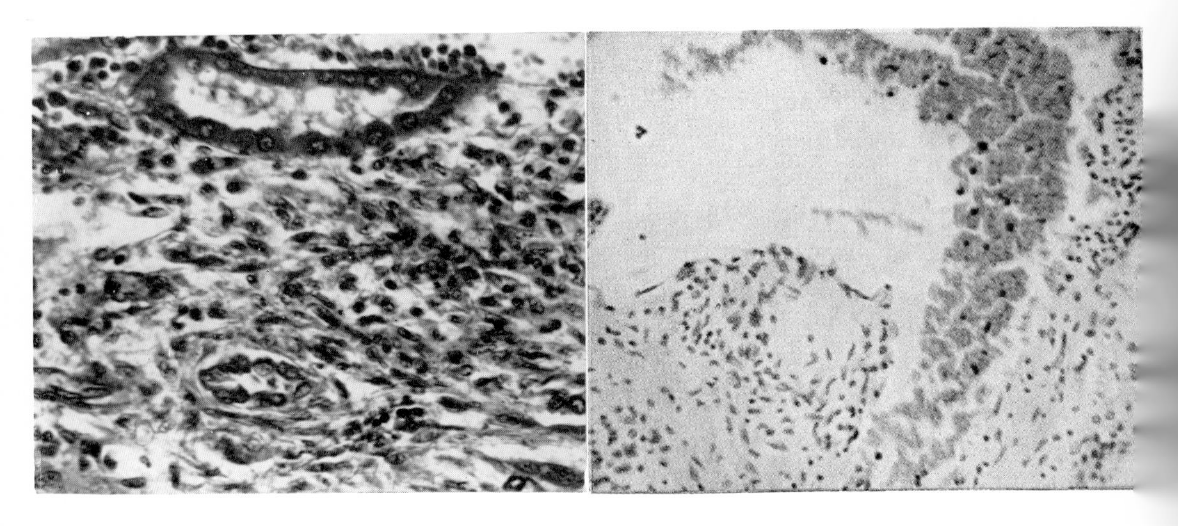

FIGURE 17. (*Left*) Severe granulomatous inflammatory reaction between the straight tubules. No trace of an extruded cast persists. *Stain:* Masson trichrome. X 250

FIGURE 18. (*Right*) *Stain:* Hematoxylin and eosin. Wall of a vein showing a hyaline mass resembling an extruded cast projecting into the lumen with a surrounding granulomatous reaction. X 150

paragraph was found; beneath others were well-developed granulomas with or without traces of hyaline material. The vein walls were frequently invaded by lymphocytes, polymorphonuclear leukocytes, or eosinophils, apparently extending from focal concentrations of the interstitial infiltrate, such concentrations being characteristically clustered about these veins.

Summary of Histologic Findings in Chronologic Sequence

The earliest change noted in the "shock kidney" was lipoid degeneration of the ascending limbs of the loops of Henle, which usually made its appearance about 18 hours after injury, progressed in severity until the third day, then tended to wane. Precipitation of the hemoglobin-like pigment in the distal convoluted and collecting tubules was infrequently observed short of 24 hours and was inconstant before 48 hours. The pigment at first stained like hemoglobin but later lost this characteristic. Moderate dilatation of the proximal convoluted tubules was evident following the development of pigment casts.

By the third and fourth days, an interstitial inflammatory infiltrate and frank necrobiotic changes in the cells of the ascending limbs were occasionally seen, and from the fifth day onward both of these findings were constant. Rarely on the third or fourth day, but usually by the fifth, tubular rupture with extrusion of nonpigmented casts was apparent, and coincidentally stromal granulomas were found in moderate numbers. From the fifth day onward, thrombophlebitis of the small veins was found in an increasing proportion of the cases.

Gross Pathology

The kidney might or might not show gross abnormalities (Figs. 19, 20, 21, and 22). Enlargement was noted as early as the second day but was not usual before the fourth. It tended to become more frequent and more extensive with duration of the lesion; the largest pair of kidneys observed, 625 grams, was found in Case 93 with the unusual survival period of 13 days. In patients with from 7- to 10-day survival periods, kidneys weighing up to 500 grams were usual (Figs. 20 and 21).

Enlarged kidneys were almost without exception pale, whereas kidneys of normal size, regardless of duration of the lesion, were usually congested. On section it became apparent that the enlargement was chiefly due to swelling

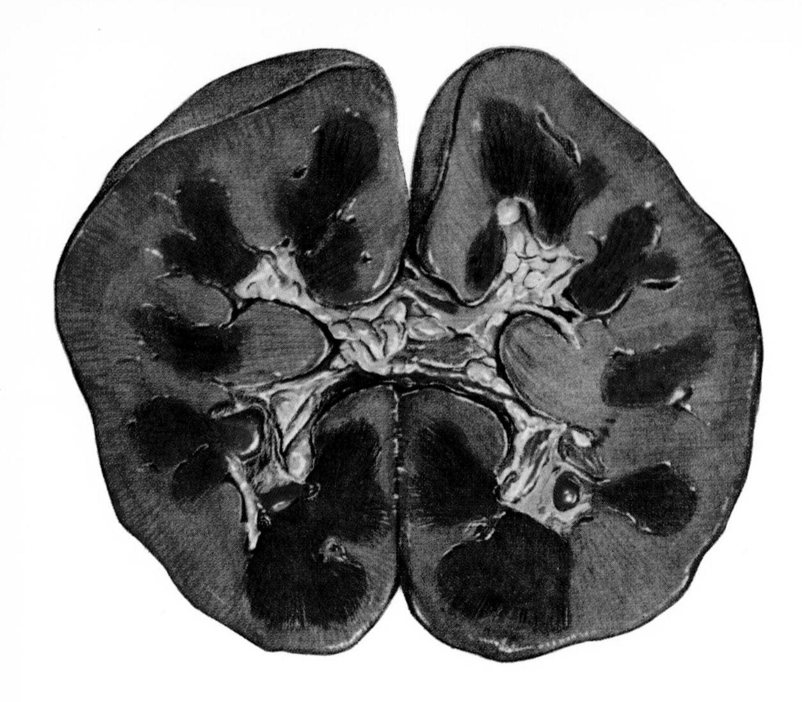

Gross Appearance of the Crush Kidney

FIGURE 19. Kidney from Case 70. Death from crush syndrome 4 days after injury. The pyramids are dark in color, resembling mahogany. The kidney is normal in size and not swollen.

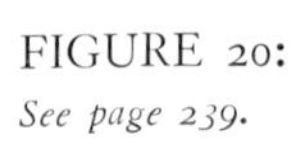

FIGURE 20:
See page 239.

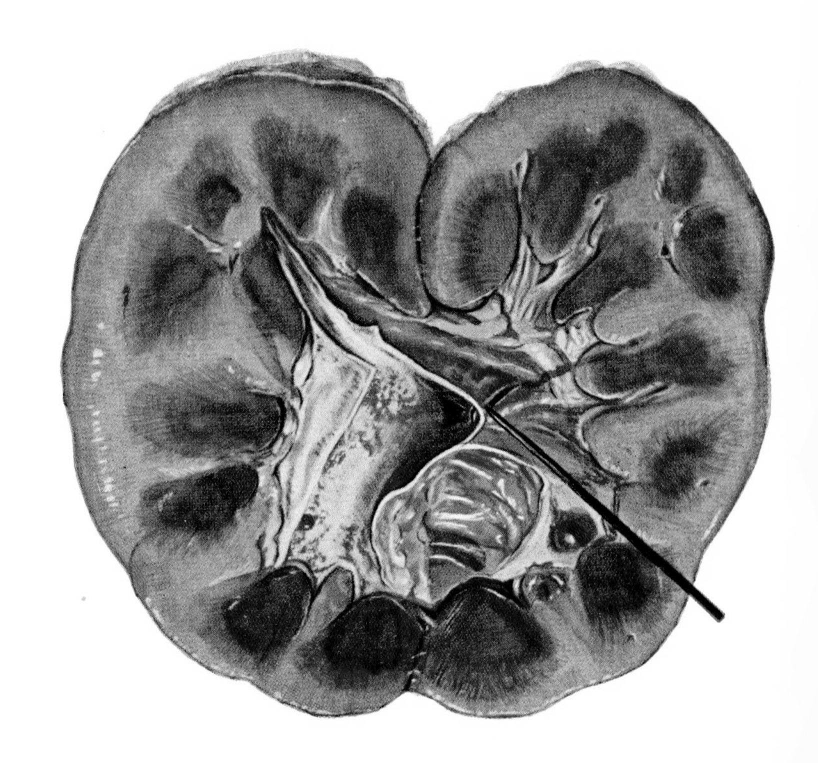

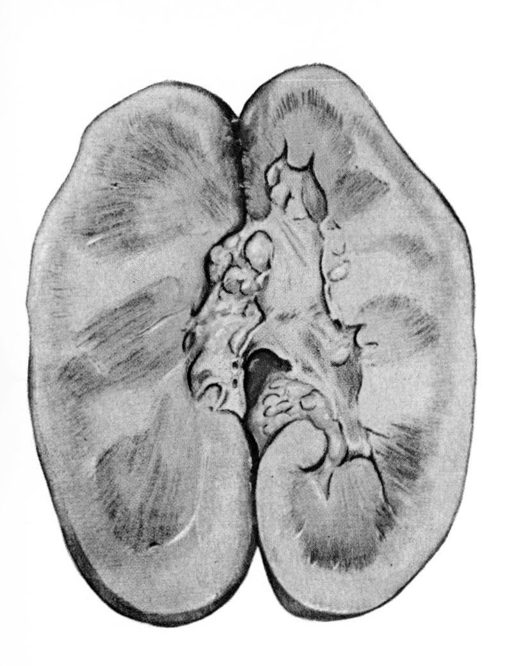

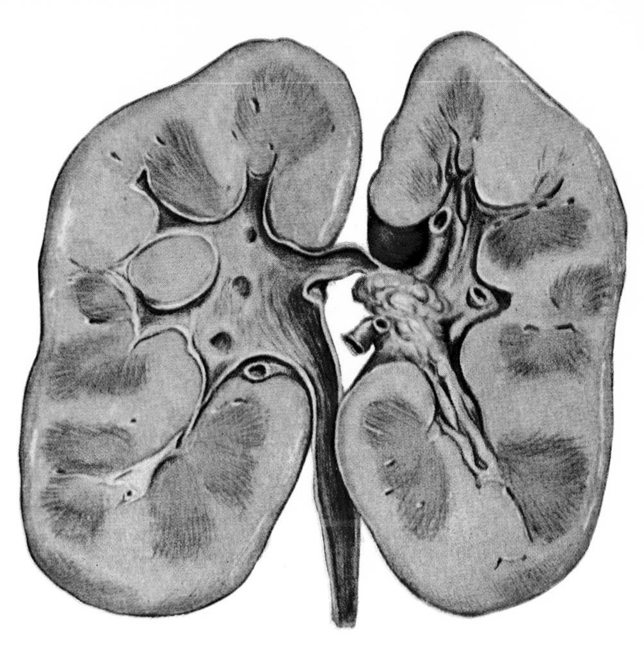

FIGURE 21. (*Left*) Kidney from Case 47 after brief fixation in Kaiserling's fluid. The patient died of pigment nephropathy 8 days after wounding. The pallor of the organ is slightly exaggerated by the fixation. The cortex is swollen and the pyramids are almost chocolate in shade.

FIGURE 22. (*Right*) Left kidney from case of mismatched transfusion (Case 9) after similar fixation in Kaiserling's fluid. Gross appearance is identical with that of Case 47 except for size. The enlargement of this left kidney was partly due to a congenital hypoplasia of its mate.

of the cortex, which would measure from 9 to 12 microns in thickness. The corticomedullary junction was unusually sharp, since the cortex was pale and the pyramids either unchanged or darker than normal. A zone of intense congestion sometimes further intensified the distinction. A constant finding was the unusual wetness of the freshly cut cortical surface.

Petechial hemorrhages beneath the pelvic mucosa were the only other gross manifestation which was at all frequent (Fig. 20). They were commonest in cases of long duration with high grades of azotemia and are reminiscent of similar hemorrhagic changes in advanced "decompensated" nephrosclerosis with renal insufficiency. They may be merely a phenomenon of the uremic state.

FIGURE 20. Kidney from Case 69. Death from crush syndrome 10 days after injury. The organ is markedly swollen. The pallor of the cortex is in striking contrast to the still dark pyramids. Fine hemorrhages are apparent beneath the mucosa of the renal pelvis. *Page 238*

Pathogenesis

Shock

Two factors which are evidently of outstanding importance in the development of the renal lesion may appear in severely traumatized persons. One is pigment excretion in the urine and the other is the physiologic state known as shock. A survey of the first hundred cases of pigment nephropathy studied at the 15th Medical General Laboratory provided interesting figures regarding the relative frequency of the lesion in different types of Army hospitals. In base hospitals (station and general hospitals), nephropathy was found in only 6 percent of the necropsies, in evacuation hospitals the percentage rose to 18, and in the field hospitals (to which only the most severely wounded, non-transportable cases were admitted) to 30 percent. Clearly pigment nephropathy occurred in direct relation to severity of injury and, by implication, to the profundity of shock.

The cases studied by the Board offer more direct evidence. Whenever possible, a clinician who was a member of the Board made the examination and recorded his impression regarding the presence and severity of shock. When shock was recognized, it was classified as slight, moderate, or severe. In 183 cases so classified pigment nephrosis was proved at necropsy in thirty-seven. (There were actually 38 proved cases in the Board's entire series, but 1 had not been classified as to degree of shock.) Their distribution in the various shock categories is shown in Table 92.

The decreasing frequency of renal involvement from those with marked shock to those with lesser degrees of shock is apparent, but the six patients

TABLE 92.—RELATIONSHIP OF PROVED PIGMENT NEPHROPATHY TO DEGREE OF SHOCK

Degree of Shock	Number of Cases	Fatal Nephropathies	Percentage
Severe	57	20	35.1
Moderate	55	7	12.7
Slight	37	4	10.8
None	34	6	17.6

who were not considered to be in shock confuse the picture. This group, which consists of Cases 9, 22, 69, 70, 120, and 132, is therefore considered in detail.

"No Shock" Group.—Case 9 is an example of a frank transfusion accident. Between 100 and 125 cc. of group A blood had been given in error to a group O recipient before a characteristic reaction developed and the transfusion was interrupted. Hemoglobinemia and hemoglobinuria were demonstrated. This case belongs in a different category and requires no further consideration.

The patient in Case 22 did not present evidence of shock at the time of entry to the hospital 3 hours after wounding, or at any subsequent period of observation. He belonged to blood group A and received 2 units of blood, presumably group A, not from the theater blood bank and not checked by any member of the Board. There was no clinical evidence of reaction to these transfusions which were given on the fourth day of disease, only 2 days before his death. On the following day the nonprotein nitrogen level in the plasma was 294 mg. per 100 cc., so the renal lesion must have antedated these transfusions. The three early transfusions on the day of wounding were of the usual theater bank blood and were given without incident. The Rh reaction of the patient was not determined. No etiology for a hemolytic reaction was discovered, yet large amounts of free hemoglobin, 193 mg. per 100 cc., were found in the bladder urine at the time of necropsy.

Cases 69, 70, and 132 are examples of the crush syndrome with severe grades of myoglobinuria. Judged by the usual clinical criteria—blood pressure, pulse, pallor, coldness of extremities, anxiety—these patients did not impress the examiner as being in shock. Each of them, however, clearly exhibited one phenomenon which is emphasized by many students of shock: hemoconcentration, as shown by hematocrit values of 71, 80, and 57, respectively. If shock itself was not present, there is no doubt that a closely allied physiologic abnormality was.

In Case 120 the patient was wounded in the right thigh by a shell fragment which completely transected the femoral artery, vein, and nerve. Hemorrhage was severe and he was given 1,000 cc. of plasma en route to the hospital. On arrival he seemed in good condition and was operated upon without further preparation, but 1,500 cc. of whole blood were given during the operation. Immediately after operation the blood pressure was 110 mm. Hg systolic and 62 diastolic, but 7 hours later it dropped to 70/40 and throughout the day the systolic level ranged between 60 and 70 millimeters of mercury. Nevertheless the patient's color was good and his skin remained warm. The pathologist has the temerity to suggest that in consideration of this case also shock can scarcely be excluded.

Pigment Excretion

In Chapter IV it was shown that *all* patients with clinical evidence of renal involvement following traumatic injury excreted benzidine-positive pigment in the urine, although the amounts varied widely. In excellent correlation with this observation is the histologic evidence of pigment precipitation in the lower nephron segments of all patients with fatal nephropathy. These related phenomena deserve further consideration.

The Nature of the Pigment

Numerous clinical studies[9 10 11] have established the two pigments found in the urine as hemoglobin and the closely related myoglobin. In histologic sections they react identically with all methods employed (the benzidine reaction, hematoxylin and eosin, Masson's trichrome and Mallory's phosphotungstic acid hematoxylin stains). It has generally been considered a safe inference that the pigment casts found in the tubules were precipitates of the same material spectroscopically identified in its soluble form in the urine, though the possibility that they might be oxidized or otherwise chemically altered forms could not be excluded. Harrison et al.[12] provided spectroscopic proof that in the lesions produced in dogs by arsine hemolysis the casts consisted predominantly of methemoglobin. No pigments such as hemochromagen or hematin which would be insoluble at the pH of urine were formed.

Efforts to identify myoglobin by chemical means in the kidneys of patients who died of the crush syndrome were disappointingly unsuccessful. (See Ap-

[9] Bywaters, E. G. L.; Delory, G. E.; Rimington, C., and Smiles, J.: Myohaemoglobin in urine of air raid casualties with crushing injury. Biochem. J. **35**: 1164–1168, November 1941.

[10] Maegraith, B. G.; Havard, R. E., and Parsons, D. S.: Renal syndrome of wide distribution induced possibly by renal anoxia. Lancet **2**: 293–296, September 8, 1945.

[11] Minami, S.: Über Nierenveränderungen nach Verschüttung. Virchow's Arch. f. path. Anat. **245**: 246–267, 1923.

[12] Harrison, H. E.; Bunting, H.; Ordway, N. K., and Albrink, W. S.: The pathogenesis of renal injury produced in the dog by hemoglobin or methemoglobin. J. Exp. Med. **86**: 339–356, October 1947.

pendix C for the method used.) The data are presented in the following tabulation.

Extraction of Myoglobin from Kidneys

Type of case	*Case No.*	*Gm. of myoglobin per Kg. of tissue*
Control (sudden death)	A	0.40
	B	0.50
Shock, no pigment casts	19	2.45
	77	1.80
Shock, pigment nephropathy	65	1.18
	66	1.30
	80	1.50
Crush syndrome	69	0.45
	70	0.60
	78	0.93

It is obvious that the kidneys in the crush cases, which one might reasonably expect to be loaded with myoglobin, did not show significantly more than those in cases of sudden death selected as controls; actually they contained considerably less myoglobin than did the kidneys in shock cases with or without nephropathy in which the urine never contained myoglobin. It seems probable that this failure to recover myoglobin correlates with the fairly rapid alteration in the staining reactions of the pigment in the lower nephron segments already described and may be attributed to a chemical degradation. Under field conditions it was impractical to attempt further identification of these products.

Acidity of the Urine and Precipitation of Pigment in the Tubules

One widely accepted explanation of the development of a pigment nephropathy is that the pigment is precipitated from solution when the glomerular filtrate becomes acid in reaction upon reaching the distal convoluted tubule. It is of interest to compare the acidity of the initial pigment-containing urines from patients in whom nephropathy was proved with those from patients with no evidence of a renal lesion other than pigment excretion. A control group in which the urine was consistently free from benzidine-positive material is also compared in Table 93 with the two pigment-containing groups.

956507 O—52——17

The ranges overlap widely, and the differences in the means are slight and not significant. Acidity of the urine can be eliminated as the determining factor in precipitation of pigment in the lower nephron. With acidity eliminated, we are left without explanation for the phenomenon of pigment precipitation. Presumably it is due to some change in renal physiology, particularly prone to occur in, but not limited to shock. Possibly it is nothing more remarkable than stagnation of the glomerular filtrate secondary to the renal ischemia which is known to be present. Possibly it is due to increased concentration of some unknown, perhaps abnormal, metabolic product as suggested by Oliver.[13]

TABLE 93.—URINE pH IN PIGMENT GROUPS AND CONTROL GROUP

Type of Case	Number of Specimens	Range of pH	Mean pH
Nephropathy	35	5.0 to 6.9	5.84±0.48
Pigment without Nephropathy	27	5.0 to 8.4	6.17±0.63
No Pigment or Nephropathy	39	5.2 to 8.2	6.25±0.61

One is tempted to speculate upon the possibility of a reciprocal relationship between the degree of shock and pigment concentration in relation to nephropathy: When pigment excretion is great, as in the crush syndrome, some burns, and transfusion accidents, little or no shock is necessary; when shock is severe and prolonged, minimal pigment excretion may be required. Many of our data would appear to support this concept, but the exceptions are too numerous and striking to permit such a conclusion.

Clinicopathologic Correlation

Any attempt to correlate form and function in the kidney is hazardous in the extreme, but its fascination is irresistible. The first effect of shock upon the function of the kidney is oliguria, followed quickly by retention of metabolic products which are both nitrogenous, such as urea and creatinine, and inor-

[13] OLIVER, J.: New directions in renal morphology; method, its results and its future. Harvey Lect. (1944-1945) 40: 102–155, 1945.

ganic, such as phosphates. Both of these effects were manifested within a few hours of the onset of shock, whereas the first recognizable morphologic change, the appearance of lipoid vacuoles in the ascending loops, developed about 18 hours after onset, and pigment casts appeared still later. The initial renal insufficiency is, therefore, functional rather than structural in basis. The studies of Cournand and his associates[14] have established the early onset of renal ischemia in shock and adequately explain the initial functional changes.

Ischemia with consequent anoxemia also serves as a logical explanation of the appearance of demonstrable lipid in the parenchymal cells. As will be shown in Chapter XII, a similar phenomenon in shock was found in the liver, the heart, and other organs in which the relationship of fatty degeneration to anoxemia has received more attention. Further knowledge of renal circulation and of the relative susceptibility of various portions of the nephron to anoxemia is necessary to an understanding of the localization of the changes. The hypothesis of Trueta et al.[15] that blood is shunted from the cortex into the vasa recta of the pyramids is not a satisfactory explanation, since the degenerative changes were maximal in the very areas which, according to his theory, receive the largest quantities of blood.

The lipoid vacuolation became more intense on the second and third days after the onset of shock. This, however, cannot be interpreted as evidence that the initial causative factor necessarily persisted. A form of "chain reaction" which required time for its complete development may have been inaugurated by the initial insult.

An interesting feature of the development of the "shock kidney" is the apparent delay in the appearance of the pigmented casts. Pigment casts were present in significant numbers in only two of the nine Board cases in which death occurred within 48 hours of injury. Even in Cases 32 and 34, in which death occurred between the second and third days, only traces of pigment could be found. It is obvious from examination of the histories of this group that none of them, with the possible exception of one (Case 34), was ever adequately resuscitated from shock. In the case records of scores of other fatal shock cases

[14] Cournand, A.; Riley, R. L.; Bradley, S. E.; Breed, E. S.; Noble, R. P.; Lauson, H. D.; Gregersen, M. I., and Richards, D. W.: Studies of the circulation in clinical shock. Surgery **13**: 964–995, June 1943.

[15] Trueta, J.; Barclay, A. E.; Daniel, P.; Franklin, K. J., and Prichard, M. M. L.: Renal pathology in the light of recent neurovascular studies. [Preliminary communication.] Lancet **2**: 237–238, August 17, 1946.

reviewed in the Pathology Section of the 15th Medical Laboratory as controls, unless there had been a transfusion accident, pigment casts were seldom recorded when death had occurred short of 24 hours, although in one burn case they were numerous at 14 hours. They were not seen with any regularity until from 36 to 48 hours had elapsed since injury.

A simple explanation for this phenomenon which invokes no new mechanism would be the suppression of glomerular filtration during shock, either because of the depressed systemic blood pressure or because of specific renal ischemia. The presence of pigment casts, therefore, may logically be considered histologic evidence of glomerular function, either continued or at least temporarily resumed.

Functional Significance of the Pigment Casts

Although it is certain that the pigment casts play no role in the initiation of renal insufficiency following shock, no such dogmatism is possible in defining their possible effect in the later stages of the lesion. Controversy has hinged on the thesis that the casts cause suppression of urine primarily by mechanical blockage of the tubules. The morphologic evidence for this is inconclusive. It is suggested by the high proportion of apparently blocked tubules in many cases and by the dilatation of portions of the nephron proximal to the cast. In our cases dilatation of moderate degree was a fairly constant phenomenon from the third day onward. It was not seen in the absence of casts, and the possibility of a mechanical block cannot be denied. The number of pigmented casts varied widely from case to case, but their number was difficult to estimate in routine sections and we did not use serial sections or microdissection to confirm our impressions of the proportion of occluded nephrons. It is doubtful that they were numerous enough to explain the almost complete urinary suppression in certain cases. Experimental evidence that the glomeruli of nephrons whose tubules are plugged with pigmented casts are nonfunctional was provided by Harrison et al.[16] in the study on dogs previously cited.

It is interesting that in other forms of renal disease, chronic glomerular nephritis and lipoid nephrosis for instance, casts form in the nephrons but are readily swept in great numbers into the urine. In pigment nephropathy, al-

[16] See footnote 12.

though casts may regularly be found in the sediment, it is rare that large numbers of them are passed.

Tubular Degeneration

The initial evidence of tubular degeneration has invariably been fat vacuoles in the ascending limbs of Henle's loops and less regularly in the distal convoluted tubules. This change evidently antedated and was independent of pigment precipitation, since it was frequently seen in the absence of the latter. By the fourth and fifth days lipid tended to disappear from the tubules, but frank necrosis and regeneration of the epithelium became evident and affected the same segment of the nephron. These phenomena were never observed in the shock cases in the absence of pigment precipitation, although in sulfonamide injury to the kidney they were occasionally seen without pigment. Although the pigment deposit appears to be a sine qua non, the mechanism of its effect is obviously indirect, since the maximal degenerative change occurred at a higher level in the nephron than did the first pigment deposits. Degeneration was most pronounced in the ascending limbs, whereas pigment deposits began in the distal convoluted tubules.

The functional significance of this tubular degeneration is of interest. In lipoid nephrosis extensive tubular degeneration is associated with oliguria. It has been suggested that the injured tubular cells permit rediffusion of the glomerular filtrate back into the vascular system. In pigment nephropathy tubular degeneration was constant, and such a mechanism may be involved in this syndrome as well. One point of difference between the two syndromes should be noted, however, before accepting the hypothesis. In lipoid nephrosis the gravity of the urine is well maintained or even concentrated above usual limits. In pigment nephropathy fixation at a low level is almost constant. This could be readily explained by the theory of mechanical blockage, since only a few unobstructed nephrons can still function.

The focal rupture of tubules, so frequently noted from the fifth day onward, has, in the author's opinion, little functional significance. It is a late phenomenon, whereas the entire syndrome—oliguria, azotemia, pigment excretion, and hypertension, together with fixation of gravity—is established before it appears. Furthermore, if actual extravasation of glomerular filtrate occurred through these ruptures, it seems inevitable that interstitial edema would be a more conspicuous feature of the histologic process.

SUMMARY

A clinicopathologic survey of necropsy findings in 60 severely wounded casualties provided 38 examples of lower nephron nephrosis in all stages of development. The initial change, appearing from 18 to 24 hours after injury, was found to be lipoid degeneration of a segment of the nephron, particularly the ascending limb of Henle's loop, less markedly the distal convoluted tubule. The second stage was the precipitation of pigment, either hemoglobin or myoglobin, in the distal convoluted and collecting tubules, seldom occurring short of 24 hours after injury, more commonly between 32 and 72 hours. Moderate dilatation of proximal and sometimes distal convoluted tubules followed pigment precipitation. Sometimes on the third, regularly on the fourth and fifth days, necrosis and regeneration of epithelium in the ascending limbs and distal tubules became evident, and simultaneously lymphocytes appeared between the tubules and about the vessels. From five days onward, rupture of tubules with herniation of their contents into the stroma and consequent granuloma formation became frequent. The last development in many cases was the formation of nonocclusive mural thrombi in many of the small, thin-walled veins.

In clinicopathologic correlation it was shown that two factors were constant in the nephropathy cases, inconstant in the remainder. These are (1) the excretion of benzidine-positive pigment in the urine, and (2) (with one apparent exception) a state of shock or, at least, a related physiologic abnormality.

Renal insufficiency was found to antedate all structural change, but was never progressive in the absence of a demonstrable pigment nephropathy. The effects of myoglobin and of hemoglobin precipitation upon the kidney were indistinguishable. Our evidence does not support the hypothesis that acidity of the urine is the factor responsible for pigment precipitation in the nephrons.

Although pigment precipitation is an essential factor in the development of the "shock kidney," the mechanism of its effect upon the kidney remains unexplained. The possibility that it is in part mechanical cannot be disregarded, but the complex chain of degenerative and inflammatory phenomena demands another explanation. Controlled experimentation will be necessary before many of these uncertainties can be resolved.

For Cases of Special Interest in this chapter, see page 282.

CHAPTER X

Sulfonamides in Relation to "Shock Kidney"

No discussion of renal failure in the wounded of World War II would be complete without consideration of the possible role of sulfonamide injury of the kidneys. Two forms of this type of injury are generally recognized. One is the purely mechanical process of crystalluria, with precipitation of the crystals in the ureters, renal pelves, and perhaps in some instances in the collecting tubules. The second is a more complex process involving true parenchymal damage to the kidney; it appears to be relatively independent of dosage and is believed by many to belong in the category of hypersensitive reactions along with other recognized sulfonamide lesions such as dermatitis, myocarditis, and pneumonitis.

The problem is difficult because this renal lesion is a characteristic lower nephron nephrosis, usually although not invariably associated with the precipitation of hemoglobin-like products in the tubules and hence indistinguishable from transfusion kidney, crush kidney, or shock kidney. With present knowledge, distinction is impossible on the basis of renal morphology.

Sulfonamide Therapy in Battle Casualties

During the period in which the cases studied by the Board were collected, sulfonamides were still extensively used in forward installations (aid stations, collecting stations, and clearing stations) in the Fifth Army Area, although their use in hospitals had greatly diminished with the arrival of large supplies of penicillin. In the aid stations a sulfonamide dressing almost universally was applied. This might or might not be supplemented by indeterminate amounts of sulfonamide powder dusted onto or into the wounds, and more of the drug by mouth, the most frequent total oral dose being 4 grams. In the field and evacuation hospitals, sulfonamide therapy usually was stopped and penicillin substituted. Notable exceptions, however, were in some cases of abdominal wounds with incipient peritonitis. Many surgeons placed from 5 to 10 Gm. of sulfadiazine in the abdominal cavity before closing it, and some continued sulfonamide treatment by mouth for several days. There was no standard practice since this was considered a matter for individual surgical judgment.

Blood Sulfonamide Levels

Relationship to Sulfonamide Intake

Blood sulfonamide levels were determined in 50 of our patients. The tests were made for free sulfonamide only, whereas the total of free and acetylated blood sulfonamide would probably have been a more valuable index of sulfonamide retention by the kidney. As would be expected, there seemed to be a general relationship between the blood levels of the drug and the quantity administered, as shown in Table 94. However, the fluctuations within each group are too great and the number of cases is too small to justify further analysis. It is noteworthy that no patient tested failed to show at least a trace of sulfonamide in the blood stream, and in two of six patients with no recorded chemotherapy, levels of 7.0 and 10.6 mg. per 100 cc. were observed. Furthermore, characteristic sulfonamide crystals were found at necropsy in the renal tubules in several other patients with no history of exposure to sulfonamide

TABLE 94.—BLOOD SULFONAMIDE LEVELS IN 50 PATIENTS

Mode of Therapy	Number of Cases	Blood Sulfonamide Level mg. per 100 cc.		
		Minimum	Maximum	Mean
Dressing only	12	0.2	* 2.4	1.4
Dressing and powder	7	0.2	5.0	1.9
Dressing, powder, and 4 Gm. orally	12	0.2	9.7	2.5
Intraperitoneal	5	3.8	27.0	12.2
Continued oral	8	3.5	51.6	11.8
No history of therapy	6	0.1	10.6	3.7

* The maximum was actually 9.7 in one case, but this case is excluded from the average because the figure is completely out of line and it seems certain that the patient must have received oral sulfonamide medication which was not recorded.

and no records of chemical tests for it. The only possible conclusions are that the records were grossly unreliable so far as sulfonamide therapy was concerned, and that, regardless of their histories, virtually all of these patients must have received some sulfonamide therapy.

Relationship to Renal Insufficiency

The 50 patients on whom blood sulfonamide levels were determined were classified on the basis of urinary suppression and nonprotein nitrogen level (with or without high azotemia). In the upper two quarters of Chart 38 the patients have been divided into those with normal urinary output and those with oliguria. In the lower two the separation is on the basis of nitrogen retention.

CHART 38. BLOOD SULFONAMIDE LEVELS IN 50 PATIENTS CLASSIFIED ACCORDING TO URINE OUTPUT AND NITROGEN RETENTION

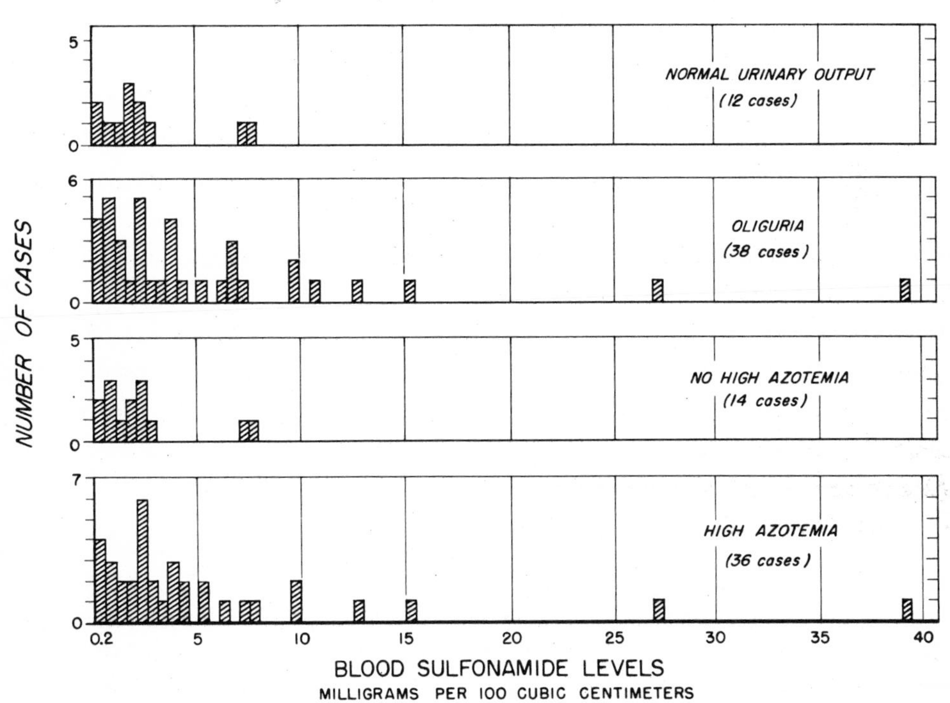

Two cases in the high azotemia group are not shown on the chart. Determinations in both cases were above 40 mg. per 100 cc., the maximal level reached being 51.6 mg. per 100 cubic centimeters.

956507 O—52——18

It is evident that blood sulfonamide levels above 8 mg. per 100 cc. were observed only in patients suffering from oliguria, or high azotemia, or both. Attempts at closer analysis are disappointingly inconclusive. The average blood sulfonamide level in 36 azotemic patients was 5.7 mg. per 100 cc. as compared with 2.3 mg. per 100 cc. in the control group of 14, but again the variations are too wide in proportion to the number of samples to warrant statistical analysis. The mean blood sulfonamide level in 38 oliguric patients was 5.4 and in 12 without oliguria, 2.5 milligrams per 100 cubic centimeters.

The results are similar when the cases are divided, in an attempt to exclude the influence of variation in dosage, into two groups as follows: Group A, those patients who had external medication only, and Group B, those who received internal medication (oral, intraperitoneal, or intravenous). Eight patients could not be classified because of inadequate information regarding therapy. Of the 18 patients in Group A, 12 were azotemic, 6 were not. The mean blood sulfonamide level in the former was 1.7 mg. per 100 cc., with a standard error of ±1.1; of the latter 1.32 with a standard error of ±0.8. Obviously the difference is not significant. In Group B, 17 azotemic patients showed a mean blood sulfonamide level of 7.8 mg. per 100 cc., with a range of 0.4 to 39; and 7 patients with no azotemia, a level of 3.7 mg. per 100 cc., with a range of 0.2 to 7.8. With a range of this magnitude in such a small number of cases, the calculation of standard errors has little meaning. Similar results followed efforts to establish any correlation of average blood sulfonamide levels with oliguria.

Very high blood sulfonamide levels (10 mg. per 100 cc. or higher) were seen only in patients with symptoms of renal insufficiency. Nothing in this relationship serves to distinguish between cause and effect. It is obvious, however, that with continued administration of a drug eliminated almost solely by the kidney, its level in the blood must mount with the onset of renal insufficiency. Two cases are worthy of individual attention.

Cases in Point

Case 21.—This patient was not a battle casualty. As treatment for a urethral discharge, the patient medicated himself with 12 Gm. of sulfathiazole in 24 hours. The following day ureteral colic developed. Crystalline concretions were observed in both ureteral orifices on cystoscopy. He was treated by pelvic lavage and had no further symptoms. It is evident that his trouble was purely mechanical.

Case 90.—This patient was a battle casualty; a severe abdominal wound had resulted in evisceration of several loops of bowel, perforation of the diaphragm, and lacerations of the liver and right kidney. The patient was in moderate shock on entry to the hospital. For the first week postoperatively he voided adequate quantities of urine and did not show nitrogen retention, but he was febrile. On the ninth day signs of consolidation developed in the lower lobe of the left lung. He was given 66 Gm. of sulfadiazine between the seventh and twelfth days. Within 24 hours the plasma nonprotein nitrogen level rose to 143 mg. per 100 cc. and later to 166 mg. per 100 cc., and the blood sulfonamide level to 51.6 mg. per 100 cc. (free sulfonamide 34.4, acetylated 17.2). Following cessation of sulfonamide therapy, the nonprotein nitrogen level fell to 41 mg. per 100 cc. in the course of 17 days. Oliguria did not develop during the period of nitrogen retention. It is possible that this may have been a case of sulfonamide injury of the renal parenchyma, but the relative importance of the simultaneous spreading infection cannot be assessed.

One other line of argument must be explored before conclusion. As was stated in the introduction, there are reasons for believing that the sulfonamide form of lower nephron nephrosis is dependent upon hypersensitivity. One reason for this belief is the frequent association of this lesion with inflammatory lesions of other tissues and organs; for example, dermatitis, myocarditis, interstitial pancreatitis, hepatitis, arteritis, and a form of pneumonitis. In the present series of cases, the only such associated lesion observed was pneumonitis. It is the personal opinion of the writer (T.B.M.) that pneumonitis can occur in uremia independently of sulfonamide treatment and that, therefore, its presence cannot be accorded great diagnostic weight.

SUMMARY

Grounds have been found for believing that the records of sulfonamide therapy in the group of battle casualties upon which this report is based were grossly inaccurate, but that it is a reasonable assumption that few if any patients escaped exposure to the drug. Very high blood sulfonamide levels were observed only in patients with renal insufficiency. Except for these extreme instances, the variation in the blood sulfonamide levels was too great in all categories studied to yield reliable correlation between blood level and renal insufficiency. In only two cases did clinical evidence point toward a sulfonamide etiology. A strong argument against such a causative mechanism was the failure to observe any instance of other forms of sulfonamide injury such as arteritis, myocarditis, dermatitis, hepatitis, or pancreatitis.

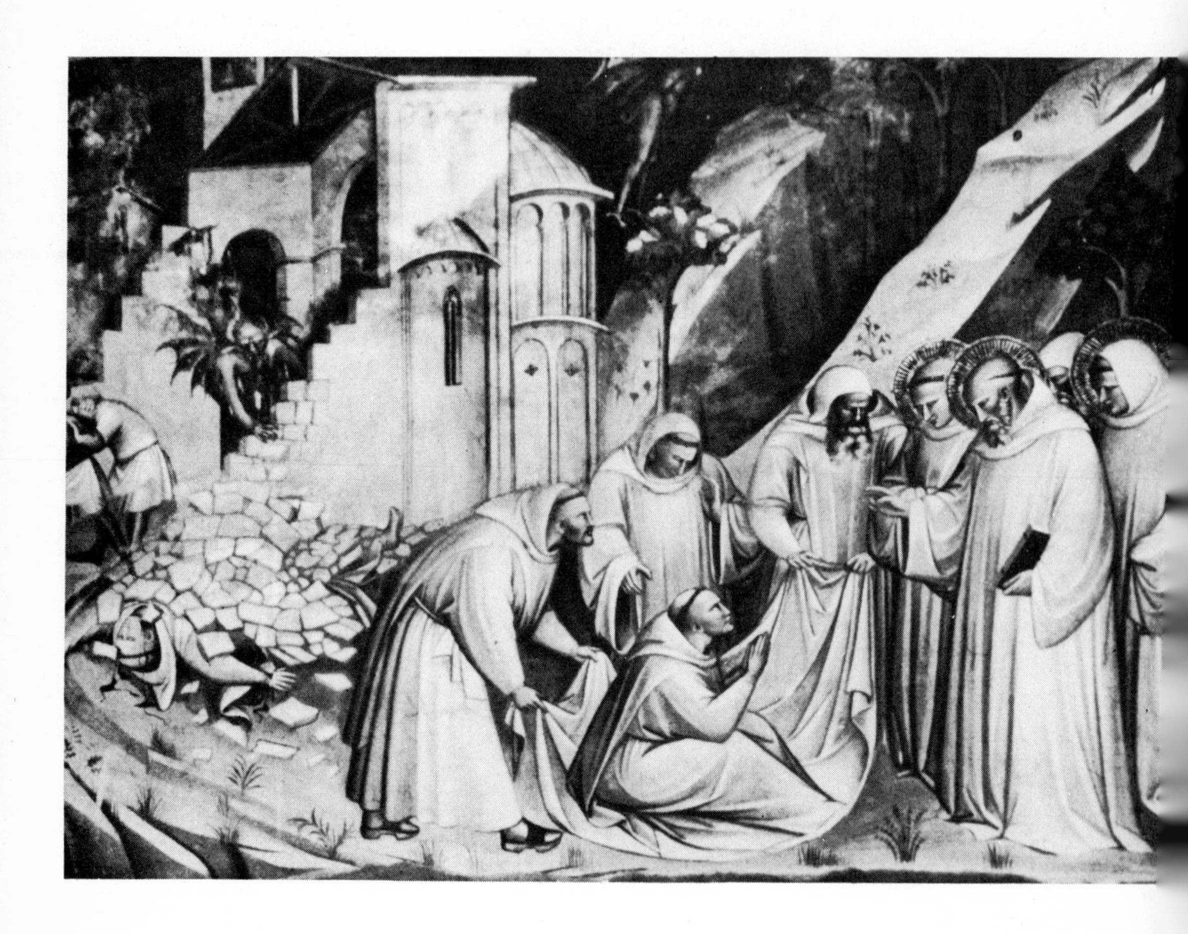

AN EARLY CRUSH CASE. This fresco in the Basilica of San Miniato al Monte, Florence, Italy, by Spinello Aretino, 1387 A.D., depicting construction of the Abbey at Monte Cassino, is perhaps the earliest record of treatment of crush injury. The devil has pushed a wall onto a monk who is then revived by St. Benedict. "Our ministrations were less effective."

CHAPTER XI

The Crush Syndrome in Battle Casualties

In preceding chapters examples of the crush syndrome have been included, frequently with little or no distinction from the more usual types of battle casualties. This group of cases, however, presents certain distinctive features which require separate consideration. Moreover, though cases were reported in the German literature among casualties of World War I, and though Bywaters[1] and others[2,3] have made careful clinical and biochemic studies of many civilian casualties during the "Battle of Britain," few thoroughly studied cases have been recorded among the battle casualties of World War II.

In this chapter the clinical, physiologic, biochemic, and pathologic features and the results of treatment will be discussed on the basis of nine cases, five of which were fatal. All of the patients were crushed within stone houses typical of the Italian countryside. (It is perhaps not a coincidence that the first known description of the syndrome came from Italy in 1908 as a report of casualties of the earthquake at Messina.) Five of the buildings in which the injuries occurred, one of them housing a medical collecting company, were struck by artillery shells. Two of the casualties resulted when a demolition charge exploded and the remaining two were incurred when a house about two hundred yards from our laboratory was struck by a bomb from a German raider at dawn. It was consequently possible to observe the patients virtually from the moment of release from the rubble in which they were partially buried. All nine are listed, together with pertinent data, in Table 95.

[1] Bywaters, E. G. L.: Ischemic muscle necrosis; crushing injury, traumatic edema, crush syndrome, traumatic anuria, compression syndrome: a type of injury seen in air raid casualties following burial beneath débris. J.A.M.A. **124**: 1103–1109, April 15, 1944.

[2] Douglas, J. W. B.: Incidence of signs of renal injury following prolonged burial under débris in an unselected series of 764 air-raid casualties admitted to hospital. Brit. J. Urol. **17**: 142–147, December 1945.

[3] Dunn, J. S.; Gillespie, M., and Niven, J. S. F.: Renal lesions in 2 cases of crush syndrome. Lancet **2**: 549–552, November 8, 1941.

TABLE 95.—DATA CONCERNING 9 PATIENTS WITH CRUSH SYNDROME

Case No.	Age of Patient	Duration of Crush	Time from Release to Hospital Arrival	Time from Release to Administration of First Intravenous Fluid	Parts Affected	Operation	Time from Release to Operation	Patient's Outcome
	yrs.	*hrs.*	*hrs.*	*hrs.*			*hrs.*	
56	25	6	6	<6	Left shoulder, pelvis, both hips .	None	....	Lived.
69	21	3.7	0.3	7.2	Left arm, right forearm, both thighs, left chest wall.	. . . do	....	Died.
70	25	3.8	0.5	9.3	Both buttocks, both thighs . .	. . . do	....	Do.
73	34	3	2	10	Back, right thigh, and leg . . .	. . . do	....	Lived.
78	19	9	22	14	Left thigh, left forearm, right thigh, and leg.	Fasciotomy, right leg.	96	Died.
93	32	8	13	13.2	Chest, abdomen, both legs, left arm.	None	....	Do.
99	23	<5	10.3	Nothing I.V. . . .	Left thigh, fracture of right zygoma.	Elevation of right zygoma.	120	Lived.
124	23	1	6	8	All of body except both legs below knee.	None	....	Do.
132	22	1.5	4.8	Immediate therapy	Left shoulder, neck, scalp laceration.	Exploration and drainage, neck and shoulder; tracheotomy.	14	Died 56 hours after release.

Clinical Features

The clinical features of crush syndrome can be divided into two categories: primary and secondary. The primary features, comprising the direct effects of crushing injury, were common to all nine cases. The secondary features, seen only in the five fatal cases, were the usual signs and symptoms of posttraumatic renal insufficiency described in Chapters IV and V.

Primary Phase

Shock.—Shock, as judged by the usual clinical criteria, was not characteristic of the majority of our patients with the crush syndrome and was never seen in patients observed within 10 hours of release from the compressing agents. One patient (Case 70), for instance, looked so well when examined 30 minutes after release that he was evacuated to the rear without treatment. He nevertheless died 4½ days later. Only one patient (Case 93) was in shock when first examined and this was 13 hours after release. He had had no previous medical attention. A diagnosis of slight shock was made in Case 78 twenty hours after release, and though diagnoses of shock were never made in Cases 69 and 132, transitory episodes of impalpable pulse and unmeasurable blood pressure were recorded in the case histories (at 19 hours in Case 69 and at 14 and 23 hours in Case 132). In Case 70 and in all the surviving patients, hypotension was never observed.

Nausea and Vomiting.—Nausea or vomiting was recorded in only three cases, all of which terminated fatally. Nausea with hiccuping was observed in one patient (Case 70). This occurred on the first and second days after release when the nonprotein nitrogen concentration was 83 to 104 mg. per 100 cc. of plasma. Vomiting was recorded twice. One patient (Case 93) vomited while he was still pinned down by masonry but not afterward. The second patient (Case 78) had troublesome vomiting on the second and third days after release from compression. On those days the nonprotein nitrogen of the plasma was 92 mg. per 100 cc. and occasionally higher.

Local Changes.—Commonly the appearance of the skin gave no indication of the changes in the underlying muscle. In some patients, however, there were bruises and areas of ecchymosis and lividity of the overlying skin (Fig. 23). Immediately after release from compression the affected parts began to swell. The swelling took place first within the fascial compartments and resembled

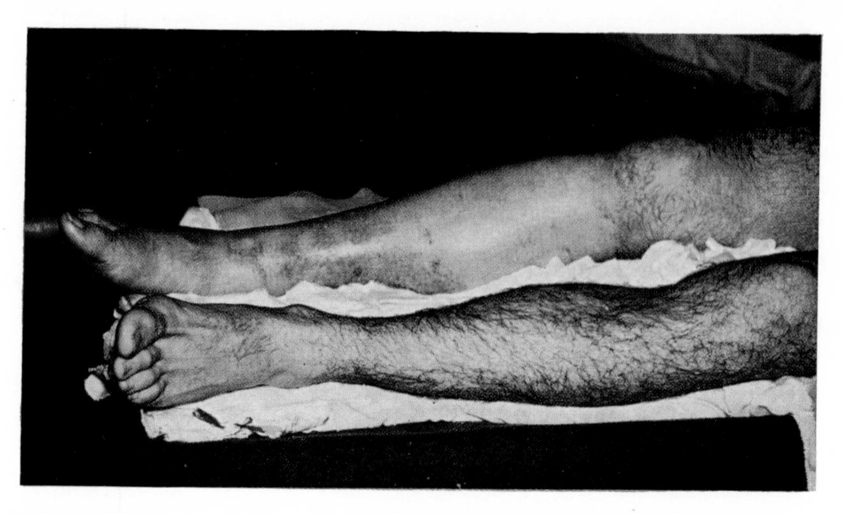

FIGURE 23. Bruising, ecchymosis, and swelling of extremity (Case 78).

the swelling of the calf muscles following interruption of the popliteal artery. The affected areas became hard, tense, and brawny. Only later, usually after the third day, did soft, pitting subcutaneous edema appear. Distribution of lesions was variable. The extremities were most often involved, particularly the legs, and the muscles of the buttock were frequently included. In one patient (Case 132) the muscles of the shoulder and neck were most affected, and edema of the neck was so great that a tracheotomy proved necessary.

During the first few days of the syndrome, the patients might have no complaints or they might complain of stiffness, soreness, aching, and tenderness in the involved areas. Symptoms were often inversely proportional to the severity of injury. In relatively mild lesions, pain was elicited by pressure on the affected area; more severe lesions were insensitive to pressure. Some patients complained of numbness of the skin of the toes and over the involved muscles. Examination revealed patchy areas of hypesthesia or anesthesia of the skin, a "stocking" type of anesthesia of the limbs, and absent reflexes. Involved muscle groups were paralyzed or sometimes temporarily spastic. It was sometimes impossible to feel pulsations in the arteries of the affected limbs, reminding one of the early phase of Volkmann's contracture. In one patient (Case 78) a fasciotomy was done for that reason. The leg was so insensitive that it was possible to perform the operation without anesthesia.

Fractures.—Rather surprisingly, in view of the nature of the initial trauma, no major fractures were observed. The only fracture recorded (of the zygoma) could be considered only coincidental.

Secondary Phase

One patient (Case 132) died 56 hours after release from compression; the other four lived from 4 to 13 days after release. One died suddenly, apparently of acute cardiac failure, the others more slowly, with progressive lethargy and drowsiness but no typical uremic coma. Drowsiness was particularly marked in one patient (Case 78) who had been treated with magnesium. None of the patients in this group had convulsions at any time during their illness. The mechanism of death appeared to be pulmonary edema, except in one patient (Case 93) in whom lobar pneumonia developed on the thirteenth day shortly after the appearance of a diuresis had led to hope for his recovery.

All of the patients who died showed the usual signs and symptoms of a lower nephron nephrosis previously described (Chapters IV and V). The initial urine specimens were deeply pigmented and reacted positively with the benzidine test; oliguria was marked and, except in Cases 69 and 93, progressive (see Table 97). The urine, with one exception, was persistently acid and the specific gravity was constantly low from the third day onward. The nonprotein nitrogen level in the plasma rose progressively, and on the third or fourth day mild hypertension developed. Details of the chemical abnormalities of the blood and urine follow.

Physiologic and Biochemic Features

Blood

Blood Volume.—The blood volume was determined immediately upon arrival at the hospital in only two patients with crush injury. The first (Case 93) was the only patient of the group thought to be in severe shock. He had lost one-third of his total blood volume, apparently entirely in the form of plasma, for he showed no evidence of diminution of the total hemoglobin or red-cell mass. The hemoconcentration might have been partly responsible for the clinical picture of shock, as severe shock was generally associated with a loss of circulating blood greater than one-third of the normal volume. The second patient

CHART 39. HEMATOCRIT VALUES* IN FATAL CRUSH SYNDROME

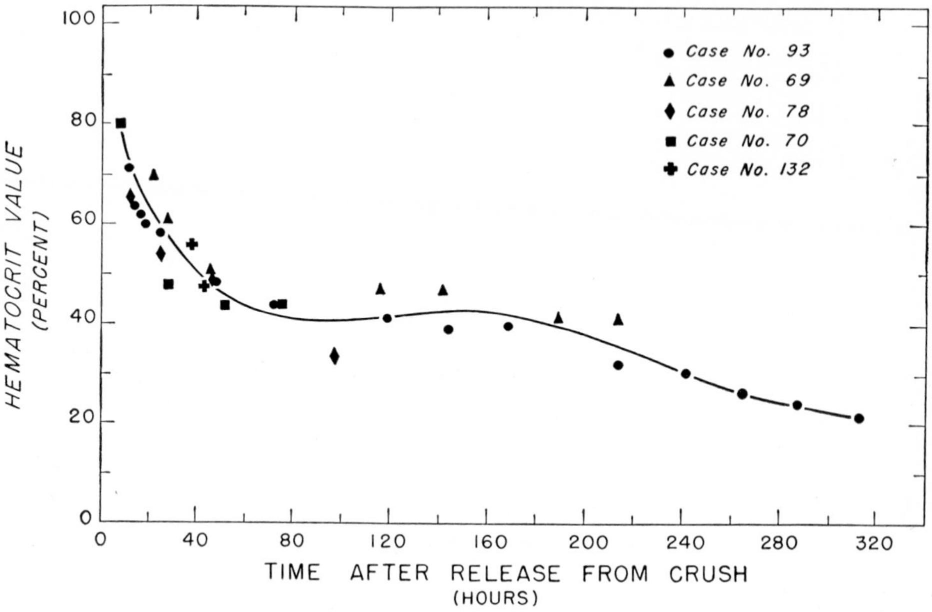

* Normal: 47. Range: 42–52.

(Case 124) showed no evidence of shock clinically and no decrease was found in the volume of circulating blood.

In three patients (Cases 69, 78, and 93) the blood volume was determined during their course. It was abnormal in only one of them (Case 78), being increased by about two liters 24 hours after the patient's release from compression. During that period he had received 600 cc. of plasma (2 units), 400 cc. of 4-percent sodium bicarbonate, and 1,000 cc. of 5-percent dextrose in isotonic saline solution intravenously. He had taken 800 cc. of liquids by mouth and had voided 350 cc. of urine. He died 3 days later with severe pulmonary edema. In Case 93, the patient received no more fluid intravenously than was necessary to correct his blood volume deficit. He died of lobar pneumonia 13 days after release. The blood and plasma volumes in Case 69 were within normal limits on the second and ninth days. In retrospect, from rough fluid-balance calculations, this patient was given perhaps 2,000 cc. more parenteral fluid, including large doses of sodium bicarbonate, than optimal. The fact that severe peripheral edema developed indicates that total body water, if not circulating blood volume, was probably increased.

CHART 40. HEMATOCRIT VALUES* IN NONFATAL CRUSH SYNDROME

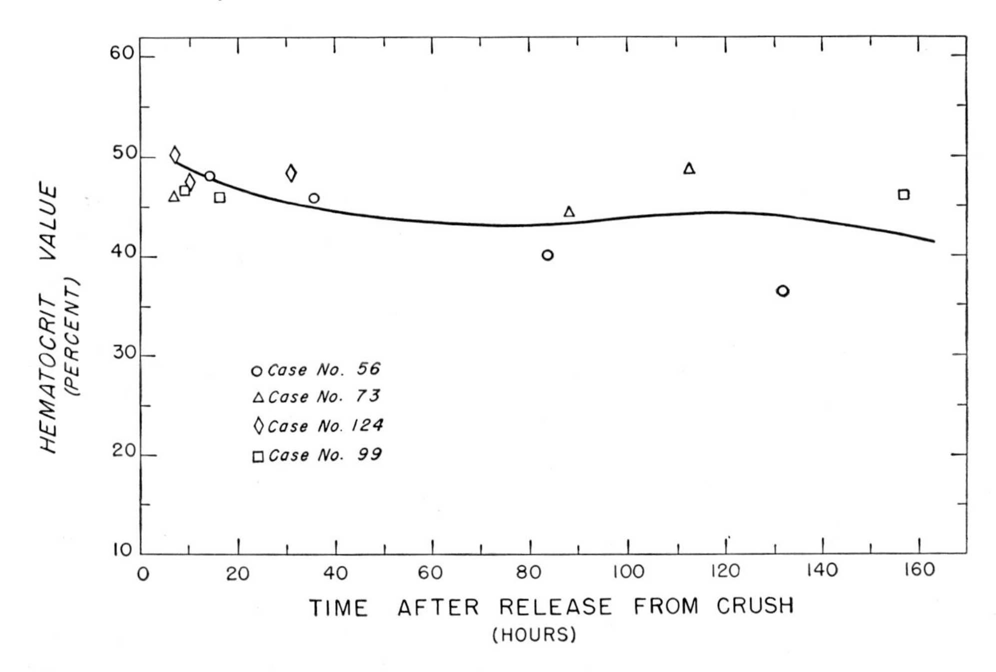

* Normal: 47. Range: 42–52.

Hematocrit Value and Plasma Proteins.—The most striking feature of the immediate findings in the blood of patients with the crush syndrome was the hemoconcentration in those who subsequently died. It was chiefly among these patients with the crush syndrome that hemoconcentration was found in our series of seriously wounded. In one patient (Case 70) the hematocrit value was 80 percent 9 hours after his release from the crushing force. It is noteworthy that the clinical evaluation of this man failed to reveal evidence of shock. All of our patients with crush syndrome who died had initial hemoconcentration (Chart 39 and Table 96). It was, however, transitory and the hematocrit value was within normal limits by the end of the second day. None of those who survived had hematocrit levels above normal limits[4] (Chart 40 and Table 96).

Plasma proteins were within normal limits[5] in six of the eight patients on whom early determinations were made. One initial determination in a patient who lived and four determinations made in the first 24 hours after release

[4] Normal: 47. Range: 42 to 52 percent.

[5] Normal: 6.5. Range: 6 to 7 Gm. per 100 cc.

TABLE 96.—HEMATOCRIT VALUE IN RELATION TO PATIENTS' COURSE

Fatal Cases

Case No.	Hours after Release	Hematocrit Value * cc. cells in 100 cc.	Case No.	Hours after Release	Hematocrit Value * cc. cells in 100 cc.
70	9.0	80.0	70	52.0	44.0
78	12.0	65.0	93	72.5	43.5
93	13.0	71.0	70	76.0	44.0
93	14.5	63.0	78	96.0	34.2
93	16.0	61.5	69	117.5	47.0
93	16.5	59.9	93	119.5	41.1
69	21.5	70.0	69	141.5	47.0
93	23.0	59.0	93	144.0	39.0
78	24.0	54.1	93	167.5	39.8
69	27.0	61.0	69	189.5	41.6
70	28.0	48.0	69	214.0	42.0
132	37.5	57.0	93	215.5	32.9
132	45.0	47.0	93	240.5	30.5
69	46.0	51.7	93	265.0	26.5
78	47.0	49.0	93	287.5	24.5
93	48.0	48.0	93	311.5	21.9

Nonfatal Cases

Case No.	Hours after Release	Hematocrit Value * cc. cells in 100 cc.	Case No.	Hours after Release	Hematocrit Value * cc. cells in 100 cc.
73	7.0	46	56	35.5	45.7
124	7.0	50	56	83.5	40.0
99	9.0	46.8	73	88.5	44.4
124	10.0	47.7	73	112.5	48.5
56	14.0	48.0	56	131.5	36.7
99	16.5	46.0	99	157.0	46.2
124	31.0	48.0	56	203.5	39.0

* Normal: 47. Range: 42–52.

from compression in a fatal case were moderately elevated (Table 97). Again, as was the case in the hematocrit values, the elevated plasma protein concentration soon returned to normal. Although our data are too few to permit of interpretation, it is probable that a consistently high plasma protein concentration in the first 24 hours is indicative of a poor prognosis.

In these crush cases the initial concentration of red blood cells was relatively greater than the concentration of plasma protein, as may be seen in Chart 41. These findings suggest that with release of compression and re-establishment of circulation to the injured areas, there is prompt outpouring of plasma into

TABLE 97.—PLASMA PROTEIN CONCENTRATION IN RELATION TO PATIENTS' COURSE

Fatal Cases

Case No.	Hours after Release	Plasma Protein * Gm. per 100 cc.	Case No.	Hours after Release	Plasma Protein * Gm. per 100 cc.
93	13.0	8.2	78	96.0	6.1
93	14.5	7.7	69	117.5	5.4
93	16.5	7.3	93	119.5	6.2
69	21.5	6.8	69	141.5	4.7
93	23.0	7.3	93	144.0	6.2
78	24.0	6.5	93	167.5	6.1
69	27.0	6.4	69	189.5	4.5
70	28.0	6.1	69	214.0	5.1
69	46.0	6.3	93	215.5	5.9
78	47.0	5.6	93	240.5	6.1
93	48.0	6.2	93	265.0	5.9
70	52.0	6.9	93	287.5	5.8
93	72.5	6.2	93	315.5	5.8
70	76.0	6.5	...	...	...
Nonfatal Cases					
124	7.0	6.7	56	35.5	6.4
73	7.0	6.8	56	83.5	5.5
99	9.0	6.8	73	88.5	5.8
124	10.0	6.0	73	112.5	7.1
56	14.0	7.9	56	131.5	6.0
99	16.5	6.7	99	157.0	6.7
124	31.0	6.3	56	203.5	6.8

* Normal: 6.5. Range: 6–7.

the affected tissues, manifested clinically by the rapid development of swelling in the affected parts. With the loss of plasma from the circulating blood, the concentration of the red blood cells is increased. If, as is likely, the plasma lost into the tissues contains less protein than normal plasma, an explanation of the early increases in the concentration of plasma proteins in some severe cases is afforded. The rapid disappearance of the hemoconcentration (and of the elevated plasma protein level in two instances) is in part accounted for by the intravenous administration of plasma and crystalloids, but this is not the only factor, for the dilution occurred in the absence of intravenous therapy. The effect could be explained by the reabsorption of extravasated plasma.

During the later stages of the syndrome in the fatal cases, the hematocrit

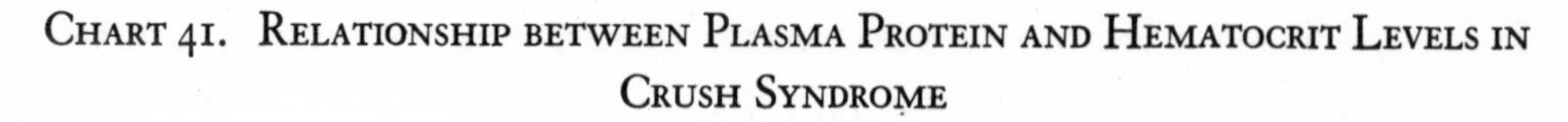

CHART 41. RELATIONSHIP BETWEEN PLASMA PROTEIN AND HEMATOCRIT LEVELS IN CRUSH SYNDROME

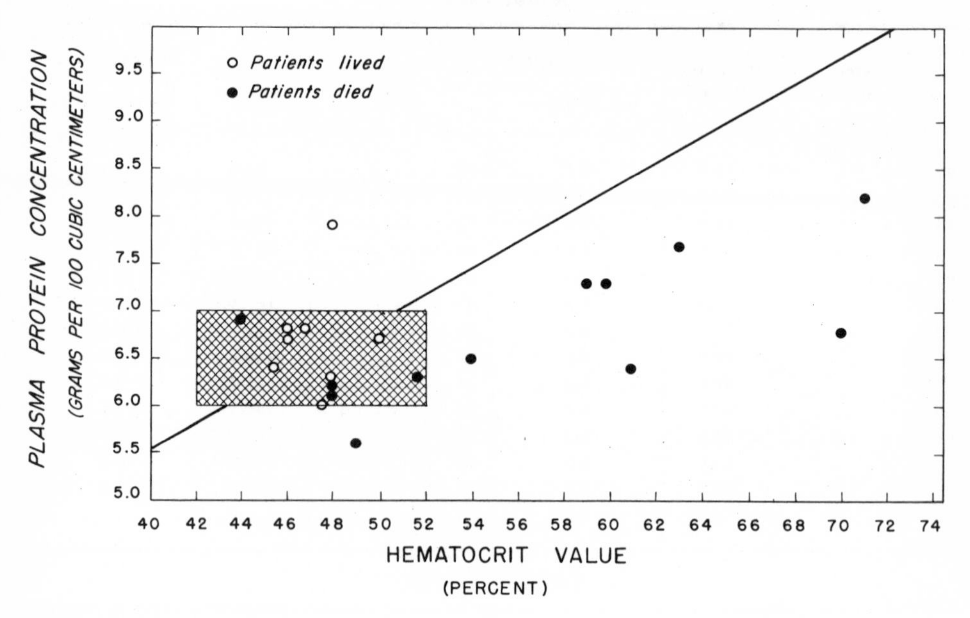

The diagonal line indicates the locus of a point representing equal dilution or concentration of the red blood-cell mass and the plasma protein. Data on first 3 days after injury. The line is theoretical and obviously does not represent the relationship that would obtain if increments of a crystalloid solution were added to whole blood.

value remained within low normal limits except in Cases 78 and 93 in which it fell below 40, eventually dropping to 21.9 on the day of death in the latter case. There was greater variability in the concentration of the plasma proteins during the course of the disease. Two determinations in patients who survived and seven determinations in patients who died dropped below 6 Gm. per 100 cc., three of them being below 5.5 (Table 97).

Plasma Nonprotein Nitrogen.—Among the patients who survived, concentration of the nonprotein nitrogen in the plasma was essentially normal throughout the course of the illness. Among those who died, it was elevated from the start and rose progressively at an almost linear rate (Chart 42). No determinations were made in one fatal case. The concentration of phosphorus in the plasma rose more slowly and appeared to reach its asymptote earlier.

Plasma Chlorides.—The plasma chloride concentrations were essentially normal among the patients who survived. Among those in whom fatal crush

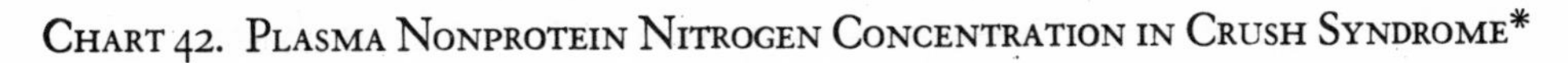

CHART 42. PLASMA NONPROTEIN NITROGEN CONCENTRATION IN CRUSH SYNDROME*

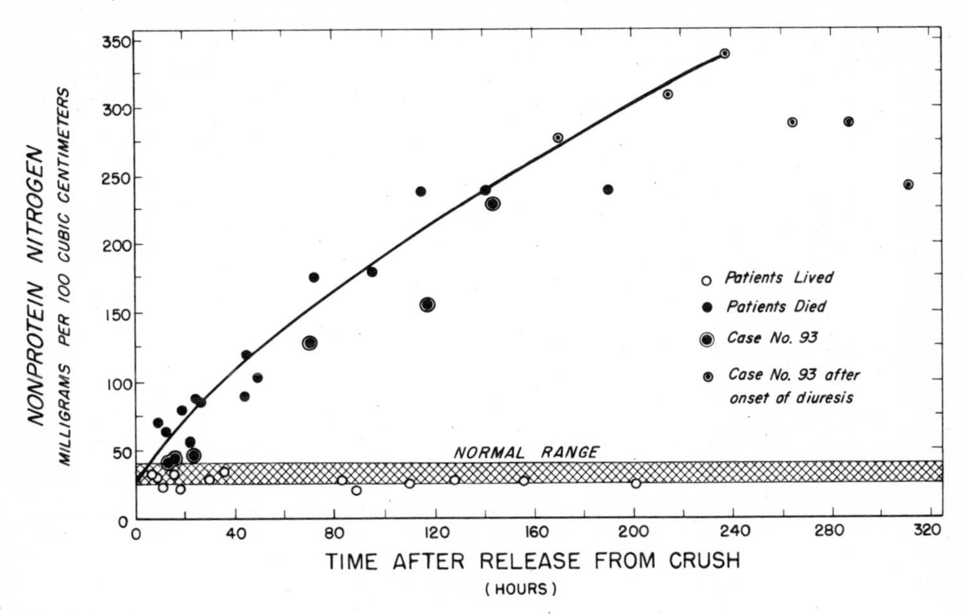

* Data on 4 fatal and 4 nonfatal cases. In Case 93, plotted separately on the chart, a "recovery" diuresis was well started before the patient died of pneumonia on the thirteenth day after injury.

syndrome developed, however, there was a progressive drop in the concentration of plasma chlorides except in one patient (Case 93) who developed a diuresis and showed evidence of improving renal function although he subsequently died (Chart 43). At necropsy lower nephron nephrosis and lobar pneumonia were demonstrated. No determinations were made in one fatal case. Concomitant with the fall in plasma chloride level, there was generally a fall in the alkali reserve of the blood as suggested by the lowering of its CO_2 combining power. These changes in plasma carbon-dioxide combining power and chloride levels were entirely comparable to those seen in renal insufficiency following other types of trauma (Chapter V).

Plasma Pigment.—Blood specimens taken shortly after release from compression revealed abnormal quantities of a free pigment in the plasma which reacted positively to the benzidine test. Blood samples were collected in carefully dried, but not oiled, syringes and needles. With this technique, a free plasma "hemoglobin" concentration up to 15 mg. per 100 cc. was considered within the normal range. Chart 44 shows the values obtained in the first 5 days after injury both in the patients who died and in those who survived. All but

CHART 43. PLASMA CHLORIDE CONCENTRATION* IN CRUSH SYNDROME

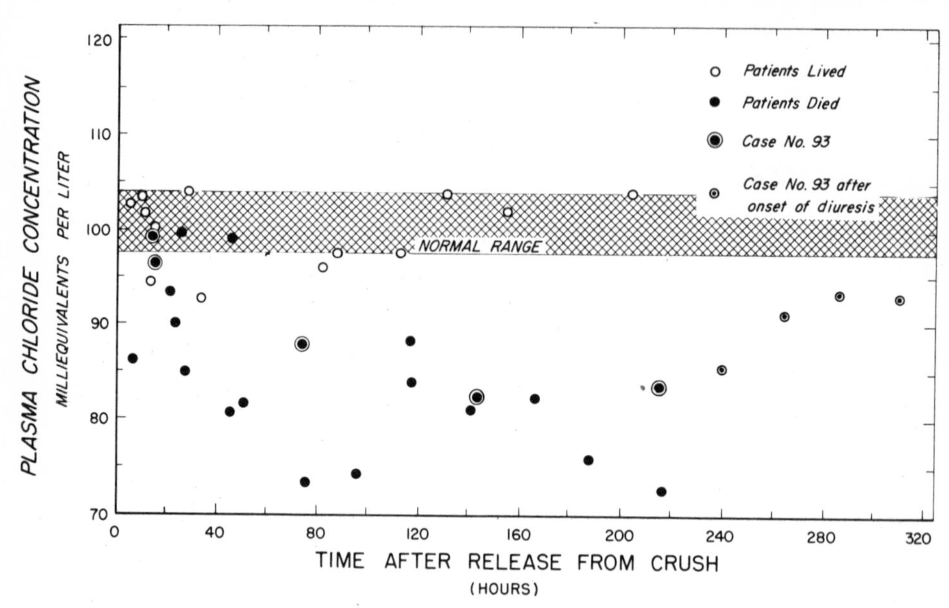

* Normal: 100. Range: 97.5–104. Data on 4 fatal and 4 nonfatal cases.

two of the determinations we were able to obtain during the first 24 hours were above the limits accepted as normal; the exceptions were determinations made in Case 99, nine and sixteen hours after release. Only one of the patients showed a heme concentration of over 40 mg. per 100 cubic centimeters. Data were available on eight cases. Of particular interest, from those data, is that, like the return of the hematocrit level and the plasma protein concentration to normal, the concentration of the free benzidine-positive substance in the plasma tended to be within normal limits by the end of the second day. As in the case of the hemoconcentration, then, the presence of free benzidine-positive substance in the plasma might have been missed if specimens had not been collected soon after the patients' release from the crushing force.

The nature of this substance, free in the plasma and giving the reaction of a heme, could not be settled. The quantities present were not large enough to make spectroscopic analysis possible in the instrument available to us. Chemical examination of the urine of these patients (Chapter VIII) showed that both hemoglobin and myoglobin were excreted in large amounts, the proportions of each varying widely from case to case. It is reasonable to assume, therefore, that both pigments were represented in the plasma as well.

CHART 44. FREE BENZIDINE-POSITIVE SUBSTANCE IN PLASMA IN CRUSH SYNDROME*

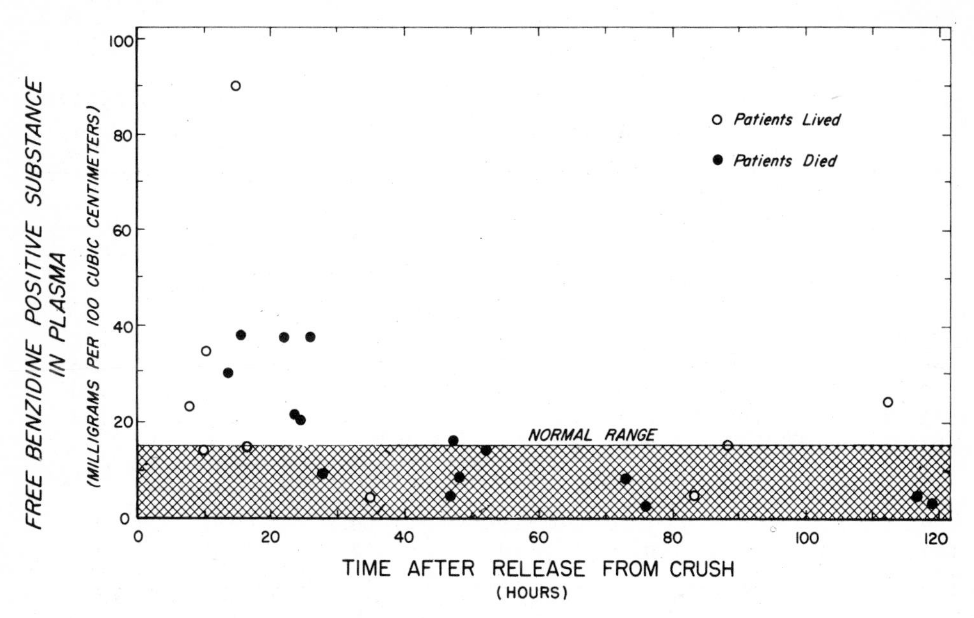

* Data on 4 fatal and 4 nonfatal cases.

Urine

Gross abnormalities were found only in the urine specimens collected soon after release from the compression force. Table 98 indicates the duration of some of the abnormalities in the urine. It will be observed that myoglobin was not found in the urine more than a day and a half after release from the crushing force. Abnormality in the color of the urine lasted somewhat longer (up to 3 days), and albuminuria to a significant degree was detected for as long as 9 days after release from the crushing influence.

Output.—None of the patients who survived the injury had any diminution in volume of urinary output below the limits of normal. In all of those who died (Table 99) urinary output was diminished from the start. All had oliguria. In one instance (Case 70) anuria (an output of less than 100 cc.) was recorded during the 24 hours beginning the day after release. Two other patients were oliguric until the second 24-hour period, when the output dropped below 100 cc. a day. The remaining two patients (Cases 93 and 78) were oliguric but never became anuric. In one (Case 69) diuresis had just begun to develop when he suddenly died; in another (Case 93, Table 99) an excellent diuresis was established and the patient might have survived the injury had he not died of lobar pneumonia.

TABLE 98.—DURATION (DAYS) OF ABNORMALITIES IN THE URINE OF 9 PATIENTS WITH CRUSH SYNDROME

Case No.	Color Abnormality	Albumin	Benzidine-Positive Substance		Patient's Outcome
			Hemoglobin	Myoglobin	
70	3	4	4	1.5	Died.
69	2	9	9	1	Do.
78	2	4	....	....	Do.
132	2	2	....	....	Do.
93	3	* 7	** 4	1	Do.
73	1	1	....	....	Lived.
56	1	1	1	0	Do.
99	1 (?)	0	0	0	Do.
124	0	0	0	0	Do.

0 =none present.
* Beyond this time the urine in this patient showed only negligible traces of albumin.
** Beyond this time only traces or faint traces of hemoglobin were recorded.

TABLE 99.—URINARY OUTPUT IN 5 FATAL CASES OF CRUSH SYNDROME

Time after Release from Compression	Urinary Output (cc. per 24 hours)				
	Case 69	Case 70	Case 78	Case 93	Case 132
Day of release	....	200	....	150	——
First day after release	230	30	350	160	300
Second day after release	50	85	500	165	30
Third day after release	45	75	250	130	——
Fourth day after release	100	35	160	130	——
Fifth day after release	100	....	....	292	——
Sixth day after release	80	....	....	410	——
Seventh day after release	150	....	....	800	——
Eighth day after release	100	....	....	1,305	——
Ninth day after release.	450	....	....	1,935	——
Tenth day after release	....	....	....	2,760	——
Eleventh day after release	....	....	....	4,135	——
Twelfth day after release	....	....	....	3,050	——
Thirteenth day after release	....	....	....	890	——

Color.—Yellow and straw color were considered to be the normal colors of urine. An amber color was considered on the borderline of abnormality. All of the patients who died had abnormal urinary color varying from red to red-brown, or mahogany to dark amber; this lasted 2 or 3 days. Among the patients who survived, the color varied from "ruddy" to amber; but this did not persist longer than 1 day.

Benzidine-Positive Pigment.—The grossly abnormal color of the urine in patients with the crush syndrome was found to be caused by the presence of a pigment which reacted positively to the benzidine test. By the technique described in Appendix C, this pigment was thought to consist of myoglobin as well as hemoglobin in three of the five patients who died of the crush injury. In the fourth patient no attempt was made to distinguish between the two pigments, and in the fifth patient the benzidine test was not made on the dark-amber urine. Results of the tests for myoglobin were never positive in urine specimens obtained later than 24 to 36 hours after release from the crushing force. Benzidine-positive substance was found later than the second day and up to the eighth day after release, but in such small amounts that it was impossible to employ the test to distinguish between myoglobin and hemoglobin. Qualitative spectroscopic examinations suggested the presence of myoglobin in the specimens obtained in fatal Cases 69, 70, and 93.

Albumin.—Two of the patients who survived showed some albuminuria. In neither case did it last more than 1 day, and in only one (Case 56) of the two was it of any degree of severity. All of the patients who died had marked albuminuria. Up to 4 or 6 days it persisted unchanged or with increased severity. If the patient lived longer, the degree of albuminuria then decreased, as in Cases 69 and 93. In the latter the urine contained only a faint trace of albumin by the time the patient died of lobar pneumonia 13 days after release from the crushing force.

Sediment.—The urinary sediment was remarkable because findings were so scarce. In one patient who survived (Case 124), no record was made of the examination of the organized sediment. Of the other three patients who lived, only one (Case 73) showed casts in the urinary sediment. On the first day after injury his urine showed occasional coarse and finely granular casts; 2 days later the sediment was normal. Two of the five patients who died had no casts in the urine, although a rare red blood cell and a few white blood cells were found; three did show coarse and finely granular casts in the urinary sediment, but these casts were not abundant, even in centrifuged specimens.

Specific Gravity.—For the first day or two of the illness, the specific gravity of the urine was normal in all cases. After the second to fourth days, however, the specific gravity of the urine fell and appeared to become fixed at 1.012 to 1.013. Urine concentration tests were not done in these patients, but as in other cases of posttraumatic renal insufficiency early impairment of ability to reabsorb water by the renal tubules is surely a characteristic feature (Chapter V).

Reaction.—With one exception, the patients passed acid urine at all times throughout the illness. This one exception (Case 69) was a patient whose urine was on the alkaline side of neutral (pH 7.2) on two occasions on the seventh and eighth days of the illness. At all other times the urine of this patient was acid, despite administration of sodium bicarbonate in doses thought adequate for alkalinization of the urine (16 to 36 Gm. per 24 hours). As had been found in the study of patients who had renal insufficiency from other causes, alkalinization of the urine by means of administration of sodium bicarbonate was inconsistent with safety.

CHART 45. BROMSULFALEIN EXCRETION IN PATIENTS WITH FATAL CRUSH SYNDROME

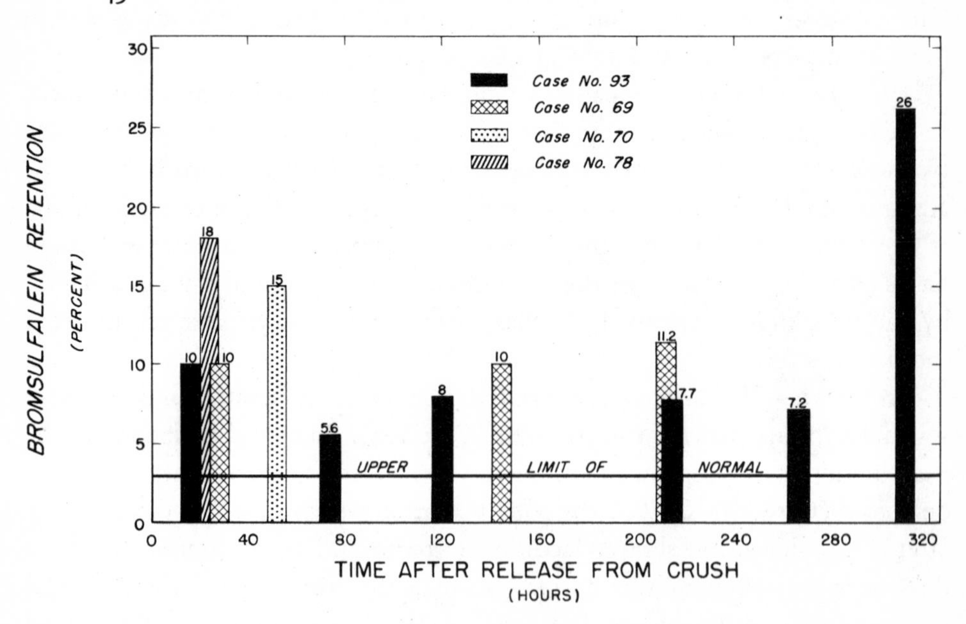

One value in each of 2 cases was estimated for a 45-minute period, as the figures had been recorded at 30 and 60 minutes.

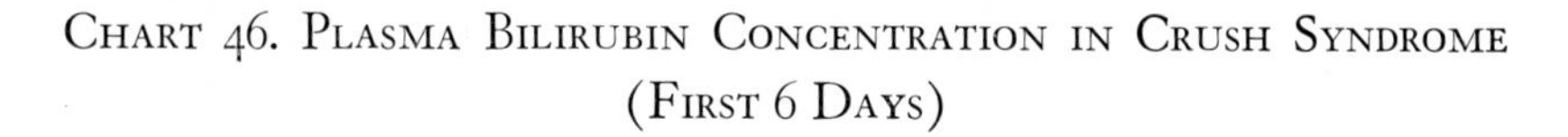

CHART 46. PLASMA BILIRUBIN CONCENTRATION IN CRUSH SYNDROME (FIRST 6 DAYS)

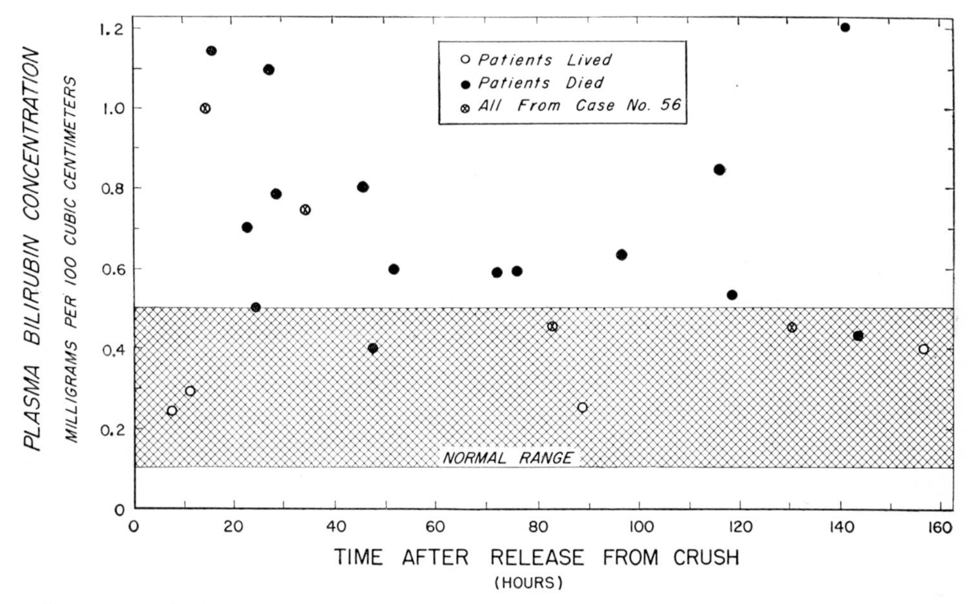

All values in the fatal cases were above normal though still below the level at which clinical jaundice would appear (2 mg. per 100 cc.). Values for patients who survived were within normal limits with the exception of Case 56, plotted separately on the chart. Data on 4 fatal and 4 nonfatal cases.

Liver Function

The function of the liver was tested in one of the four patients who survived and in four of the five patients who died. The examination consisted of a test of the ability of the liver to excrete bromsulfalein injected intravenously. Dosage was calculated on the basis of 5 milligrams of bromsulfalein per kilogram of body weight (Chapter II). By this method, retention of the dye up to 3 percent of the injected dose after 45 minutes was considered the upper limit of normal. In the patient who survived the function of the liver was found to be normal as tested by this method. In all of the patients who died liver function was found to be impaired (Chart 45). The average dye retention in the four fatal cases was 12.77 percent, exclusive of one determination made in Case 93, which showed 26-percent retention on the day the patient died of lobar pneumonia.

The concentration of bilirubin in the plasma was increased in those patients in whom fatal crush syndrome developed and in one patient (Case 56) who survived (Chart 46). Data were obtained on eight cases. Sufficient information was not available to distinguish between increased production of bilirubin and decrease in its elimination.

Pathology

The important findings at postmortem examination were confined to the lungs, the liver, the skeletal muscles, and the kidneys.

Lungs.—All of the five fatal cases showed slight to extensive pulmonary edema, both grossly and microscopically. The weight of the two lungs together was recorded in four of the five fatal cases. The weights varied from 1,075 to 1,600 grams. Blood as well as edema fluid appeared on cut surfaces of the lungs in Case 132 and, microscopically, large numbers of alveoli were packed with red blood cells. This patient had had a tracheotomy and the blood may have been aspirated. Another patient (Case 78) was unusual in that even the visceral pleura was edematous. Fluid poured from the cut surfaces without the necessity of compression, and the tracheobronchial tree was filled with nonbloody fluid. In Case 93 death was due primarily to lobar pneumonia involving the left upper lobe. Microscopically, in addition to the typical pneumonia process, some areas showed edema with spreading pneumonic involvement.

Liver.—In view of the decreased liver function, as measured by ability to excrete bromsulfalein and as indicated by the elevated plasma bilirubin and the abnormally low ratio of urea nitrogen to total nonprotein nitrogen, some histologic changes were expected in the liver. Surprisingly few were found. The liver was microscopically normal in Case 70, and showed only scattered vacuoles in Case 132. In Case 69 occasional mitotic figures were observed in hepatic cells, and in Case 93, in which there had been terminally a rising bilirubin concentration in the blood and a terminal bromsulfalein retention of 26 percent, the only histologic changes found were mild nuclear atypicality in the cells at the centers of the lobules.

Skeletal Muscles.—The gross changes in the involved muscles were conspicuous. In the involved areas the normal pigment had disappeared, leaving muscle bundles with the appearance of fish or rabbit flesh. Sometimes an entire muscle was decolorized, more commonly only segmental areas, particularly re-

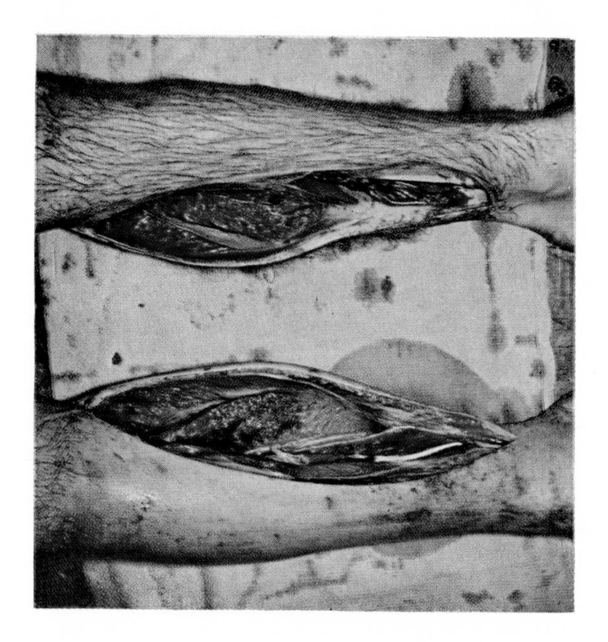

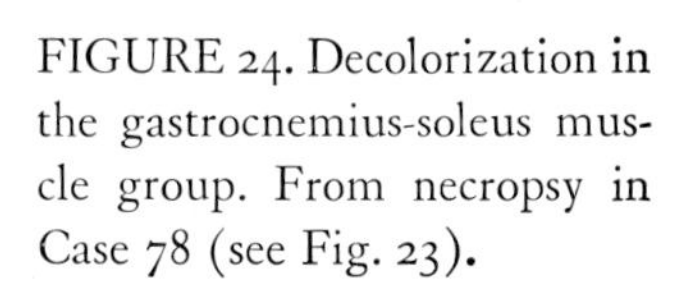

FIGURE 24. Decolorization in the gastrocnemius-soleus muscle group. From necropsy in Case 78 (see Fig. 23).

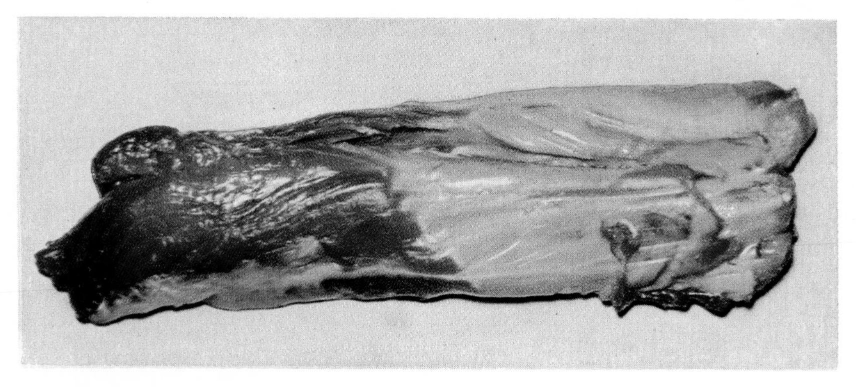

FIGURE 25. Decolorization in the left brachioradialis muscle in Case 93. Note the "fish flesh" appearance, the sharp line of demarcation, and the distinct white band at the junction of the depigmented and normally pigmented muscle.

gions close to major bony structures (Fig. 24). In Figure 25 (Case 93) complete depigmentation of the distal half of the forearm muscles is apparent, whereas the proximal half is normally colored. The transition from normally colored to depigmented areas was sharp, particularly in the cases of longer survival, and in Case 93 (13 days' survival) the junction was marked by a narrow white band 2 to 3 mm. broad (Fig. 25). In spite of the loss of color, the tissue remained moist, capillary oozing appeared from cut surfaces, and no thrombi could be discovered in any grossly visible vessels. Hemorrhage and edema were extremely irregular in extent and intensity, absent from some lesions, and marked in others. The gross depigmentation correlated with chemical assays showing almost complete loss of myoglobin in the affected areas (Table 100).

Microscopic sections were available from four cases 4, 5, 10, and 13 days respectively after injury. In the acute cases hematoxylin and eosin stains showed relatively inconspicuous changes. Evidences of muscle-cell degeneration were, however, present. Some cells were swollen, hyaline, and more strongly acidophilic than normal. More commonly the cells stained less intensely than normal, cross-striations were exaggerated, occasional fractures and clefts were present, and the sarcolemma nuclei appeared decreased in number (Fig. 26). Though edema and hemorrhage were apparent in some areas, there was no inflammatory reaction, either polymorphonuclear or histiocytic. With the Masson and phosphotungstic acid hematoxylin stains, the changes were far more conspicuous. Some of the swollen hyaline fibers stained intensely red with the Masson, or blue with the phosphotungstic stain, but the great majority responded feebly or not at all to the specific staining reactions. In sections across the border of a depigmented area it was evident that the loss of specific staining reaction corresponded closely with the margin of depigmentation (Fig. 27 a). It was of interest that the cells with exaggerated cross-striations usually failed to stain specifically.

TABLE 100.—MYOGLOBIN CONTENT OF MUSCLE AND KIDNEY IN 4 PATIENTS WHO DIED FROM CRUSH SYNDROME

Tissue	Myoglobin Content *Gm. per Kg. of Wet Tissue*			
	Case No. 69	Case No. 70	Case No. 78	Case No. 93
Normal muscle	* 2.10	3.60	4.20	3.74
Depigmented muscle	1.00	0.27	0.83	0.54
Partly depigmented muscle	1.86	....	3.00	....
Kidney	0.45	0.60	0.93	....

* The low value was probably caused b y the extensive interstitial edema in this case.

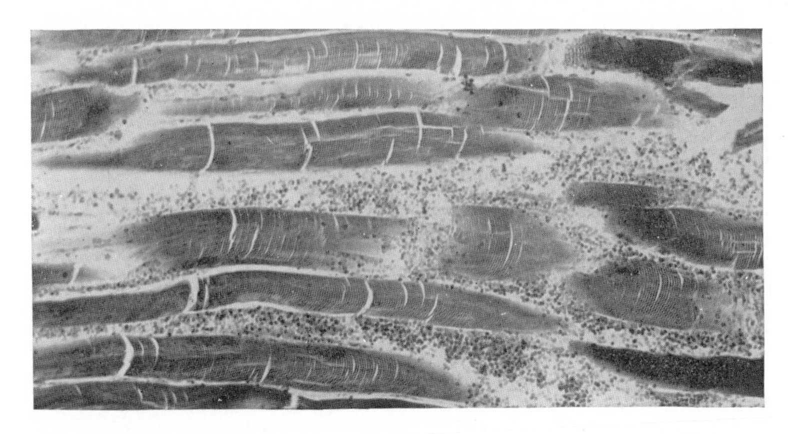

FIGURE 26. Decolorized muscle from Case 70. The patient died 4 days after injury. The muscle cells, which should stain intensely with the phosphotungstic acid hematoxylin, employed stain weakly. Cross-striations are exaggerated and numerous transverse clefts have appeared. An occasional cell has become hyalinized and lost all evidence of striation. There is much hemorrhage into the interstitial connective tissue.

In the cases of longer duration (10 and 13 days), changes were conspicuous with all staining methods but particularly with hematoxylin and eosin. Many swollen, necrotic muscle cells had become intensely basophilic owing to the precipitate of innumerable fine granules staining like calcium throughout the sarcoplasm (Fig. 27 c and d). In other cells the precipitate was intense in the central portion but absent at the periphery (Fig. 28 a). Another common type of degenerative change was a coarse hydropic vacuolation which frequently produced an appearance suggestive of vegetable cells (Fig. 27 d). Other degenerating cells showed varying degrees of infiltration with histiocytes (Figs. 27 b and c). The sarcolemma nuclei in many cells showed amitotic division, with chains of touching nuclei 5 to 10 elements in length (Figs. 27 b and 28 b). About many of these, viable cytoplasm was present in long, slender masses suggesting regeneration of muscle cells. The interstitial connective tissue was slightly edematous and densely infiltrated with histiocytes (Fig. 28 b). No definite evidence of fibroblastic proliferation could be made out. Blood vessels still remained free from thrombi or inflammatory reaction.

Kidneys.—In all but one patient (Case 70) the kidneys were enlarged at necropsy. In three of the five fatal cases the combined weights of the two kidneys were recorded; they were respectively 500, 550, and 625 grams. The capsules stripped easily. In some there were ecchymoses beneath the capsule. Focal

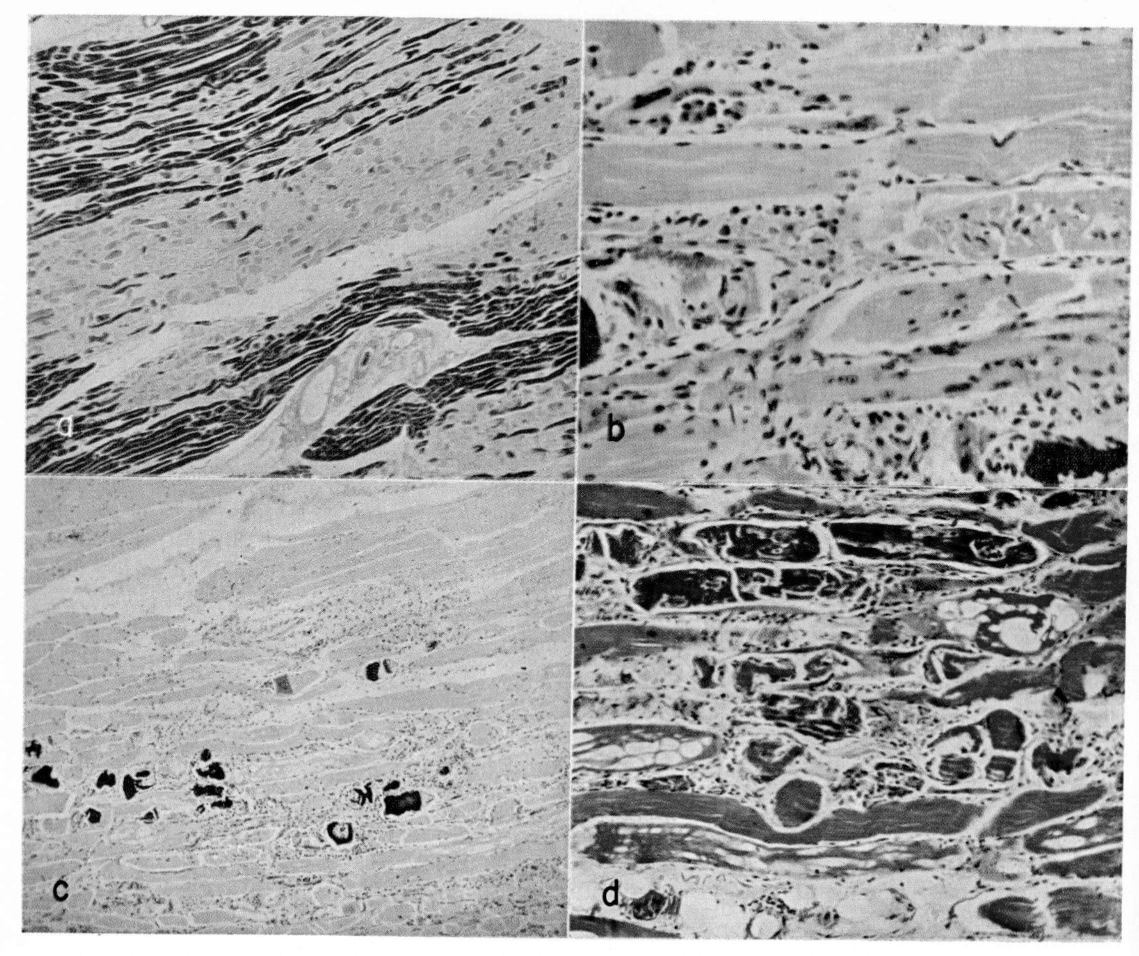

FIGURE 27, *a*. Muscle from Case 70 (4 days' survival). Phosphotungstic acid hematoxylin stain. Section taken from a partially depigmented area. In the more severely involved areas necrotic muscle cells stain only a faint brown instead of an intense purplish-blue. Even the surviving cells stain irregularly and striations are difficult to see. The interstitial tissue is edematous but shows little inflammatory infiltration.

b. Case 70 (see also *a* and Fig. 26). Hematoxylin and eosin stain. At the top are three swollen muscle cells which have lost striations. Beneath them are two necrotic cells which have been invaded by histiocytes. At upper right and lower left are fragments of surviving muscle which show chains of touching nuclei. Two foci of calcification are present. The interstitial tissue shows fibrosis and inflammatory infiltration.

c. Muscle from Case 69 (10 days' survival). Hematoxylin and eosin stain. This low-power view shows focal calcification and vascular degeneration of muscle cells as well as chronic inflammatory infiltration and fibrosis of the interstitial tissues.

d. A higher magnification from the same section shown in *c*. Masson trichrome stain. Coarse vascular degeneration of muscle cells producing vegetable-cell appearance is evident. Several muscle cells no longer stain red in normal fashion and have been invaded by histiocytes. Fibrosis and histiocytic infiltration of the interstitial tissue is apparent.

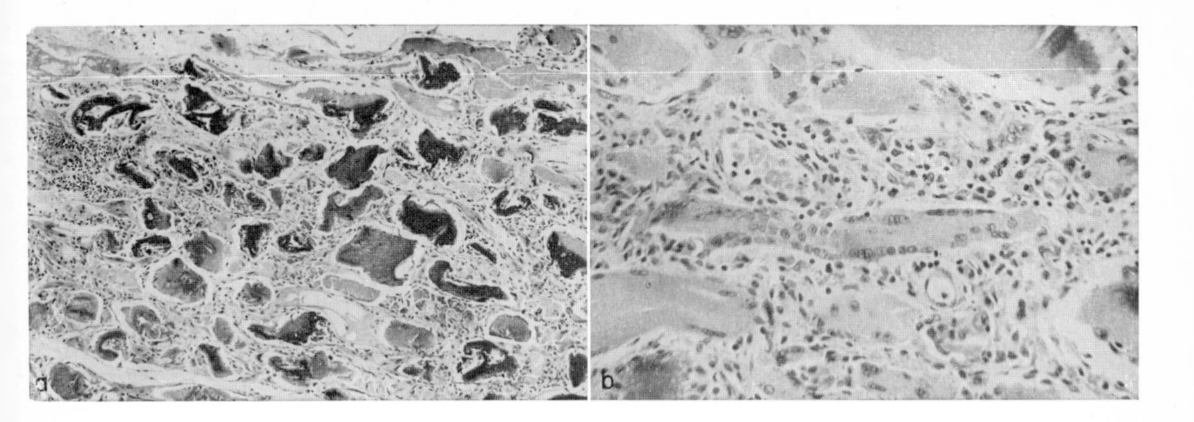

FIGURE 28, *a*. A focus of intense calcification involving almost every muscle cell. There is marked increase in interstitial fibrous tissue with an occasional focus of lymphocytic infiltration. Section from Case 93 (13 days' survival).

b. Section from the same case. Hematoxylin and eosin stain. A regenerating muscle cell shows long chains of touching sarcolemma nuclei. The fibrosis and the patency of the blood vessels are noteworthy. Partial calcification of some muscle cells at the periphery of the field is evident.

hemorrhages and fibrin deposits were commonly found beneath and on the epithelium of the renal pelvis (see Fig. 20 in Chapter IX). When the kidneys were cut, with one exception (Case 70), the renal parenchyma pouted through the cut, rolling outward and forming a rounded instead of a sharp edge.

Characteristically, the cut surface of the parenchyma showed pallor of the cortex and darkening of the pyramids to a dark brown or mahogany color (Figs. 19 to 22 in Chapter IX). The thickness of the cortex was normal or increased, never decreased.

The microscopic appearance of the kidneys from patients who died from crush syndrome have been described and illustrated in Chapter IX as a "lower nephron nephrosis," and it will be sufficient merely to list the salient features here.

Microscopic Features of the Kidney.—Most conspicuous was the presence of densely pigmented casts in the distal convoluted and the collecting tubules. These could not be distinguished in stained or unstained sections from the pigmented casts in Case 9, a known transfusion reaction. Proximal to the pigmented casts, usually in the ascending limbs of Henle's loops, hyaline nonpigmented casts were numerous. In cases with survival periods of 4 days, these hyaline casts were frequently extruded into the stroma and formed foci for granulomatous reactions. Degenerative changes in the renal parenchyma were limited to the lower nephron segments, usually the ascending limbs, less often the distal convoluted tubules.

Glomeruli were uniformly normal except for the presence of granular precipitate in the capsular space. The proximal convoluted tubules were sometimes moderately dilated and their lumens contained granular precipitate, but the epithelial cells were normal and brush borders were well preserved. Interstitial inflammatory reaction was always present at the corticomedullary junction, and in two cases of 10 and 13 days' duration, a narrower zone of interstitial inflammatory reaction was seen beneath the capsule. In the same two cases nonocclusive thrombi were present in some of the veins at the corticomedullary junction.

Treatment of Crush Syndrome

The results of treatment of patients with crush syndrome were disappointing. (Our ministrations were certainly less effective than those of Saint Benedict, whose successful treatment of a monk crushed beneath the masonry of a wall at Monte Cassino is depicted on page 254.) In general, efforts during the first 48 hours were directed toward correction of the hemoconcentration and attempts at alkalinization of the urine. Subsequently the treatment was that for renal insufficiency as described for patients with renal insufficiency from other causes (Chapter VI).

Correction of Hemoconcentration.—Hemoconcentration was treated by administration of plasma and crystalloid solutions during the first 48 hours. Beyond this time, the degree of hemoconcentration was no longer a serious problem, for reabsorption had probably begun to exceed transudation. Only two of the nine patients received whole blood. One of the two (Case 69) received only 250 cc. of blood, administered before the hemoconcentration had been recognized. The other (Case 132) was given 1,500 cc. of whole blood when he became pulseless and no blood pressure could be determined in his extremities.

Alkalinization of the Urine.—According to Bywaters'[6] hypothesis, alkalinization should be started at the time the casualty is found, immediately after or even before release from compression. This was not possible in any of our patients. The seriousness of the injury was not recognized by the aid-men. As a matter of fact, the diagnosis was not made by the medical officers until, through an educational campaign, they had been made aware of the possibility of the syndrome in any crush injury.

[6] See footnote 1.

CHART 47. EFFECT OF ALKALI THERAPY IN A PATIENT WITH CRUSH SYNDROME (CASE 69)

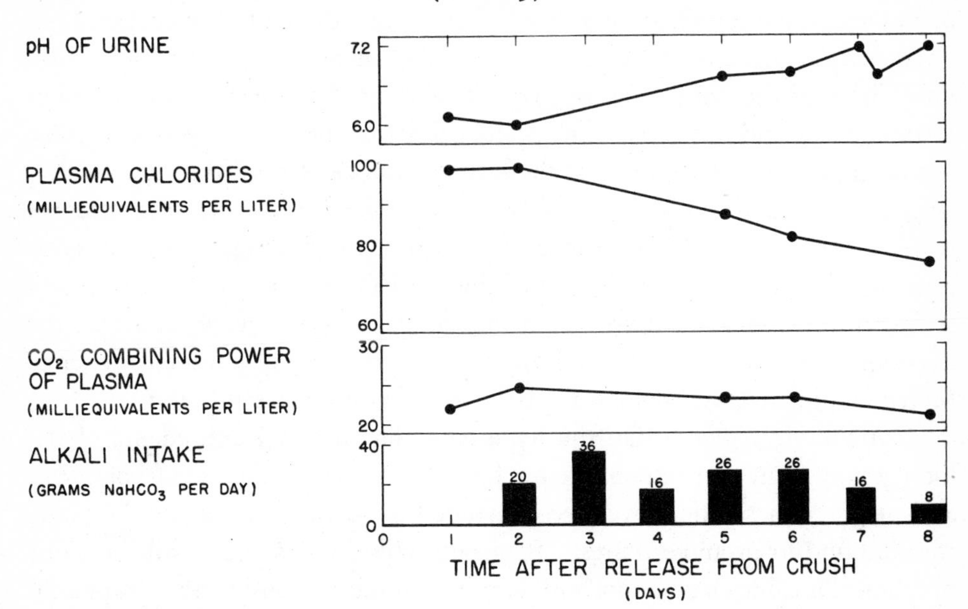

After admission to the hospital, however, all but two of the nine patients received alkali therapy. Four of the five patients who died were treated with alkali, one starting promptly upon admission to the hospital, one starting during the first 24-hour period after release from the crushing force, and two during the second 24-hour period. No beneficial effects were observed that could be attributed to the alkali. As a matter of fact, the most striking feature was the failure, in the fatal cases, to succeed in alkalinizing the urine. A pH of 7.2 was attained in only two specimens of urine in Case 69 (Chart 47). This patient had received larger doses of sodium bicarbonate than the other patients. One patient in this group (Case 124) did have an alkaline urine (pH 8.4) 4 hours after intravenous administration of sodium bicarbonate, and it was kept alkaline by the administration of 3 Gm. of the bicarbonate every 4 hours. This patient had a minimal renal lesion and survived. Administration of sodium bicarbonate was done cautiously or abandoned altogether, because of unfortunate experiences with vigorous attempts at alkalinization in patients with renal insufficiency from other causes (Chapter VII).

Diuretics.—Alcohol was used with the hope that it would promote blood flow through the kidney and serve as a diuretic. It was used intravenously (total dose: 50 to 100 cc. of 95-percent ethyl alcohol as a 5-percent solution in dextrose or isotonic saline solution), and as whiskey by mouth (60 to 180 cc. per day). No beneficial effects were detected that could be attributed directly to the alcohol. Three of the patients were given 10-percent dextrose in distilled water intravenously, and one received 50-percent dextrose intravenously as a diuretic, but no effect was noted in any of them that could be attributed to the medication. The failure of both alcohol and hypertonic solutions of dextrose to promote urine flow or improve kidney function confirmed the findings in patients with renal insufficiency from other causes (Chapter VI). Not only did concentrated solutions fail to induce a diuresis, but in three cases (Cases 70, 78, and 132) the hypertonic dextrose solution may have hastened the onset of pulmonary edema. Mercurial diuretics were not tried in patients with the crush syndrome.

Dehydrating Agents.—On the hypothesis that swelling and edema of the kidney may be in part responsible for failure of function, the use of potassium and magnesium solutions was recommended by Barker[7] to reduce the tissue swelling and to promote diuresis. Potassium chloride was not available to us for clinical use, but magnesium sulfate was used intravenously and intramuscularly. It was employed in three cases (Cases 69, 78, and 93) in doses of 4 to 8 Gm. daily for 3 to 5 days, which was sufficient to elevate the concentration of magnesium in the blood as indicated in the two patients in whom such analyses were made (Cases 78 and 93). In these three patients there was no definite effect upon urinary output, and it is impossible to attribute any beneficial effect to the use of magnesium. Undue drowsiness in Case 78 could well have been caused by the magnesium therapy, for his serum concentration of magnesium was 5.8 milliequivalents per liter at necropsy. The serum magnesium reached a level of 6.8 milliequivalents per liter at one stage during the course of treatment in Case 93. For the same reasons stated in Chapter VI, it is our opinion that neither magnesium nor potassium solutions should be used in the treatment of this syndrome.

Other Measures.—Study of these nine patients taught us little as to possible means of preventing anuria or inducing diuresis. Generally accepted methods failed. On the hypothesis that injury to the kidney may be produced when reabsorption of extravasated fluid takes place, pressure bandages were considered worthy of trial and were applied in one case (Case 78) without apparent effect.

[7] BARKER, MARION H.: Personal communication.

In this case, however, serious extravasation into the tissues had already occurred before the patient reached the hospital. Cold applications might prevent rapid flooding of the kidney with large quantities of muscle-breakdown products, inasmuch as cold is known to inhibit the flow of lymph from the periphery into the general circulation. This therapy was not tried. Again, however, to be effective it would have to be started immediately after release from compression. Therapeutic amputation of the involved extremities was thought to be out of the question for the same reason.

What was learned from the patients with crush syndrome, as well as from those with renal insufficiency from other causes, was that it is very easy to bring about an increase in plasma volume in these patients by too vigorous attempts at inducing a diuresis with intravenous crystalloids. Once oliguria or anuria is established, it is best to withhold fluid, allowing, preferably by mouth, just enough fluid to compensate for loss from the gastrointestinal tract, and for insensible loss through the skin, from the lungs, and from the sweat glands. Under ordinary circumstances, these requirements can be met by 1,000 cc. or less of fluid daily; more must be allowed if excessive extra-renal losses occur. In general, patients with renal insufficiency have been found to be over-hydrated rather than under-hydrated, and this accounts for the fact that pulmonary edema is a common cause of death.

SUMMARY AND CONCLUSIONS

A laboratory and clinical study was made of nine patients who received crushing injuries; four of the patients survived, five died. It is emphasized that the crush syndrome develops insidiously in patients who appear well when first seen. All patients who have suffered compression interfering with the circulation of muscle masses for periods of an hour, and perhaps even less, should be observed carefully for development of features of the syndrome; namely, tense swelling of the affected parts, hemoconcentration, benzidine-positive pigment (presumably myoglobin) free in the plasma and urine, and oliguria or anuria. If examinations are not made within 24 or 48 hours, the hemoconcentration and the myoglobinuria may be missed. The volume of urinary output should be watched closely, for significant oliguria may easily be overlooked.

The principal pathologic findings are in the compressed muscles and in the kidneys. In the former the normal pigment, myoglobin, was rapidly mobilized and absorbed, and extensive necrosis of muscle developed which tended to heal with calcification if the patient survived a week or longer. In the kidney a pigment nephropathy was found, which was indistinguishable from that which develops following other forms of severe trauma. A common terminal finding was severe pulmonary edema.

The treatment applied to these nine cases has been described. In the presence of oliguria or anuria, it was impossible to alkalinize the urine with doses of sodium bicarbonate which could be administered without danger of producing severe metabolic alkalosis. It is particularly important not to flood the circulatory system with intravenous solutions in an attempt to induce diuresis, once oliguria or anuria have become established. When excessive fluid is administered, the patients may die of pulmonary edema before fatal uremia develops.

That a recovery diuresis may develop in these cases is evidenced by two patients in this series in whom recovery diuresis had begun before death; in one of them it was well developed.

CASES OF SPECIAL INTEREST IN THIS CHAPTER

Fatal

69 70 78 93 132

Nonfatal

56 73 99 124

CASES OF SPECIAL INTEREST IN CHAPTER IX

Nonfatal

13	29	44	60	72	87	109	125	133	150
27	37	54	71	81	104	112	130	138	

Fatal

9	25	47	65	85	97	117	123	A-30
12	26	49	66	86	98	118	129	
22	31	52	74	88	108	120	131	
24	41	55	80	95	116	122	136	

Crush Syndrome

69 70 78 93 132

CHAPTER XII

General Pathology of Traumatic Shock

To demonstrate a relationship between a parenchymal degenerative change or pattern of changes and the clinical state of shock several conditions must be satisfied. The lesions must first be sufficiently distinctive, so that there can be no possibility of confusion with postmortem degeneration or the artefacts of poor fixation and faulty histologic technique. Second, they must be clearly distinguishable from the group of agonal changes seen in the tissues of any person whose death has not been instantaneous or at least relatively rapid. Specificity of individual lesion cannot reasonably be expected, but the changes should be demonstrable in a high proportion of shock cases, absent in cases of sudden death, and relatively infrequent in cardiac, metabolic, or cerebral deaths in which shock-like states are comparatively uncommon. There should be a demonstrable time-relationship between the onset of shock and appearance of the lesions, and conversely between recovery from shock and their disappearance. So far as could be ascertained, no pattern of lesions which fulfills these conditions[1] in man has been described in the literature.

The anatomic changes associated with shock may be usefully divided into (1) those which occur concomitantly with the state of shock and therefore are of interest in relation to its pathogenesis and (2) those which follow shock and therefore may be considered as its consequences. In studies of the pathology of human shock attention has heretofore been concentrated primarily on the former. In the present work attention is particularly devoted to the latter, but two brief sections dealing with pulmonary edema and with fat embolism have been included because of the extensive consideration given to them by previous investigators.

In our own preliminary investigations, the search for possible sequelae of

[1] Moon, V. H.: Analysis of shock. Brit. M. J. 1: 773–779, June 10, 1944.

956507 O—52——22

shock seemed fruitless for many months. The postmortem material of several hundred battle casualties was vainly examined for any lesion or combination of lesions which would fulfill the imposed conditions. The organs of patients dying after 4, 8, or 12 hours of prolonged shock showed little evidence of histologic change and none which could not readily be duplicated in a series of non-shock cases. When, however, the range of investigation was broadened to include material from casualties who lived more than 18 hours after injury, and when frozen sections stained for fat with Sudan IV were substituted for paraffin sections, a fairly constant pattern was disclosed. Evidence was obtained that approximately 18 hours after a shock-producing injury, fat vacuolation appears in the parenchymal cells of the heart, liver, and kidneys. These changes increased in frequency and severity up to 96 hours after injury, then progressively declined with longer periods of convalescence from the episode of shock, unless complicating factors, such as fat embolism or severe infection, prevented resolution of the process.

The pancreas and adrenal were also studied in the same group of cases. In the pancreas no lesion was recognized which appeared to correlate with shock. In the adrenal gland a series of changes was readily demonstrable: swelling of the cortex, pseudotubular degeneration, and depletion of stainable lipid, particularly of doubly refractile lipid. Since these changes did not differ qualitatively and were less marked quantitatively than those seen in cases with infection and in other types of control material, their significance is questionable. Only one factor, the depletion of doubly refractile lipid elements, showed a tendency to reversibility with increasing time intervals following resuscitation from shock.

Material

The nucleus of material for this section of the study was provided by the necropsy protocols and corresponding microscopic preparations from 60 cases that had been studied clinically by members of the Board. As the work progressed, the importance of sepsis as a complicating factor became apparent. Additional cases were therefore selected from the files of the 15th Medical General Laboratory in which the clinical data were sufficiently detailed to establish the diagnosis of shock and in which major sepsis could be excluded. Numerous additional examples of acute shock were included in order to cover a wider time-range than was provided by the Board's cases. In the tables to follow, these supplementary cases have been included unless the tables are designated as "Board Cases."

Control material was drawn both from the 15th Laboratory and from the Army Institute of Pathology. This included several groups of cases: (1) instantaneous or sudden deaths, such as homicides and motor vehicle accidents, (2) "medical deaths" unselected except for elimination, as far as possible, of "shock-like" states (the group included cerebral, cardiac, and infectious diseases), (3) deaths primarily due to starvation (from necropsies done in a German concentration camp), and (4) deaths from aplastic anemia. Not all organs were available for fat stains in all of these cases; consequently the number of controls varies somewhat from one section to another. The starvation and aplastic anemia groups were selected because of the known frequency with which fatty vacuolation of various organs occurs under these conditions.

The majority of necropsies on the combat soldier had been performed under field conditions by an officer of a field or evacuation hospital whose experience in pathology was often limited. (In the original 60 cases, one of the Board members was usually present at the necropsy.) Deaths were most numerous at times of heightened military activity when hospital staffs were overworked in caring for the living. Necropsies were sometimes conducted in hospital operating rooms but more often in tents without benefit of flooring, heat, or adequate illumination. Scales were rarely available. The examinations and records were inevitably incomplete. The central nervous system was rarely examined, the intestinal tract seldom opened, and wounds of the extremities were given but cursory attention to determine the presence or absence of gross infection, major vascular involvement, or extensive necrosis of muscle. Blocks of representative tissues were fixed in formalin, occasionally in Zenker's solution, and transmitted to the Pathology Section of the 15th Medical General Laboratory where they were sectioned and the histologic findings were reviewed by the author.

Findings

Lungs

The Board's cases include no examples of sudden death; hence the lungs were never normal. Congestion was described in every case; edema in approximately 85 percent; atelectasis in 70 percent; fat embolism in 65 percent; intra-alveolar hemorrhage in 55 percent; interstitial hemorrhage in 25 percent, and pneumonia in 30 percent. Because two of these lesions, pulmonary edema and fat embolism, have received considerable attention in relation to the mechanism of shock, their significance is worth examining in more detail.

Pulmonary Edema.—Estimation of the severity of pulmonary edema is difficult from the available data in view of the large number of prosectors and the few lung weights recorded. A rough classification into three grades has been attempted for 47 cases in which adequate information was recorded in the necropsy protocols: Grade I, little or no edema (classified as "slight") with lung weights probably below 800 Gm.; Grade II, moderate edema with lung weights between 800 and 1,200 Gm.; Grade III, severe edema with lung weights from 1,200 to 1,800 grams. Fifteen cases were Grade I (slight), 14 Grade II (moderate), and 18 Grade III (severe).

Several factors might influence the development of pulmonary edema in these patients. It has been suggested[2] that pulmonary edema is a constant and integral part of the shock mechanism. It is certainly a common sequela of renal insufficiency, from which a large proportion of the patients in this series suffered. It could be due to myocardial failure and evidence will be presented later in this chapter that myocardial degeneration actually was present in many cases. It might be influenced by fat embolism and finally it could be brought about, or at least intensified, by over-enthusiastic intravenous fluid therapy.

In Table 101 the degree of pulmonary edema is compared with the period of survival in 47 shock cases. The patients dying in less than 48 hours represent by and large the group in which resuscitation was unsuccessful. One patient (Case 22) briefly appeared to be resuscitated only to develop two secondary attacks of circulatory failure, in the last of which he died. These patients may fairly be considered to have died in, perhaps of, severe and prolonged shock. Five had minimal, 2 moderate, and only 3 severe edema. All had received repeated infusions of plasma and whole blood.

In the patients who survived into the third or fourth days, it is safe to assume that shock had disappeared. In the majority of these, incipient renal insufficiency was manifest, and only one patient failed to show a nephropathy at

[2] Moon, V. H.: Shock, its mechanism and pathology. Arch. Path. **24**: 642–663 (November) and 794–813 (December), 1937.

TABLE 101.—SEVERITY OF PULMONARY EDEMA AND SURVIVAL PERIOD IN 47 SHOCK CASES
Board's Cases

Pulmonary Edema	Survival Period *Number of cases*				Total Cases
	Less than 48 Hours	3 or 4 Days	More than 4 Days		
			Uremic	Non-uremic	
Grade I (Slight)	5	3	4	3	15
Grade II (Moderate)	2	2	6	4	14
Grade III (Severe)	3	7	7	1	18
Total	10	12	17	8	47

postmortem examination. They were oliguric or anuric, and the plasma nonprotein nitrogen had climbed to levels of 90 to 130 mg. per 100 cc., though few or no symptoms of uremia were manifest. In nine of these cases there was a moderate or severe pulmonary edema, but since in five of them there was also histologic evidence of myocardial degeneration, it would be impossible to assess the relative importance of cardiac and renal factors.

The 25 patients dying from the fifth day onward have been divided into uremic and non-uremic groups. Pulmonary edema of moderate degree was present in 6, and of severe degree in 7 of the 17 cases in the former group despite the fact that many of these patients were treated in consultation with clinical members of the Board and the intake of fluid was rigidly restricted. Since there was histologic evidence of myocardial injury in only 3 patients of this group, the evidence points strongly to renal insufficiency as the primary cause of the pulmonary edema. In the non-uremic group, 4 of 8 patients showed moderate and only 1 severe edema. In this group the most frequent cause of death was peritonitis.

In summary, pulmonary edema was less frequent and less severe in patients who were never successfully resuscitated from shock than in those patients who did recover from the acute stage of shock but subsequently displayed evidence of renal insufficiency. Our anatomic data offer no confirmation for the hypothesis that loss of fluid into the alveoli is an important factor in the development of shock.

Pulmonary Fat Embolism.—Pulmonary fat embolism is a very frequent complication of battle casualties, as the 65-percent incidence in the present group of cases shows. Its significance is extremely difficult to assess. In the early stages of World War I, much attention was given to it and it was considered by some investigators[3] to be an important, perhaps the most important cause of shock. Further experience failed entirely to substantiate the hypothesis, the theories of Bayliss and Cannon[4] became dominant, and fat embolism was forgotten.

Frozen sections were cut and stained for fat in all of the present series of cases in which lung tissue was available (51 cases). An attempt was made to estimate the severity of the embolism in three grades as follows: In Grade I only an occasional droplet is seen. In Grade II droplets are fairly numerous; they are found chiefly in large vessels or arterioles and seldom have passed into the capillaries of the alveolar walls. In Grade III a considerable proportion, a quarter to half or more, of the arterioles are plugged, and in numerous areas capillaries are filled as if by an injection mass. Systemic fat embolism of significant grade was never found in association with Grades I and II but was present in about a fifth of the cases in Grade III. Judged by experience covering several hundred battle casualties, the author considers it improbable that Grades I and II of pulmonary fat embolism are functionally significant.

In Table 102 the grade of fat embolism is compared with the degree of shock. It is apparent from inspection of the table that Grade III fat embolism was present in only 8 of the 39 cases of moderately severe or severe shock. Conversely, of 10 patients with significant fat embolism, 8 were estimated to have moderate or severe shock. It is evident that fat embolism is not the cause of shock in any considerable proportion of cases. Conversely, severe pulmonary fat embolism was always associated with shock, usually of moderate or severe

[3] PORTER, W. T.: Fat embolism, a cause of shock. Boston M. & S. J. 176: 248, February 15, 1917.

[4] GREAT BRITAIN. MEDICAL RESEARCH COMMITTEE. Special Report Series, No. 26. Traumatic Toxaemia as a Factor in Shock. Oxford, His Majesty's Stationery Office, 1919. IV. CANNON, W. B., and BAYLISS, W. M.: Note on muscle in relation to shock, p. 19–23. V. BAYLISS, W. M.: Further observations on the results of muscle injury and their treatment, p. 23–26. VI. CANNON, W. B.: Some characteristics of shock induced by tissue injury, p. 27–32.

degree. To determine whether or not this relationship is causal would require the study of a much larger series of cases than the present one.

TABLE 102.—FAT EMBOLISM AND SHOCK IN 51 BOARD CASES

Degree of Shock	Grade of Fat Embolism *Number of cases*				Total Cases
	0	I	II	III	
None	5	....	2	....	7
Slight	1	2	....	2	5
Moderate	3	3	2	3	11
Severe	8	11	4	5	28
Total	17	16	8	10	51

Fat Embolism and Pulmonary Edema.—In Table 103 the grade of pulmonary fat embolism is compared with the degree of pulmonary edema. It is obvious that there is no correlation.

TABLE 103.—FAT EMBOLISM AND PULMONARY EDEMA IN 44 BOARD CASES

Degree of Pulmonary Edema	Grade of Fat Embolism *Number of cases*				Total Cases
	0	I	II	III	
Slight	5	5	1	3	14
Moderate	5	5	2	2	14
Severe	4	4	4	4	16
Total	14	14	7	9	44

Heart

Material was available from 45 of the Board cases and 61 cases from the supplemental series, the latter including 10 shock cases and 51 control cases. Fat vacuolation was found in 24 of the cases from both series. This consisted

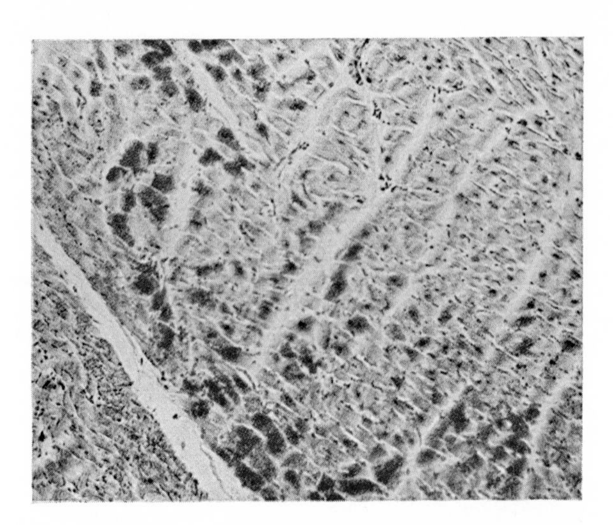

FIGURE 29. Frozen section of myocardium stained with Sudan IV. The patient died 48 hours after a shock-producing wound. Many cells are apparently filled with minute vacuoles, from 2 to 3 microns in diameter, which appear as bright red granules. The affected cells are not swollen and the nuclei appear normal. X 70

of very minute vacuoles, seldom more than 2 microns in diameter, arranged in parallel rows between the myofibrils (Fig. 29). When present in a cell, the vacuolation was apparent throughout the cell's entire length and breadth, rarely segmentally or focally. It was entirely independent of the amount of lipochrome demonstrable at the nuclear poles. The affected cell often seemed slightly swollen in the frozen section but this change could not be recognized with certainty in the paraffin sections. Sometimes single cells, more often groups of from 10 to 50 adjacent fibers, were affected. Vacuolation was never diffuse throughout the myocardium. In appearance it was strongly reminiscent of, though usually less severe than the patchy fat vacuolation seen in severe anemia. However, no gross changes suggestive of "tigering" were ever noted.

The severity of the change, estimated by the number and size of the vacuoles per cell and the proportion of cells involved, was roughly quantitated on a zero to 3-plus scale. The degree of involvement is compared with the survival period in Table 104. It is evident that fat vacuolation of cardiac muscle cells was not observed in previously healthy young men who developed shock following trauma but failed to survive at least 18 hours. In patients manifesting shock who lived from 18 to 96 hours, fat vacuolation of the myocardium was found in 75 percent. With longer periods of survival the incidence dropped sharply to 17 percent, and there were no cases of grade 3+ severity.

TABLE 104.—MYOCARDIAL FAT VACUOLATION IN 55 SHOCK CASES*

Survival Period	Number of Cases	Grade of Fat Vacuolation *Number of cases*				Percent Positive
		0	1+	2+	3+	
Less than 18 Hours . .	10	10	0	0	0	0
18 to 96 Hours	16	4	4	2	6	75
More than 4 Days . . .	29	24	2	3	0	17

*45 Board cases and 10 from the supplemental series.

Focal fat vacuolation of cardiac muscle cells has been noted frequently by the author in cases of systemic fat embolism with embolization of the myocardial capillaries. In only two of the group under consideration was this complication present. These two men died on the fifth and sixth days after injury. If they are excluded, the incidence of fat vacuolation in the patients surviving more than 4 days falls to 11 percent.

In Table 105 the degree of shock and the severity of fat vacuolation are compared in 14 patients among those dying within the 18- to 96-hour period who had been examined during life by a clinical member of the Board. The number of cases is small, but increasing intensity of fat vacuolation is apparent as shock becomes more severe.

TABLE 105.—DEGREE OF SHOCK AND FAT VACUOLATION OF MYOCARDIUM IN 14 BOARD PATIENTS WHO SURVIVED FROM 18 TO 96 HOURS

Degree of Shock	Grade of Fat Vacuolation *Number of cases*			
	0	1+	2+	3+
Slight	0	0	1	0
Moderate	1	2	1	1
Severe	2	1	0	5

Control Cases.—A group of 51 non-shock control cases is shown in Table 106. They include a number of instances of sudden death and a miscellaneous group of medical conditions. Since fat vacuolation can be produced in experimental animals by short periods of starvation,[5, 6] it seemed appropriate to study some cases of starvation deaths from prison camps. And, because fatty change in the myocardium has long been recognized as a sequela of severe anemia, a series of cases of aplastic anemia was included. Analysis of the material from the point of view of the presence or absence of peritonitis, an important factor in relation to liver and adrenal lesions, yielded no evidence that infection was important in the production of the myocardial changes.

TABLE 106.—FAT VACUOLATION OF MYOCARDIUM IN 51 CONTROL CASES

Type of Case	Number of Cases	Grade of Fat Vacuolation *Number of cases*				Percent Positive
		0	1+	2+	3+	
Sudden Deaths	15	15	0	0	0	0
Starvation Deaths	12	12	0	0	0	0
Deaths from Aplastic Anemia	9	6	0	2	1	33
Miscellaneous "Medical" Deaths	15	11	2	1	1	27

Summary.—Fat vacuolation of cardiac muscle fibers is a pathologic process not seen in previously healthy persons who die suddenly or who die following a shock-producing injury in a period of less than 18 hours. It is found in 75 percent of individuals who have survived a similar injury for periods of 18 to 96 hours, but becomes unusual in those living more than 4 days after injury. In a small sample group the degree of fatty change appeared to parallel the severity of shock. Though the lesion is found inconstantly in a variety of medical conditions, particularly those associated with severe grades of anoxemia, the frequency is considerably below that observed following shock.

[5] DIBLE, J. H.: Fat mobilization in starvation. J. Path. & Bact. 35: 451–466, May 1932.

[6] DIBLE, J. H., and LIBMAN, J.: Further observations on fat mobilization in starvation. J. Path. & Bact. 38: 269–284, May 1934.

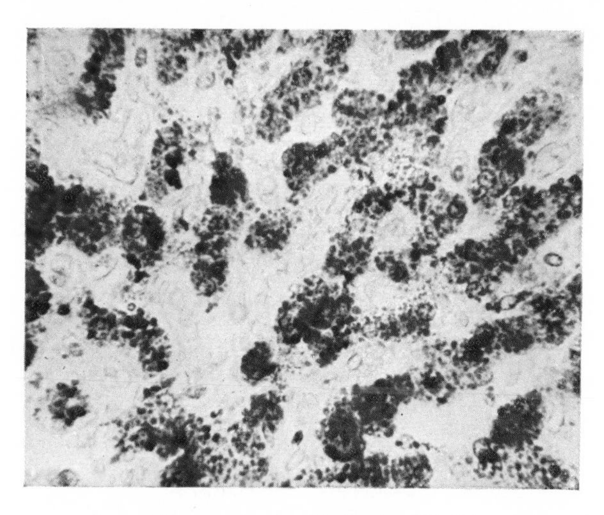

FIGURE 30. Frozen section of liver stained with Sudan IV. The patient died 72 hours after a shock-producing wound. The illustration shows the center of a lobule with some fine fat vacuolation of all visible liver cells. X 400

Liver

Fat vacuolation of the liver appears in such a variety of conditions and may be present in so many apparently normal individuals that one is often tempted to regard it as not significant unless the amount is very great. The usual form observed consists of vacuoles of considerable size, ranging from 5 to 20 microns in diameter. Such vacuoles are readily visible in paraffin sections with low magnification (from 16- to 30-mm. objectives) inasmuch as they occupy the full thickness of the section and appear as sharply outlined holes. Because of their large size there are never many vacuoles in a single cell.

Fat vacuolation of this type was rarely seen in shock cases, and when found probably existed before the shock-producing injury. Extensive fat vacuolation was nevertheless readily demonstrable in shock if sufficient time had elapsed for its development. This form of fat vacuolation consisted almost entirely of very fine droplets in the range from 2 to 4 microns in diameter (Fig. 30). Even when the process was severe, though slightly larger droplets were found, there was little tendency for them to fuse, and as many as 15 or 20 might be present in a single cell. The vacuolation is readily seen in paraffin sections if the 4-mm. lens is used. Few of them extend through the thickness of the section, but two or more layers can be seen by varying the depth of focus. Because of the small size of the vacuoles, some difficulty may be experienced in frozen sections in distinguishing them from the normal pigment which is often slightly sudanophilic. The fat vacuoles are a little larger than the pigment granules and are rounder. Very often they show a crescentic intensification of the stain on one margin.

The affected cells in the initial stages were always centrally located in the lobule; with increasing severity the involvement spread to the periphery. There was little evidence of swelling of the cells and the organ as a whole was not enlarged, yellow, or greasy. For this reason it seems improbable that the amount of fat in the liver could have been greatly increased, though a check by chemical methods would be necessary to decide this point.

The occurrence of small-droplet fat in relation to the survival period in 51 Board cases is shown in Table 107. It is evident that in shock patients surviving from 18 to 96 hours, moderate to severe fat vacuolation was an almost constant finding. With longer survival periods, the proportion of cases with mild or no fat vacuolation increased but instances of severe vacuolation were still found. In reviewing the group of 31 patients who survived more than 4 days, it became apparent that severe fatty changes were particularly frequent in patients with peritonitis, the only common cause of prolonged sepsis in this series. This is also shown in the table.

Table 107.—Fat Vacuolation in the Liver in 51 Shock Cases,* and Influence of Peritonitis in Patients Surviving Longer than 4 Days

Survival Period	Number of Cases	Grade of Fat Vacuolation *Number of cases*				Percent Grades 2+ and 3+
		0	1+	2+	3+	
18 to 96 Hours. . . .	20	1	1	3	15	90
More than 4 Days. . .	31	12	4	6	9	48
With Peritonitis . .	14	3	1	3	7	71
No Major Infection .	17	9	3	4	1	29

*Board cases only.

Since 26 of the 51 Board cases were complicated by peritonitis, the significance of the figures in Table 107 is open to doubt. In Table 108, which includes 28 supplementary cases from the 15th Laboratory, all cases of peritonitis or other major sepsis have been excluded. In this selected series, it is apparent that fat vacuolation of more than minimal degree was seldom seen in shock patients who failed to survive at least 18 hours. Of those who survived from 18 to 96 hours, 87 percent showed the presence of fat, 59 percent in moderate or severe degree. With survival beyond 96 hours, the tendency to return to normal is seen, the total dropping to 47 percent and that for the more severe grades to 29 percent.

TABLE 108.—CENTROLOBULAR FAT VACUOLATION OF LIVER CELLS IN 53 SHOCK CASES UNCOMPLICATED BY MAJOR INFECTION*

Survival Period	Number of Cases	Grade of Fat Vacuolation — *Number of cases*				Percent Positive	Percent Grade 2+ or 3+
		0	1+	2+	3+		
Less than 18 Hours	14	11	2	1	0	22	8.2
18 to 96 Hours.	22	3	6	4	9	87	59
More than 4 Days.	17	9	3	4	1	47	29

* Includes 25 Board cases and 28 supplementary shock cases.

Control Cases.—Since fat vacuolation of the liver is such a common phenomenon and can be produced by so many etiologic factors, numerous control cases seemed necessary. Seventeen instances of sudden death were selected at random from the laboratory files. Fifteen cases of "medical" deaths (cardiac, cerebral, nephritic) without obvious shock-like states, 20 instances of death from aplastic anemia, and 38 starvation deaths were included—a total of 90 control cases. The incidence of *centrolobular* fat vacuolation in 36 shock cases and 90 controls is shown in Table 109.

The occurrence of moderate or severe fat vacuolation in 24 percent of the sudden-death group is worthy of comment. This group was compiled largely from motor-vehicle accident and homicide cases in base-section troops. The proportion of limited-service personnel and older men was higher in such troops than in combat organizations. Two of the men in the group studied had been intoxicated at the time of death and had enlarged, grossly fatty livers suggestive of chronic alcoholism. In contrast, the acute-shock group, with survival periods shorter than 18 hours, was made up almost entirely of battle casualties, all previously healthy and vigorous young men, and therefore represents a better control group than the "sudden deaths." The relatively high incidence (40 percent) in the miscellaneous medical deaths is not surprising in view of the multiple etiology of fat deposit in the liver, but is still not as high as the frequency (59 percent) in the 18- to 96-hour shock group. The low incidence in the anemia group proved surprising in view of the known frequency of myocardial fat vacuolation in such conditions. The starvation cases provided a most interesting contrast to the shock material. Although fat was present in the majority of these cases, it was always manifest at the periphery, never at the center of the lobule.

TABLE 109.—CENTROLOBULAR FAT VACUOLATION OF LIVER IN SHOCK CASES AND CONTROLS

Type of Case	Number of Cases	Grade of Fat Vacuolation *Number of cases*				Percent Grades 2+ or 3+
		0	1+	2+	3+	
SHOCK CASES						
Less than 18 Hours' Survival	14	11	2	1	0	8.2
18 to 96 Hours' Survival	22	3	6	4	9	59
CONTROLS						
Sudden Deaths . . .	17	8	5	2	2	24
Miscellaneous "Medical" Deaths.	15	3	6	3	3	40
Deaths from Aplastic Anemia	20	10	6	1	3	20
Starvation Deaths . .	38	0	0	0	0	0

Summary.—Eighteen hours after a shock-producing injury, fat vacuolation was demonstrable in the liver cells at the center of the lobule in 87 percent of 53 cases uncomplicated by major infection and was of moderate or severe grade in 59 percent. After the fourth day it tended to disappear in cases uncomplicated by peritonitis. The incidence in the 18- to 96-hour cases was somewhat higher than in any of the control group studied.

Kidney

The histologic changes in the kidney following shock have been described in detail in Chapter IX. Fat vacuolation in the ascending limb of Henle's loop (see Figures 9 and 10, Chapter IX) was shown to be the first definite histologic evidence of renal injury. In the present analysis, only this feature of the numerous renal changes which may develop will be considered. The findings in 90 cases are summarized in Table 110. Supplementary shock cases, as previously described, have been added to the Board's cases.

TABLE 110.—FAT VACUOLATION OF ASCENDING LIMBS OF HENLE IN 90 SHOCK CASES

Survival Period	Number of Cases	Grade of Fat Vacuolation *Number of cases*				Percent Positive	Percent Grade 2+ or 3+
		0	1+	2+	3+		
Less than 18 Hours	20	17	2	1	0	15	5
18 to 24 Hours.	11	5	1	4	1	55	45
24 to 96 Hours.	26	4	1	4	17	85	81
More than 4 Days.	33	13	6	7	6	58	39

As in the heart and liver, fat vacuolation was rarely found in shock patients surviving less than 18 hours after injury. It was already present in 55 percent of the 18- to 24-hour group and was evident in 85 percent of those surviving from 1 to 4 days. With survival beyond that period it decreased somewhat in frequency to 58 percent, and considerably in severity, the 2+ and 3+ grades dropping from 81 percent to 39 percent. In the kidney as in the heart, the severity of fat vacuolation was uninfluenced by the presence or absence of peritonitis.

Control Cases.—The degree of fat vacuolation in the ascending limbs in 55 control cases is shown in Table 111. Fat vacuolation in the ascending limbs of Henle's loop is found with sufficient frequency (43 percent of the "medical" deaths in the present group) to have led some authors[7] to consider it normal.

[7] MÖLLENDORF, WILHELM VON, ed. Handbuch der mikroskopischen Anatomie des Menschen . . . Berlin, J. Springer, 1930. vol. VII, Part I. Harn- und Geschlechtsapparat, p. 86.

Its complete absence in 19 cases of sudden death and its presence in only 15 percent of 20 shock cases representing patients who died in less than 18 hours following injury clearly indicate that it is not a normal finding in healthy young men in the 18- to 35-year age group. Dible[8 9] has shown that fat rapidly appears in this segment of the nephron in starvation experiments in rabbits. The data on starvation deaths included in our series showed an incidence of 50 percent, with 38 percent of 2+ or 3+ grade. These figures are nevertheless well below those (85 percent and 81 percent) of the 1- to 4-day shock cases shown in Table 110.

TABLE 111.—FAT VACUOLATION OF ASCENDING LIMBS OF HENLE IN 55 NON-SHOCK CONTROL CASES

Type of Case	Number of Cases	Grade of Fat Vacuolation *Number of cases*				Percent Positive	Percent Grade 2+ or 3+
		0	1+	2+	3+		
Sudden Deaths . . .	19	19	0	0	0	0	0
Miscellaneous "Medical" Deaths	14	8	3	1	2	43	22
Starvation Deaths. .	12	8	1	3	0	50	38
Deaths from Aplastic Anemia	10	8	1	1	0	25	13

Summary.—Fat vacuolation of the ascending limbs of Henle's loop is abnormal in men from 18 to 35 years of age. It was found in only 15 percent of shock patients dying in less than 18 hours but was present in 85 percent of shock patients surviving from 1 to 4 days after injury. From the fourth day onward, a decrease in frequency and severity was demonstrable, regardless of whether a hemoglobinuric nephrosis developed.

Adrenal

A normal adrenal gland is rarely seen at necropsy by the civilian pathologist who does not have opportunity to perform postmortem examinations upon

[8] See footnotes 5 and 6.

[9] DIBLE, J. H., and POPJAK, G.: Distribution of fatty change in kidneys and some factors influencing its production. J. Path. & Bact. 53: 133–146, July 1941.

persons who have died suddenly without previous disease. The adrenal gland of the healthy young male has a narrow cortex which ranges from 1.0 to 1.3 mm. in width. The cells are richly packed with lipid (stainable with Sudan IV), predominantly in the fascicular layer, but numerous vacuoles are also demonstrable in the zona glomerulosa and reticularis. Limited to the zona reticularis are large quantities of doubly refractile lipid which serve to outline this layer sharply when viewed with crossed Nicol prisms.

In our shock cases no medullary changes but a variety of cortical changes were observed. The amount of stainable lipid decreased and the optically active fraction was markedly depleted. The cortex was slightly swollen and frequently showed the pseudoacinar type of degeneration described and illustrated by F. B. Mallory in 1914,[10] more recently emphasized by Rich[11] in relation to sepsis, and noted by Mallory and Brickley[12] in the burn victims of the Cocoanut Grove disaster. The changes observed did not differ qualitatively from and were less severe quantitatively than those of sepsis or of such control conditions as aplastic anemia and starvation, though some degree of terminal infection may have complicated much of this control material. Only one feature, the doubly refractile lipid depletion, showed evidence of reversibility with recovery from shock.

In Tables 112 and 113 the stainable and the doubly refractile lipids are compared in a group of 40 shock cases free from septic complications and a control group of 18 cases of sudden death. The amount of lipid, as in other organs, was visually estimated on a zero to 3+ scale. In this instance, however, the maximal 3+ figure represents the normal and zero the stage of maximal depletion.

A moderate depletion of the total stainable fat is evident in the shock group surviving from 18 to 96 hours. There is, however, no evidence of return to normal with longer intervals of survival after recovery from shock; the process is, in fact, much intensified in the group surviving more than 4 days. In contrast to the stainable lipid, the doubly refractile fraction was occasionally below the usual level in cases of sudden death (17 percent) and was depleted in

[10] Mallory, F. B.: Principles of Pathologic Histology. Philadelphia, W. B. Saunders, 1914, p. 653.

[11] Rich, A. R.: Peculiar type of adrenal cortical damage associated with acute infections, and its possible relation to circulatory collapse. Bull. Johns Hopkins Hosp. 74: 1–15, January 1944.

[12] Mallory, T. B., and Brickley, W. J.: Symposium on management of Cocoanut Grove burns at the Massachusetts General Hospital; pathology, with special reference to pulmonary lesions. Ann. Surg. 117: 865–884, June 1943.

956507 O—52——24

TABLE 112.—STAINABLE LIPIDS IN ADRENAL CORTEX IN 40 SHOCK CASES WITHOUT INFECTION AND 18 CASES OF SUDDEN DEATH

Type of Case	Number of Cases	Amount of Lipid *Number of cases*				Percent Diminished	Percent Greatly Diminished
		3+	2+	1+	0		
SHOCK CASES							
Less than 18 Hours' Survival.	11	11	0	0	0	0	0
18 to 96 Hours' Survival	13	8	3	2	0	38	15
More than 4 Days' Survival	16	4	8	4	0	75	25
CONTROLS							
Sudden Death . .	18	18	0	0	0	0	0

TABLE 113.—DOUBLY REFRACTILE LIPIDS IN ADRENAL CORTEX IN 40 SHOCK CASES WITHOUT INFECTION AND 18 CASES OF SUDDEN DEATH

Type of Case	Number of Cases	Amount of Lipid *Number of cases*				Percent Diminished	Percent Greatly Diminished
		3+	2+	1+	0		
SHOCK CASES							
Less than 18 Hours' Survival.	11	8	2	1	0	27	9
18 to 96 Hours' Survival	13	1	4	7	1	92	61
More than 4 Days' Survival	16	3	7	3	3	81	38
CONTROLS							
Sudden Death . .	18	15	3	0	0	17	0

27 percent of shock patients dying in less than 18 hours, in one case severely depleted. In the shock cases of 18 to 96 hours' survival, this type of lipid was diminished in all but one instance (92 percent of the cases) and markedly so

in eight cases, or 61 percent. In those patients surviving more than 4 days, some evidence of a tendency to return to normal is shown by a drop in the percentage of severe depletion from 61 to 38 percent.

Control Material.—It was difficult to know what kind of control material would be suitable inasmuch as most types of illness which lead to death produce similar and even more marked adrenal changes. Four groups of control cases are listed in Table 114. It is evident that a wide variety of factors affect the storage of lipidic substances in the adrenal cortex, many of them more profoundly than does shock.

TABLE 114.—ADRENAL CORTICAL LIPIDS IN 44 CONTROL CASES

Type of Case	Number of Cases	Stainable Fat		Doubly Refractile Lipids	
		Percent Diminished	Percent Greatly Diminished	Percent Diminished	Percent Greatly Diminished
Miscellaneous "Medical" Deaths.	14	50	22	79	29
Starvation Deaths	9	78	44	100	78
Deaths from Aplastic Anemia . .	11	82	18	91	91
Fatal Cases with Infection	10	100	80	100	100

Summary.—Although numerous changes occur in the adrenal cortex following shock, they do not differ in character from, and are less severe than those seen in infection and in a wide variety of lethal disorders. The only factor which was found to change abruptly 18 hours after a shock-producing injury was the amount of doubly refractile lipid in the zona reticularis. This was diminished in 92 percent of the cases in the 18- to 96-hour group (Table 114). This factor also was the only one in which any tendency could be established to return toward normal with increasing time intervals following recovery from shock.

COMMENT

The possible roles of pulmonary edema and of fat embolism in the pathogenesis of shock in men wounded in battle have been discussed in the sections devoted to these phenomena. The pattern of parenchymal degenerative changes described in the heart, liver, kidneys, and adrenals deserves further consideration as a probable consequence of shock. None of the changes described are specific for the state of shock. Fat is known to make its appearance in one or another of these organs in response to a variety of pathologic conditions such as anoxemia, starvation, and chemical or bacterial toxic agents—and lipids disappear from the adrenal under an even greater variety of conditions. Critical examination of the data is therefore necessary before concluding that the observed changes were due to shock.

Errors of subjective interpretation in relying upon such vague changes as "parenchymatous degeneration" and "cloudy swelling," which are readily confused with postmortem degeneration and the artefacts of faulty histologic technique, have been avoided by the use of frozen sections and fat stains; general histologic experience indicates that there is no significant shift in the proportion of stainable fat up to 12 hours after death. Less is known of the behavior of doubly refractile lipids, but in the material included in this study no evidence was discovered that this fraction of the fatty substance was affected by postmortem degeneration within the same time limit. The observed variations from the normal are therefore vital phenomena.

Next in importance are the time relationships to shock. Table 115 shows the percentage of all cases with abnormal fat vacuolation in the heart, liver, and kidney, and depletion of the doubly refractile lipid in the adrenal, for each group and for the sudden-death control group. In each of the four organs studied no significant difference in demonstrable fat is apparent between the sudden-death series and the shock cases in which death occurred in less than 18 hours. Abnormal changes are evident, however, in these organs in from 75 to 92 percent of shock patients who survived from 18 to 96 hours after injury. The almost synchronous appearance of the lesions 18 hours after injury in all four organs suggests a single causative factor. The delay in appearance of the morphologic evidence of injury in many instances until shock has been relieved is not incompatible with a causal relationship. Days and even weeks may intervene between injury and reaction with such widely varying agents as diphtheria toxin and x-rays.

Of equal importance in establishing an etiologic relationship between shock and the lesions which have been described is evidence of reversibility, of return to or at least toward normal with increasing intervals after the episode of shock. As all the necropsy material in this series necessarily derived from individuals with lethal disorders, it is not surprising that a complete return to normal was not usually demonstrable. Clear evidence of a tendency to reversibility is shown in Table 116, in which the more severe grades of changes in the 18- to 96-hour group are compared with those in the group surviving 4 days or longer. It is noteworthy that the time interval before recovery was demonstrable was essentially the same for all four organs, the change becoming demonstrable on the fourth day in each instance. The possible contention that the changes described were merely agonal, like depletion of liver glycogen, is refuted by this evidence of reversibility in a large number of cases progressing to a fatal outcome due to other factors.

TABLE 115.—INCIDENCE OF ABNORMAL FAT CHANGES IN THE HEART, LIVER, KIDNEY, AND ADRENAL IN SHOCK CASES AND CONTROL CASES OF SUDDEN DEATH

Type of Case	Heart *percent of cases*	Liver *percent of cases*	Kidney *percent of cases*	Adrenal Gland (Depletion of doubly refractile lipid) *percent of cases*
SHOCK CASES				
Less than 18 Hours' Survival	0	22	15	27
18 to 96 Hours' Survival	75	87	76	92
More than 4 Days' Survival	17	47	58	81
CONTROLS				
Sudden Death	0	24	0	17

TABLE 116.—INCIDENCE OF SEVERE FATTY CHANGES IN SHOCK CASES

Period of Survival	Heart *percent of cases*	Liver *percent of cases*	Kidney *percent of cases*	Adrenal Gland *percent of cases*
18 to 96 Hours	50	59	81	61
4 Days or Longer	12	29	39	38

Though it has been repeatedly stressed that none of the changes described can be considered pathognomonic of shock, it is not impossible that the *pattern* of changes may be. This is suggested by the data shown in Table 117. The incidence of the lesions under consideration has been compared in shock patients surviving from 18 to 96 hours with three groups of control cases: a miscellaneous group of "medical" deaths, a group of aplastic anemia fatalities, and one of starvation deaths. Only in the shock group did more than three-quarters of the cases show involvement of all four organs.

Subsequent to making the observations upon the adrenal gland which we have recorded, our attention was called to the investigations of Popjak[13] on the lipids in the rat adrenal in experimental shock. He found swelling of the cortex and marked depletion of both stainable and doubly refractile lipid. This occurred regularly 15 to 24 hours after the shock-producing crush injury, a time interval essentially the same as in our human material. In his animals restoration to normal in 48 hours was the rule.

TABLE 117.—DISTRIBUTION OF LESIONS IN CONTROL GROUPS COMPARED WITH SHOCK CASES

Type of Case	Heart *percent of cases*	Liver *percent of cases*	Kidney *percent of cases*	Adrenal Gland *percent of cases*
SHOCK CASES				
18 to 96 Hours' Survival	75	87	76	92
CONTROLS				
Starvation Deaths	0	0	50	100
Deaths from Aplastic Anemia	33	20	25	91
Miscellaneous "Medical" Deaths	27	40	43	79

We have little evidence of what the significance of these lesions may be from the functional point of view. The renal lesion has already been discussed in Chapter IX. No electrocardiograms were made on these patients and no determinations of adrenal cortical hormone excretion were made. In Chapter II the results of bromsulfalein tests in shock patients were discussed. A transitory period of retention of the dye was observed, which it seems reasonable to cor-

[13] POPJAK, G.: Lipids of rat adrenal in shock caused by experimental crushing injury. J. Path. & Bact. 56: 485–496, October 1944.

relate with the fatty changes in the liver which have been described. Although no morphologic evidence of bile stasis was observed in liver sections, the possibility of a hepatic as well as a hemolytic factor must be borne in mind in interpreting the elevated plasma bilirubin often noted in these patients.

SUMMARY AND CONCLUSIONS

Two morphologic phenomena which have been implicated in the pathogenesis of shock, pulmonary edema and pulmonary fat embolism, were studied in a series of fatal battle casualties. Pulmonary edema was found to be too inconstant and too late in development to be an important factor in the initiation of shock in severely wounded men. Pulmonary fat embolism proved to be a frequent coincidental lesion. It was absent or minimal in degree in the majority of cases, and its significance in the small remaining proportion could not be established.

A standard pattern of visceral changes was found in patients with traumatic shock who survived a minimum of 18 hours after injury. This consisted of fat vacuolation of the heart, the central cells of the liver lobules, and the ascending limbs of Henle's loops in the kidney. In the adrenal gland, the doubly refractile lipid became depleted after the same time interval. In all four organs these changes persisted for 3 days after injury. From the fourth day onward in cases uncomplicated by infection, a tendency to return to normal could be demonstrated. The incidence of this pattern of changes proved higher in shock cases than in a variety of control material. It was concluded that they constitute evidence of parenchymatous injury produced by shock.

APPENDIX A

Organization and Operation of the Board for the Study of the Severely Wounded

North African (later Mediterranean) Theater of Operations, U.S.A.

ORGANIZATION

The background of events and observations leading to recognition of the need for an organized study of the severely wounded in an active theater of war has been described in the Introduction to this volume. The Chief Surgeon, North African Theater of Operations, Maj. General Morrison C. Stayer, U.S.A., discussed this problem with two members of his staff, Colonel Edward D. Churchill, MC, Surgical Consultant, and Colonel William S. Stone, MC. On their recommendation he initiated action from which stemmed the Board whose work has been presented in this volume. His memorandum to the Commanding General follows.

HEADQUARTERS

NORTH AFRICAN THEATER OF OPERATIONS

Office of the Surgeon

1 September 1944

SUBJECT: Appointment of Medical Board to Study the Treatment of the Severely Wounded

TO: Quartermaster, Ordnance, G–1, G–4 and AG

1. Outstanding progress in the treatment of the wounded has been made by the Medical Service in this theater. Many lives have been saved by this work and many individuals that would have been hopeless wrecks, if they survived, have been rehabilitated into normal or near normal individuals. Further progress in improving the Medical Service will depend upon proper and timely employment of the

skilled and experienced medical personnel present in the theater. There are several urgent problems that should have additional study if a progressive medical service is to be maintained. On the Surgical Service, there is increasing evidence that the recovery of some of the severely wounded is handicapped by renal lesions that complicate treatment or are sequelae of the original injury. In addition, there have been some observations made on wounded troops that a clinical condition which has been labeled pulmonary edema is frequently encountered. Because of the above it is considered desirable that the whole problem of resuscitation of wounded be critically studied by competent, experienced clinicians and that the results of this work be made available to the Medical Service of this and other theaters.

2. It is therefore requested that a Board be appointed by the Commanding General, NATOUSA, for the study of designated phases of the treatment of the severely wounded, the Board to operate directly under the Surgeon, NATOUSA, who will be responsible for the administration and supervision of the technical and professional details of the Board's work.

a. The Board will be made up of the following personnel:

MEDICAL PERSONNEL

Lt. Col. Tracy B. Mallory, O–518569—15th Medical Gen. Lab.
Lt. Col. F. A. Simeone, O–400993—Surgeon's Office, NATOUSA
Lt. Col. H. K. Beecher, O–526881—Surgeon's Office, NATOUSA
Major E. R. Sullivan, O–398217—6th General Hospital
Captain C. H. Burnett, O–356977—94th Evacuation Hospital

CHEMISTS

Captain S. L. Shapiro, O–509728—15th Medical Gen. Lab.

NURSES

2nd Lt. Gladys E. Maroon, N–742599—21st General Hospital
2nd Lt. Helen G. Woodman, N–741233—21st General Hospital

OFFICER Branch Immaterial (may be limited service).

One (1) Lieutenant or Captain. Request that temporary detail be made from Replacement Pool.

ENLISTED PERSONNEL Ten (10)

1 Sergeant—Showstack, Paul J., ASN 31297297—Medical Museum
2 Chemistry Technicians:
—T/4 Babb, Benjamin F., ASN 33521601—15th Med. Gen. Lab.
—T/3 Guin, Carlos F., ASN 18033517—15th Med. Gen. Lab.
1 General Laboratory Technician: 2nd Medical Laboratory
2 Clerks, Typists)
4 Enlisted Men) Qualified as drivers, tent handlers, general utilities, etc.
To be obtained on Temporary Duty from Replacement Pool.

TRANSPORTATION

2 C & R Cars
1 1½-ton personnel carrier truck
1 Mobile Laboratory (complete with equipment and supplies (as defined by the Board) to be obtained from the 15th Med. Gen. Lab.)

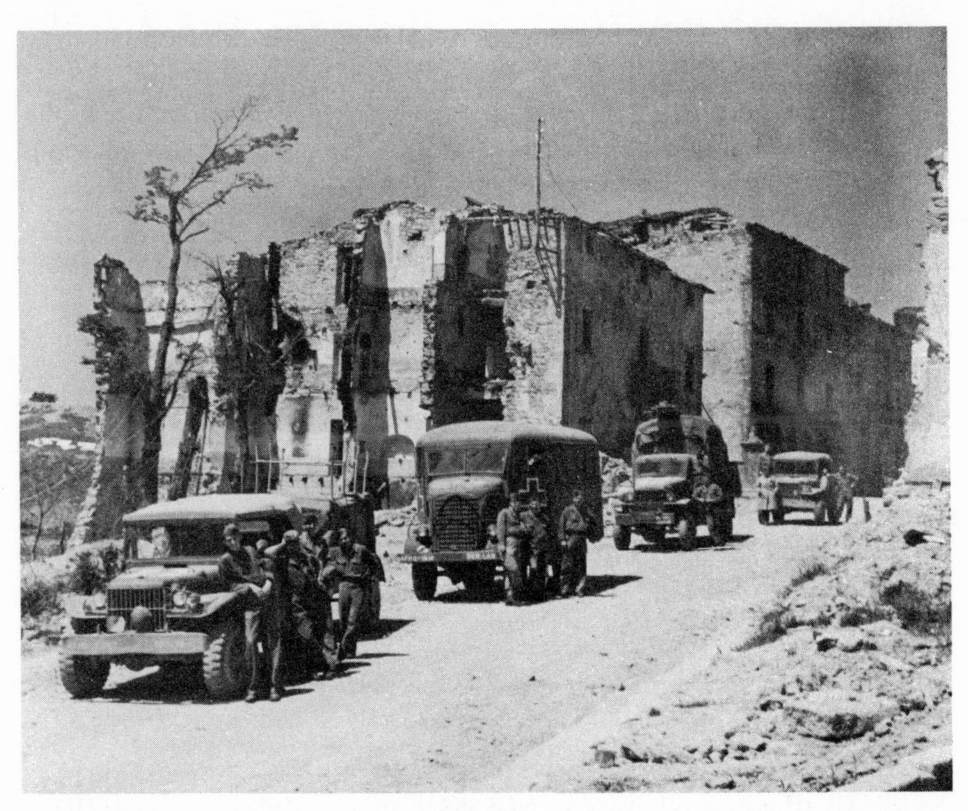

VEHICLES carrying equipment used by the Board for the Study of the Severely Wounded pause before a bomb-damaged building in Monghidoro.

TENTAGE Seven (7) Pyramidal Tents

3. Personnel involved will be on a temporary duty status while assigned to the Board and will be relieved of all other duties while so assigned. Upon completion of their work, the Board will render a report of their findings and recommendations to the Surgeon, NATOUSA. Progress reports will also be made when findings would indicate that immediate advantage should be taken of the scientific data obtained by the Board.

4. If requested by the Board, all Medical Installations coming under the jurisdiction of this Headquarters will, in every way possible, aid the Board in its work.

5. Medical supplies and equipment not obtainable at units where the Board is functioning, will be furnished, as requested by the Board, from Medical depot stocks on 90-day shipping ticket. All supplies, equipment and transportation to be returned to proper organization or depot upon completion of temporary duty.

6. Verbal concurrence has been obtained from all other Headquarters and units involved.

For the SURGEON:

E. STANDLEE, Colonel, MC

Lt. General Jacob B. Devers, Commanding General, North African Theater of Operations, recognizing that lives might be saved by means of such a study, gave his immediate support to the project. Only two days after the date of the original memorandum from his Chief Surgeon, he published the following order establishing the Medical Board to Study the Treatment of the Severely Wounded. (This title was later commonly abbreviated to the Board for the Study of the Severely Wounded.) The Board was made directly responsible to the Chief Surgeon of the Theater.

HEADQUARTERS

NORTH AFRICAN THEATER OF OPERATIONS

UNITED STATES ARMY

3 September 1944

SUBJECT: Appointment of Medical Board to Study the Treatment of the Severely Wounded

TO: All Concerned

1. A Board of Officers, consisting of the following officers:

LT COL TRACY B. MALLORY	O–518569 MC	15th Medical General Laboratory
LT COL FIORINDO A. SIMEONE	O–400993 MC	Medical Section, AFHQ
LT COL HENRY K. BEECHER	O–526881 MC	Medical Section, AFHQ
MAJOR EUGENE R. SULLIVAN	O–398217 MC	6th Gen Hosp on T/D Med Sec, AFHQ
CAPT CHARLES H. BURNETT	O–356977 MC	94th Evac Hosp, Semi-mobile
CAPT S. L. SHAPIRO	O–509728 SnC	15th Medical General Laboratory
2nd LT GLADYS E. MAROON	N–742599 ANC	21st General Hospital
2nd LT HELEN G. WOODMAN	N–741233 ANC	21st General Hospital

is appointed for the study of designated phases of the treatment of the severely wounded. Officers involved will be on a temporary duty status while assigned to the Board and will be relieved of all other duties while so assigned.

2. The Board will operate directly under the Surgeon, NATOUSA, who will be responsible for the administration and supervision of the technical and professional details of the work of the Board. Upon completion of work, the Board will render a report of their findings and recommendations to the Surgeon, NATOUSA.

By command of Lieutenant General DEVERS:

R. E. LINES, Captain, AGD
Asst. Adj. Gen.

PERSONNEL AND EQUIPMENT

In addition to the members of the Board, the nucleus of which consisted of those officers who had already been working both individually and as a team on various preliminary studies, a sizable group of full-time technical and administrative assistants was found necessary and was attached to the Board on temporary duty. First Lieutenant William H. McMahon, INF, of the 7th Replacement Depot served for a short time as administrative officer. Captain Louis D. Smith, SnC, who had been working with the Board from the beginning, was formally assigned to the Board in December.

The two nurses originally assigned to the Board, Second Lieutenants Gladys E. Maroon, ANC, and Helen G. Woodman, ANC, 21st General Hospital, were succeeded by Second Lieutenants Rose C. McDonnell and Marguerite V. Cronin, ANC, 6th General Hospital, who later were succeeded by First Lieutenants Florence L. Giberti and Phyllis G. Madden, ANC. Also attached to the Board were Second Lieutenant (then T/Sgt.) Louis Breslow, MAC, and Sergeant Paul J. Showstack, 3d Medical Detachment, Museum and Medical Art Service, the former as documentary artist and the latter as photographer.

The following enlisted laboratory technicians were assigned to duty with the Board: T/3 Carlos F. Guin, Jr. and T/4 Benjamin F. Babb, of the 15th Medical General Laboratory; Pfc. Earl R. Zea, Pfc. George L. Williams, Pfc. James A. Donaldson, and Pvts. Clyette S. Alligood, Donald M. Campbell, and Walter C. Huhn, Jr., all of the 7th Replacement Depot. T/Sgt. Carl A. Sauget, T/Sgt. Anthony N. Ashute (later replaced by T/3 Edwin A. Rooney), and T/4 Billy D. Ashley (replacing Sgt. Guin) were later added to the enlisted personnel. Sergeant Babb was chief medical technician.

Basic equipment available was as listed in the original memorandum from the Chief Surgeon. Supplies and equipment not obtainable at units where the Board was functioning were to be furnished from depot stocks on a 90-day basis. In addition, arrangements were made for a continuous supply of distilled water and standard solutions, and for replacements of supplies and expendable laboratory equipment from the 15th Medical General Laboratory via the "blood-plane" (a plane placed at the disposal of the 6713th Blood Transfusion Unit to forward blood from the base section bleeding unit to the advance distributing unit). It was planned to set up as much laboratory equipment as possible in a tent. Since, however, some delicate apparatus might be inadequately protected under canvas, the mobile laboratory truck of the 15th Laboratory was placed at the Board's disposal. Details of the organization and operation of the field laboratory appear in Appendix B.

DEFINITION OF OBJECTIVES

After discussion among Board members in consultation with Colonel Churchill and Colonel Stone, it was agreed that the major problems for investigation should be: (1) Physiologic and metabolic studies of the severely wounded; (2) adequacy of shock resuscitation therapy; (3) possible hazards of transfusion with type O blood, and (4) the mechanism of renal insufficiency following resuscitation from shock. The investigative program of the Board, although developed along diversified and varied lines, remained focused on these primary broad objectives.

MANNER OF OPERATION

It was evident that the objectives of the study as defined could be approached only by selection of a base of operations which would meet all of several essential requirements: 1. Facilities for rationing, housing, and other administrative support of the Board. 2. Access to an adequate number of severely wounded men. 3. Observation of the severely wounded at the earliest possible time after wounding but under such circumstances that patients included in the study normally would remain available for observation through the period of resuscitation (including surgery) and at least the immediate postoperative phase of treatment. 4. Utilization of an installation in the established chain of evacuation, thereby avoiding establishment of special facilities. Obviously aid stations, collecting stations, and clearing stations met only the second of these requirements. General hospitals failed to meet either the second or third. Forward hospitals, i. e., either evacuation or field hospitals as employed in the combat zone in Italy, satisfied the general requirements. The size of the research unit, however, precluded attachment to a platoon of a field hospital. It was not too great for an evacuation hospital and selection of a base was thus determined.

On 19 September 1944, therefore, with equipment loaded on a 2½-ton truck, two Command and Reconnaissance cars and the overload transported by the "blood plane," the personnel of the Board reported to Fifth Army Headquarters and proceeded to the 94th Evacuation Hospital at Pratalino, a few miles north of Florence, Italy. During the greater part of the 8-month period of the study

(September 1944 to May 1945) the Board remained with this hospital. For a 2-month period it was attached to the 24th General Hospital, and during that time two members of the Board alternated at B platoon of the 32nd Field Hospital while another was making biochemic tests at the 8th Evacuation Hospital. This was at the time of the push of the 10th Mountain Division, and illustrates one method by which extensive data were obtained on casualties in several areas during periods of maximum military activity.

A system of study gradually evolved as work poured in. The hospital provided a special ward tent in which all patients under study were concentrated following operation. The Board supplied the nursing service, but primary responsibility for professional care remained in the hands of the hospital staff. The clinical members of the Board supervised the study ward and looked over new admissions to the hospital shock ward to select cases suitable for study. Liaison was rapidly established with nearby field and evacuation hospitals whose staffs kept the Board informed of cases appropriate for inclusion in the main study. Daily trips were made by two or more members of the Board to many of these hospitals to examine patients, record intakes and outputs, keep follow-up notes, copy histories, pick up blood and urine specimens, and occasionally take part in necropsies. Suitable clinical cases were abundant and the laboratory was often hard pressed to keep up with material.

The Board functioned in a close and unified manner, with all members contributing to the whole task. Individual members assumed responsibility for various phases of the work. Lt. Colonel Mallory, who acted as chairman of the Board, was in charge of the pathologic aspects of the work and directed the laboratory. He made numerous postmortem examinations, supervised others, and from time to time took the accumulated material back to the 15th General Laboratory for histologic study. Lt. Colonel Simeone was primarily responsible for determinations of blood volume, as well as cardiovascular findings. Lt. Colonel Beecher was responsible for the liver function studies, and, with Lt. Colonel Simeone, for almost all the admission blood volume data. He was collator of the final report. Lt. Colonel Sullivan was in charge of hematologic aspects and, with Captain Smith, made the studies of blood groups and isoagglutinins, and worked with Lt. Colonel Mallory on some of the pathologic studies, particularly on pigment. Major Burnett carried out the kidney function studies and directed, with Lt. Colonel Simeone, the postoperative therapy and the collection of biochemic data. Captain Smith handled bacteriologic problems. Captain Shapiro was in charge of laboratory work and collaborated in the preparation of the biochemic data.

All medical installations within the Theater had been directed to aid the Board in its work, and everywhere the Board met whole-hearted cooperation. Since it was not administratively self-contained, the Board and its ancillary personnel were dependent on the various hospitals to which they were attached for quarters, rations, standard supplies, and other administrative essentials, including transportation beyond that immediately available. (As stated previously, special supplies were obtained from the 15th General Laboratory.) In addition, a high degree of professional cooperation was essential in selecting cases for special study and making them available for such study without interference with required treatment which remained the responsibility of the hospital staff.

DISSEMINATION OF PROGRESS REPORTS

It was recognized that observations and tentative conclusions based on the Board's work should be disseminated as promptly and widely as possible. This policy would have the double advantage of making significant findings available for immediate general application and of facilitating the Board's work as the result of understanding and interest on the part of the medical staffs from whom cooperative effort might be required. Therefore from time to time, findings were published in the Theater medical bulletin, discussed at medical meetings in the Theater, and circulated throughout other theaters and through The Surgeon General's Office by means of Essential Technical Medical Data reports. Personal contacts, however, were probably the most rapid and effective means for widespread dissemination of reports of the progress of the Board's work. For example, the 2d Auxiliary Surgical Group, attached to a hospital where the Board was working, split up in the fall of 1944 and one-half went to the support of the Seventh Army invading Southern France. The group in the European Theater kept in close contact with the Mediterranean group, through which reports of the study were received and disseminated as various phases were developed.

APPENDIX B

The Field Laboratory

Establishment of a field laboratory was manifestly essential to accomplishment of the program mapped out by the Board, since collection of voluminous and complex biochemic data was fundamental to the plan of study. The laboratory supporting the study had to be mobile and readily available wherever observations were to be made on the recently and severely wounded; that is, near the front line.

The 15th Medical General Laboratory was to serve as base of operations for the field laboratory and thus was available for the examination of such specimens as the Board might send to it. All histologic work in fact was done at this laboratory. In theory many other procedures required by the Board could have been performed at the 15th Medical General Laboratory but this system would have been totally inadequate to the need for two principal reasons: It would not have provided immediate reports on laboratory procedures which could aid in guiding treatment and evaluation of each patient, nor would it have revealed findings of particular interest which might suggest and direct special follow-up analyses. Furthermore many types of analyses, such as the van den Bergh diazo test, and determination of blood pH, phosphorus, chlorides, and sugar, must be performed very soon after the specimen is collected.

It was recognized, in addition, that the laboratory must not be a burden on the unit to which it might be attached and therefore it had to be self-sufficient, not only in the performance of laboratory procedures but also with regard to its utilities, such as electric power, heat, shelter, water supply, and disposal of wastes. A means of supply must be established which would permit the laboratory to carry only minimum essential equipment and chemicals for day-to-day operation and to be able to count on regular and dependable replacement of supplies and equipment from a base. Some of the practical difficulties encountered in operating the laboratory have been mentioned in the Preface.

956507 O—52——25

The joint considerations of mobility and self-sufficiency were reflected in the transport and major equipment initially made available to the Board. A large mobile laboratory truck was obtained on loan from the 15th Medical General Laboratory. In addition to reconnaissance cars and jeeps there also was available a 2½-ton cargo truck. On the latter were carried adequate glassware to take care of one day's run of samples, a size No. 1 International Centrifuge, two Coleman Junior Spectrophotometers, complete, a Klett colorimeter, a hot plate, a prescription balance with weights, a drying oven, and alcohol burners. A 2½-kilowatt generator, five carboys of distilled water, a typewriter, and nine pyramidal tents for the laboratory and the personnel completed the equipment, which was loaded on a 4-by-4 cargo truck.

In view of the anticipated working conditions, it was considered inadvisable to carry an analytical balance for preparation of standard solutions; therefore, as mentioned below, arrangements were made for obtaining a supply of these solutions as needed. The needs of the study did not necessitate carrying a refrigerator. A vacuum pump and a field autoclave were available in the mobile laboratory truck. A serviceable spectroscope was needed and was obtained later from the University of Rome.

Assurance of a continuous supply of reagents and other laboratory supplies necessitated special arrangements. Certain common items could be obtained from any medical unit to which the laboratory might be attached, but adequate supplies of distilled water, standard solutions, and special reagents and apparatus could not be obtained in this manner. Fortunately such items were readily obtainable from the 15th Medical General Laboratory which was the base of operations for the Board. They were delivered as needed to the field laboratory by means of the carrier "blood-bank" plane which shuttled between the General Laboratory and the forward distributing unit of the 6713th Blood Transfusion Unit.

Shortcomings in basic physical arrangements were soon evident. The mobile laboratory truck proved too small to provide space for more than one technician to perform chemical analyses. The pyramidal tents were not adaptable for use as a laboratory, so a ward tent was requisitioned from the 94th Evacuation Hospital. A tent of this size permitted three technicians to work comfortably without interference and allowed a systematic distribution of reagents and equipment, thus eliminating the rehandling necessary in a confined space.

Tables, a working cabinet, and a glassware cabinet were added. A sink was made from a truck gasoline tank, and water was piped from a 50-gallon drum. The sewage system was simple. All blood, plasma, urine, and solutions from completed analyses were poured into a slop pail, which was emptied into a prepared soakage pit. Water used in washing glassware ran into channels and soaked into the ground. The tables and equipment were distributed so that all the analytic work, the washing and drying of glassware, the storage of surplus supplies, and the administrative and clerical work were performed in the same tent. Blood typing and agglutination studies were made in the laboratory truck.

For the collection and submission of specimens, boxes were prepared in triplicate to contain approximately:

15 screw-cap, 22-ml. flat-bottom vials containing lithium oxalate to be used for collection of blood specimens.

10 screw-cap, 8-ml. flat-bottom vials containing ammonium and potassium oxalate for holding blood specimens on which determinations of hematocrit value and plasma protein concentration would be made.

5 corked test tubes for submission of clotted blood.

4 screw-cap, 250-ml. urine bottles.

12 sterile 10-ml. syringes.

3 sterile 30-ml. syringes.

2 sterile 2-ml. syringes.

10 dry 10-ml. syringes.

30 sterile 19-gage needles.

Absorbent cotton, alcohol, and rubber tubing for tourniquets.

Ampules of bromsulfalein, phenolsulfonphthalein, and a sterile solution containing 100 mg. per 100 cc. of the dye T–1824 for determination of blood volume.

The specimens were required to be labelled with the patient's name and the date and hour the sample was taken.

Analyses

The following analyses were undertaken on the Board's material:

Blood.—Volume, hemoglobin, hematocrit value, hydrogen ion, sugar, sulfonamides, methemoglobin, the bromsulfalein liver function test; plasma urea nitrogen, creatinine, lactic acid, bilirubin (van den Bergh reaction), uric acid, protein, free hemoglobin, carbon-dioxide combining power, magnesium, chlorides, phosphorus, and nonprotein nitrogen; serum sodium, calcium, and potassium.

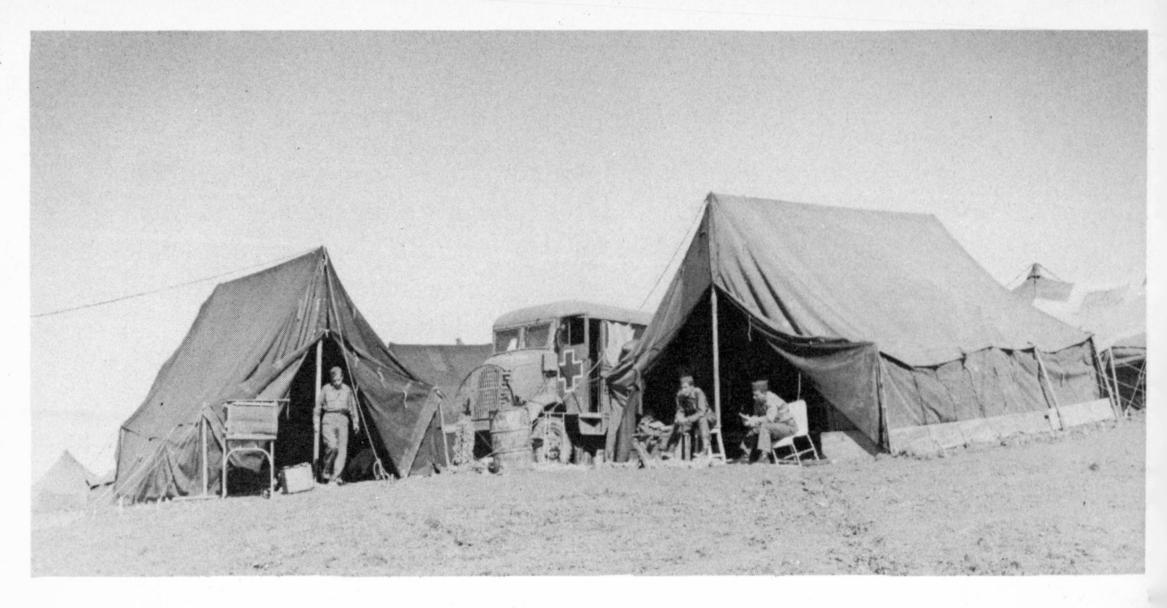

THE TWO LABORATORY TENTS and the laboratory truck used by the Board for the Study of the Severely Wounded, shown at Monghidoro, Italy, autumn of 1944. Later the laboratory tents were winterized as shown.

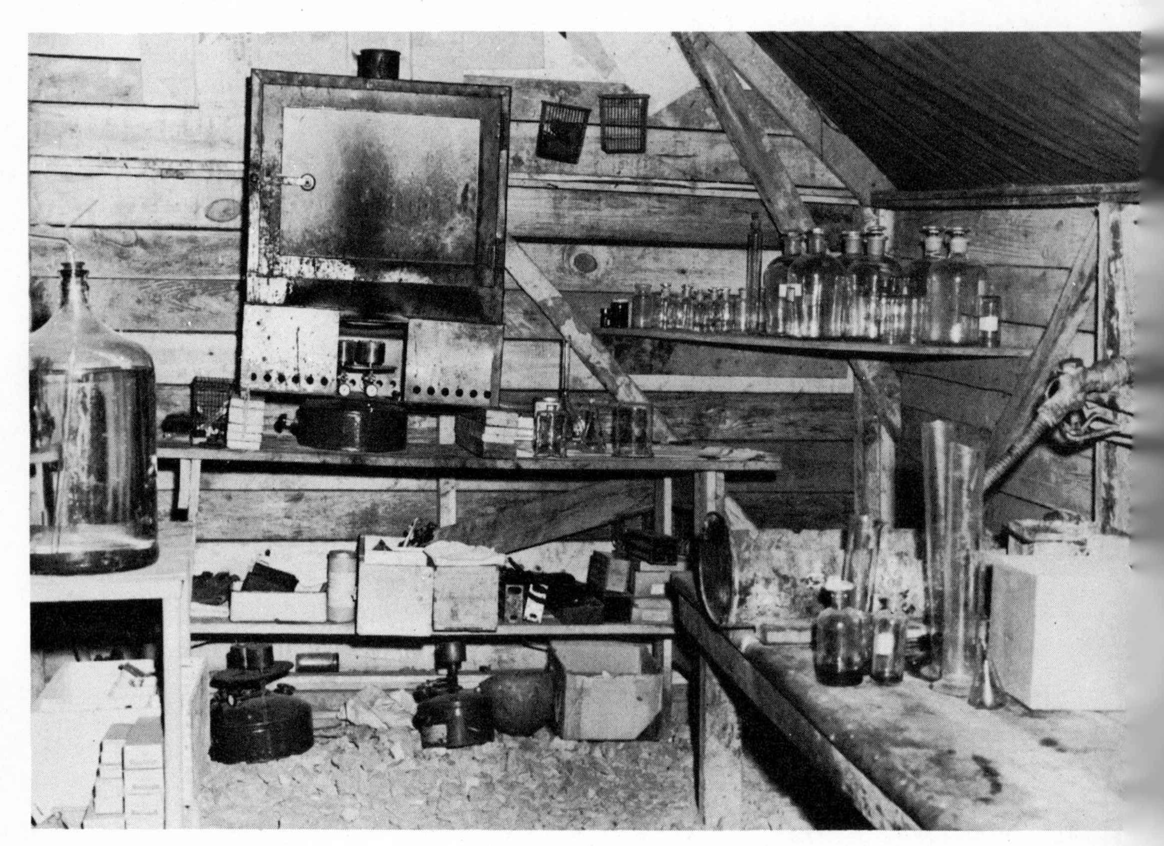

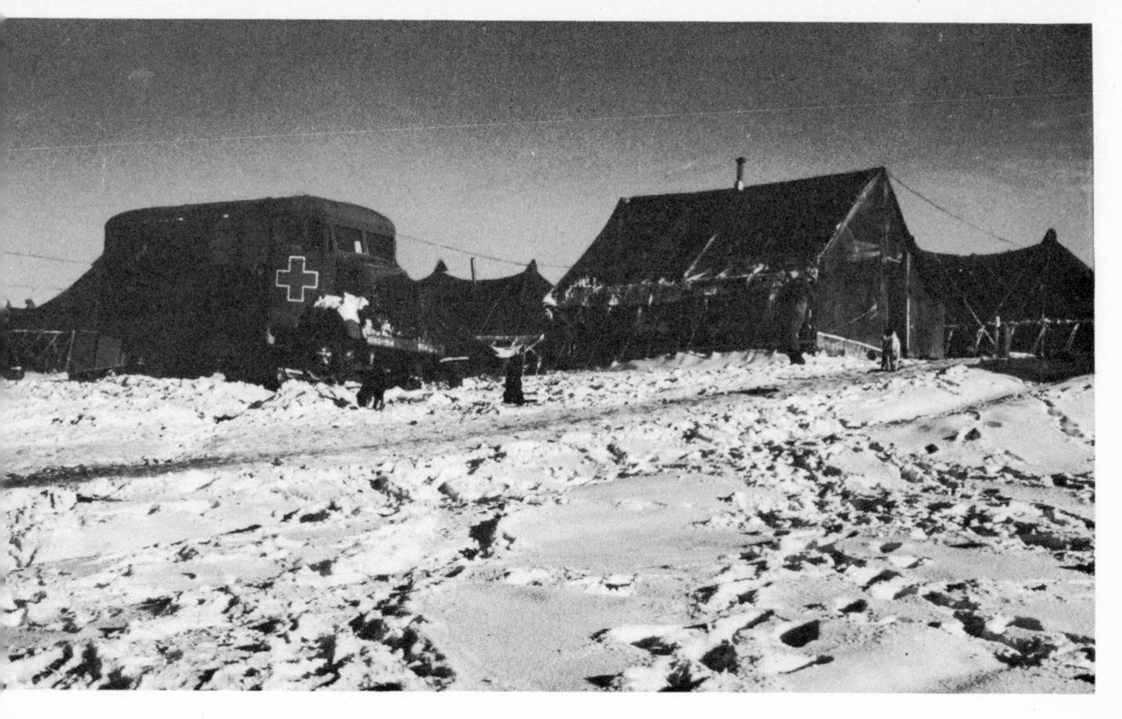

ITALY PROVIDED VARIETY OF CLIMATE. Winter snows and spring rains mired the laboratory truck and dampened equipment. Wherever possible the laboratory was housed in a building, but more often the work was done in tents.

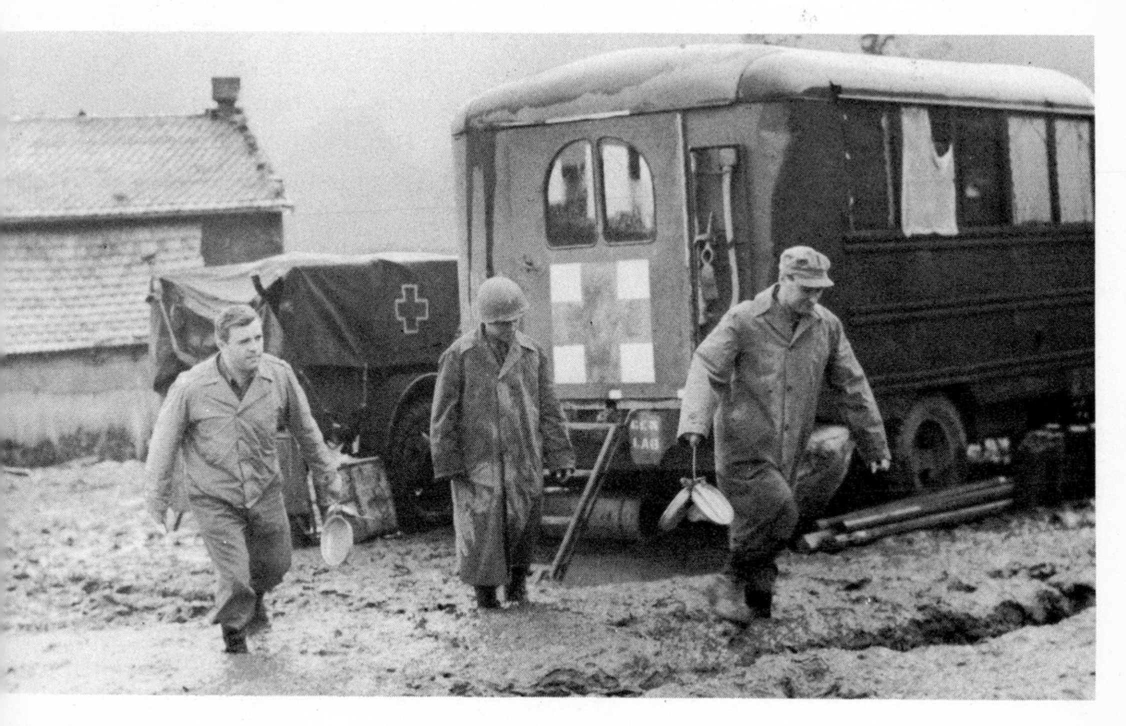

Urine.—Routine urinalysis, hydrogen ion, free hemoglobin, myoglobin, creatinine, creatine, ammonia, titratable acidity, chlorides, urea nitrogen, organic acids, magnesium, bile, urobilinogen.

Tissue.—Myoglobin.

Renal Function Tests.—Phenolsulfonphthalein excretion, mannitol clearance, para-amino hippuric acid clearance, and pituitrin concentration test.

Effort was made to synchronize the submission of specimens so that several of the same tests could be performed simultaneously; immediate analyses of single specimens were, however, made when requested.

Each technician kept a notebook in which he recorded the details of the particular determinations assigned to him. The calculations were checked, entered into the main laboratory book, and read back. After an adequate number of cases had been completed, the laboratory data were transcribed onto five copies of laboratory sheets and each set was stored in a different place (one copy being filed with the case record) in case storm, fire, or warfare would spare one or more sets. Even so, the laboratory sheets of some cases were lost in transit.

Many of the specimens submitted were irreplaceable. During the entire course of the study, no sample was sacrificed due to breakage upon centrifugation. The No. 1 International Centrifuge yielded results which far outweighed the inconveniences attached to moving and servicing it. The more easily moved table centrifuge had caused many tube breakages and was therefore not used.

The majority of the ultimate measurements made required colorimetric readings. The Coleman Junior Spectrophotometer, powered by its own 6-volt battery, contributed in several respects to improving the caliber of the work. It broadened the scope of procedures that could be carried out, it reproduced the readings accurately, and in all cases it allowed us to standardize the observations which, particularly in visual colorimetric reading of yellow, varied among technicians. Most of the color tests, except sugar and phosphorus which entailed comparison of easily-read blue colors, were set up for spectrophotometer readings. The spectrophotometer sturdily resisted the stresses and strains of repeated packing, unpacking, and moving, and no replacement of parts was necessary during the entire study.

The initial move up to the combat line was made with emphasis on care and protection of our supplies and equipment. Each subsequent move required speed. For this, boxes were prepared with individual cubicles for all the reagent bottles. The glsssware was rolled up in blankets and these blanket rolls were snugly wedged between the shelves of the glassware cabinet. The test tubes and blood-drawing equipment were kept during the working period in the same boxes in which they were moved, and the pipets were bound in groups of 10 and wedged into the working cabinet drawer. The laboratory could therefore be dismantled, packed, and loaded within four or five hours.

The first move into the field indicated that certain standards of protection in inclement weather were imperative. During the winter period the laboratory tent was winterized by completely boarding up the front and back as illustrated. A close-fitting door was installed, the floor was gravelled, and an oil stove was kept burning day and night. The final set-up during the spring was the most convenient. No stove was required and the work tables were grouped about the center of the tent. To eliminate the discomforts of heat and the roar of the ovens, the dishwashing, drying, and autoclaving were done in a pyramidal tent adjacent to the chemistry tent.

The need of conservation of electricity made it quite obvious that drying could not be effected by electric oven nor could hot plates be used. Alcohol burners and gasoline stoves served satisfactorily for this purpose. During one particularly dusty period it was necessary to operate the centrifuge and spectrophotometer in the mobile laboratory vehicle, and it was often necessary to plug with cotton all the flasks and cylinders and to box the tubes and pipets to keep them dust-free.

In the 8 months of the study, the laboratory moved seven times, and over 12,000 biochemic analyses representing 56 different types of tests were made: 8,269 on blood (31 types), 3,961 on urine (22 types), and 58 (3 types) on tissue. The scope of these chemical analyses is shown in Appendix C where the methods used are described.

A detailed listing of the number of chemical analyses is given on page 322. All work was done in connection with the Board material except for a 3-day hepatitis survey.

The field laboratory proved its value in this study. It was shown that a mobile laboratory unit could be established and could function well close to the line of combat, and that it could do accurate and comprehensive biochemic analyses in this situation.

Chemical Analyses

Blood Chemistry

Test	Number	Test	Number
Hemoglobin	636	Sulfonamides	108
Hematocrit	636	Glucose	377
Plasma protein	639	Blood volume	207
Plasma hemoglobin	892	Bromsulfalein	451
Nonprotein nitrogen	605	Sulfate	2
Creatinine	580	Methemoglobin	15
Chlorides	591	Urea nitrogen	80
Uric acid	195	Vitamin C	8
Carbon-dioxide combining power	381	Cephalin flocculation test	119
Van den Bergh	700	Mannitol clearance	75
Phosphorus	440	Renal blood flow	40
pH	28	Total mass—hippurate	29
Sodium	174	Total mass—glucose	6
Potassium	26	Lactic acid	27
Calcium	42	Bilirubin (acetone)	2
Magnesium	158		
		Total	8,269

Urine Chemistry

Test	Number	Test	Number
Routine urinalysis	670	Ammonia	130
pH	774	Titratable acidity	130
Benzidine	662	Organic acids	91
Myoglobin	144	Urobilinogen	7
Chlorides	289	Bromsulfalein	6
Phenolsulfonphthalein	385	Urea nitrogen	96
Concentration test	43	Magnesium	65
Sulfadiazine	33	Methylene blue test	119
Hippuric acid	1	Spectroscopic examination	2
Bile	32	Titratable alkalinity	2
Creatinine	197		
Creatine	83	Total	3,961

Tissue Chemistry

Test	Number
Myoglobin	41
Sulfadiazine	6
Magnesium	11
Total	58

Total Analyses 12,288

APPENDIX C

Contents

Biochemic Methods

The biochemic procedures to be used in this study were selected on the basis of their accuracy and their applicability to the anticipated conditions in a combat area. Many procedures were modified so that the critical quantitative readings might be made on the spectrophotometer. Those described for the determination of blood volume; plasma magnesium, serum sodium; creatinine and creatine in urine; the bromsulfalein and phenolsulfonphthalein tests, and the determination of myoglobin, for example, offer generally useful modifications of standard procedures. Methods in which any changes in the standard procedure were made are described in detail.

Blood Analyses

Normal Values in the Blood Analyses

The ranges of normal values for analyses made on the blood as shown in Table 118 are essentially those given in the literature. For convenience it was often necessary to assume a single figure as representing the standard normal level for a particular analysis in order to contrast it with the average findings in certain groupings of the cases in this study. The figure used for the standard normal was selected as a result of our experience with each method.

Preparation of Blood and Plasma Protein Precipitants

Tungstic Acid Filtrate

Reagent.—Van Slyke and Hawkins tungstic acid. (Twenty-five ml. of 2/3 N sulfuric acid and 25 ml. of 10-percent sodium tungstate are combined and diluted to 225 ml. with water.) This reagent is satisfactory for 1 week. Turbidity due to precipitation of tungstic acid does not interfere with preparation of the filtrate.

Procedure.—To 1 volume of blood or plasma in a flask are added 9 volumes

TABLE 118.—NORMAL VALUES USED IN THIS STUDY

Determination or Test	Range of Normal	Range of Equivalents *mEq./L.*	Standard Normal
Blood			
Volume	8–9% of body weight	....	8.5% of body weight.
Hemoglobin	14–17.5 Gm./100 ml.	....	16 Gm./100 ml.
Hematocrit value	42–52 ml. cells in 100 ml.	....	47 ml. cells in 100 ml.
pH	7.38–7.48	....	
Plasma			
Protein	6–7 Gm./100 ml.	....	6.5 Gm./100 ml.
"Hemoglobin"	Less than 10 mg./100 ml.	....	
Nonprotein nitrogen	25–40 mg./100 ml.	....	33 mg./100 ml.
Urea nitrogen	10–20 mg./100 ml.	....	15 mg./100 ml.
Creatinine	0.5–1.2 mg./100 ml.	....	1.0 mg./100 ml.
Uric acid	1.5–3.5 mg./100 ml.	....	3.0 mg./100 ml.
Phosphorus	1.8–3.5 mg./100 ml.	1.04–2.0	3.0 mg./100 ml.
Magnesium	1.0–3.0 mg./100 ml.	0.8–2.5	1.8 mg./100 ml.
Chlorides	570–620 mg./100 ml.	97.5–104	585 mg./100 ml.; 100 mEq./L.
CO_2 combining power	53–70 vol. %	24–31	60 vol. %; 27 mEq./L.
Bilirubin (van den Bergh)	0.1–0.5 mg./100 ml.	....	
Bromsulfalein (5 mg./Kg. in 45 min.)	Less than 3%	....	
Lactic acid	10–20 mg./100 ml.	....	15 mg./100 ml.
Serum			
Sodium	320–340 mg./100 ml.	139–149	330 mg./100 ml.; 143 mEq./L.
Potassium	15–21 mg./100 ml.	3.9–5.3	
Calcium	9–11 mg./100 ml.	....	

of the tungstic acid reagent, the mixture is allowed to stand for 10 minutes and is then filtered.

TRICHLORACETIC ACID FILTRATES

Reagents.—Trichloracetic acid, 10-percent solution, 15-percent solution, and 20-percent solution. (Prepared by titration.)

Procedure.—Prepare filtrates (as required by the analysis to be performed).

Determination of Blood and Plasma Volume

Modification of Gregersen Method

Blood and plasma volume was determined in this study by modification of the method developed by Gregersen[1,2] primarily for use of the Armed Forces. The dye T–1824 was used and the basic principles of the method were followed.

The Gregersen method, in brief, consists in injecting a known quantity of dye into the antecubital vein, waiting about twenty minutes for the dye to be distributed through the circulating blood, and taking three or four samples of blood at 20-minute intervals. The plasma is separated and its concentration of dye is measured and plotted against time. The curve so obtained is extrapolated back to zero time to correct for dye lost during the mixing period. This value at zero time gives the theoretical concentration of dye that would have occurred in the plasma if uniform mixing had been effected at the instant of injection and none of the dye had been excreted. The total blood volume is calculated from the plasma volume (measured by the dye) and the hematocrit value.

Experience with the method revealed two serious objections, one practical and one technical. The practical objection was that the method was too time-consuming for use with battle casualties before operation; therefore, a more rapid procedure was sought. This will be discussed later. The technical flaw in the procedure was that the difference in turbidity between the blank, dye-free plasma and the dye-containing samples yielded spectrophotometric readings which had to be resolved as amount of dye plus or minus turbidity. Plotted points using such readings rarely indicated excretion of dye as an exponential function, and very often, when considerable variations in turbidity existed, would lead to gross errors of reading at zero time. Corresponding errors resulted in the calculation of the blood volume.

The cause of this turbidity, which varies during the course of a determination, has not been ascertained. The plasma, however, does not clear upon centrifugation. The following observations made the application of a turbidity-correction

[1] Gregersen, M. I.; Gibson, J. G., and Stead, E. A.: Plasma volume determination with dyes: errors in colorimetry; use of the blue dye T–1824. Am. J. Physiol. **113**: 54–55, Sept. 1, 1935.

[2] Gregersen, M. I.: A practical method for the determination of blood volume with the dye T–1824; survey of the present basis of the dye-method and its clinical applications. J. Lab. & Clin. Med. **29**: 1266–1286, December 1944.

factor reasonable: (1) The reading of turbidity at 620 mμ was almost the same as at 680 mμ, while (2) the dye reading at 680 mμ was ¼ the reading at 620 millimicrons.

If the dyed plasma, therefore, is less turbid than the blank, dye-free plasma, the difference in readings of the dyed plasma at 620 mμ and 680 mμ expressed as OD (optical density), multiplied by 4/3, would give the corrected value for the dye only.

Example: OD at 620 mμ . . . 0.309
OD at 680 mμ . . . 0.055
OD corrected (0.309 — 0.055) x 4/3 = 0.340

If the dyed plasma is more turbid than the dye-free plasma, which it is if the reading of optical density at 680 is more than ¼ the reading at 620, a similar correction is made.

Example A: OD at 620 mμ . . . 0.300
OD at 680 mμ . . . 0.091
OD corrected (0.300 — 0.091) x 4/3 = 0.279

Example B: OD at 620 mμ = 0.409
OD at 680 mμ = 0.188
OD corrected (0.409 — 0.188) x 4/3 = 0.295

When the dyed plasma and the blank plasma are of the same order of turbidity, no correction factor is necessary.

The application of the correction factor for turbidity materially improved the character of the blood-volume curves, and indicated that the excretion of the dye approximated an exponential function.

Practically, the use of four points to determine blood volume is too time-consuming to be used in battle casualties before operation. Therefore, a more rapid method was sought, and the accuracy of a blood volume determination based on only one blood sample was studied.

Since the excretion of the dye followed an exponential curve, and the log of the concentration of the dye plotted against time formed a straight line, it remained only to determine the constancy of the slope of the disappearance curve, and to ascertain 1 point on the line, at a specified time, to calculate the optical density (OD) at zero time. This was done in 68 cases in which blood volumes had been determined by using 3-point, 4-point, and 5-point curves to establish the optical density at zero time.

First it was necessary to consider the factor of albuminuria. Because the dye T–1824 is thought to be bound to the plasma albumin, a variability of slope according to the presence or absence of albuminuria was expected. Such a relationship was demonstrated by grouping the dye disappearance-rate slopes in 67 cases according to the amount of albumin in urine specimens obtained in these cases at about the time the blood volume was determined. The disappearance of dye from plasma was expressed by the slope factor $\frac{\text{OD 0 minutes}}{\text{OD 60 minutes}}$.

If the slope factor is divided into 1,000 and multiplied by 100, it gives the percentage of dye remaining in the plasma 1 hour after injection; subtraction of the result yields the percentage of dye lost in 1 hour. The average percentage of dye lost in 1 hour in the urines of patients with no urinary suppression and with albuminuria (Group V), as compared with the average loss in 1 hour in the other four groups combined, would indicate that the dye, bound to albumin, is lost through the urine in this manner (Table 119).

TABLE 119.—COMPARISON OF ALBUMIN LOSS IN URINE WITH PLASMA DYE LOSS—AVERAGE OF 67 CASES

Groups	Number of Cases and Urinary Findings	$\frac{\text{OD 0 minutes}}{\text{OD 60 minutes}}$	Dye Retained after 1 Hour (*percent*)	Dye Lost in 1 Hour (*percent*)
I	Average of 36 cases . . . . . . (Output normal; albumin neg. or faint trace)	1.105	90.5	9.5±0.58
II	Average of 4 cases . . . . (Output normal; albumin 1+)	1.148	87.2	12.8±2.4
III	Average of 14 cases . . . . . . (Patients anuric; albumin 2+ or over)	1.111	90.0	10±0.85
IV	Average of 4 cases . . . . (Patients oliguric; albumin 2+ or over)	1.150	87.3	12.7±2.1
V	Average of 9 cases . . . . (Output normal; albumin 2+ or over. Two patients polyuric; albumin, trace)	1.195	83.7	16.3±2.8
	Average of cases in Groups I through IV . . . . (58 cases)	1.112	90	10.0±0.46
	Average of total cases	1.128	88.7	11.3±0.62

When the cases in Groups I through IV were combined and averaged, a weighted slope of 1.112 was obtained, corresponding to a 10-percent loss of dye per hour, or a change per minute of 0.00187 or $\frac{.1112}{60}$. It was possible, then, to calculate the OD at zero time, when the OD at a specific time was known, by multiplying by 0.00187 the interval (in minutes) between injecting the dye and taking the sample, and adding 1 to this figure. The OD at zero minutes was obtained by multiplying this value by the observed OD corrected for turbidity.

Example: OD 30 minutes (corrected): 0.317
1. $30 \times 0.00187 = 0.0561$
2. $1 + 0.056 = 1.056$
3. $0.317 \times 1.056 = 0.335$ (OD zero time)

To test the validity of this procedure, the first point of each of the 68 multiple-point blood volume tests was taken and the blood volume was calculated from it and compared with the blood volume obtained by determining the disappearance curve from multiple points. The results are indicated in Table 120.

TABLE 120.—RELATION OF CALCULATION OF SINGLE-POINT TO MULTIPLE-POINT METHOD—68 CASES

Relation of Single Point to Multiple Point	Number of Cases Above Multiple-Point Value	Number of Cases Below Multiple-Point Value
Within 100 ml.	27	11
Within 101–200 ml.	8	4
Within 201–300 ml.	8	3
Over 300 ml.	4	3
Total Cases	47	21

According to these data, in 69 percent of the 68 cases the calculation of blood volumes was higher by the single-point method, in 31 percent it was lower, and was within 100 ml. in 56 percent. In 90 percent of all cases it was within 300 ml. of the calculation obtained by the multiple-point method. In this series the value determined by the one-point method was clinically unsatisfactory in one case (960 ml. too high). The second point in this case yielded a value 330 ml. too high. This series demonstrated that the blood volume determined by the one-point test compares favorably with that obtained by the multiple-point test.

Procedure for Determination of Blood and Plasma Volume

Reagents

1. T–1824 solution, 1 mg. per milliliter. (The contents of ten 5-ml. ampules of 0.5-percent T–1824 are removed and made up to a 250-ml. solution, using sterile technique.)
2. Standard copper sulfate solutions (specific gravity series for determination of hematocrit value).
3. Sodium chloride, 0.9-percent solution.

Procedure

A sterile 10-ml. syringe is filled with exactly 10 ml. of T–1824 and placed where it will be readily available. About twenty milliliters of blood are drawn from the antecubital vein with a sterile syringe, leaving the needle in the vein. Exactly 5 ml. of blood are measured into a specially oxalated bottle for determination of the hematocrit value, and the remaining blood is transferred to a lithium oxalate bottle. This is the blank tube. The syringe containing the dye is carefully attached to the needle remaining in the vein, and all the dye is injected. (Any indication of pain by the patient during the injection of the dye should be regarded as evidence that some dye is passing outside the vein, thus invalidating the analysis.) The exact time of injection is noted. After an interval of from 20 to 40 minutes, 15 ml. of blood are drawn from the antecubital vein of the opposite arm and placed into a lithium oxalate bottle. This is the dye-containing tube. Again the exact time the blood is drawn is noted.

The hematocrit value is determined from the 5-ml. sample (the blank blood), using the copper sulfate method of Phillips et al.[3] All the samples are centrifuged and the supernatant plasma is separated. The two tubes of blank plasma are pooled, at least 5.5 ml. are placed in a 19- by 150-mm. Coleman cuvette, and the same quantity of the dye-containing plasma is placed in a similar cuvette. (In the event that the amount of plasma is inadequate, dilutions

[3] Phillips, R. A.; Van Slyke, D. D.; Dole, V. P.; Emerson, K., Jr.; Hamilton, P. B., and Archibald, R. M.: Copper sulfate method for measuring specific gravities of whole blood and plasma. BUMED News Letter, U. S. Navy, June 25, 1943, p. 1–16.

are made with 0.9-percent saline solution, treating both tubes in the same manner.)

The blank tube is set to read at 100-percent transmission at 620 mμ in the spectrophotometer and the optical density of the plasma in the dye tube is noted. This procedure is repeated at 680 millimicrons. Exactly 1 ml. of T–1824 solution is diluted to 500 ml. with water, placed in a matched cuvette, and, blanking out with distilled water, the optical density at 620 mμ is determined.

Calculation

1. From the readings at 620 mμ and 680 mμ the corrected optical density (OD) is calculated as discussed previously.

2. The optical density is calculated at zero minutes, using the factor for the number of minutes after injection as previously discussed.

3. Plasma volume:

OD_o = corrected optical density at zero minutes for dyed plasma.
OD_{dye} = optical density of (1:500) dilution of dye that was injected for test.

$$\text{Plasma volume} = \frac{OD_{dye}}{OD_o} \times 500 \times 10.$$

(The figure of 500 represents the dilution factor of the dye as read in the instrument, and the figure 10 is the number of milliliters injected.)

4. Blood volume:

100 minus the hematocrit value = percentage of plasma (% Pl)

$$\text{Blood volume} = \frac{\text{Plasma volume}}{\%\ \text{Pl}} \times 100$$

Summary

1. The technique for determining the circulating blood volume by means of the dye T–1824 and a spectrophotometer is described.

2. The correction for variable turbidity of samples is described.

3. The disappearance of the dye in battle casualties was 10 percent of the injected substance at the end of 1 hour.

4. Albuminuria increased the disappearance rate.

5. The feasibility of blood volume determinations based on only one dye-containing sample is demonstrated.

956507 O—52——26

Blood Chemistry

Nonprotein Nitrogen Products

Nonprotein Nitrogen in Plasma—Modified from Koch and McMeekin[4]

Reagents

1. Sulfuric acid, 50-percent aqueous solution by volume.
2. Potassium persulfate, saturated solution. (Seven Gm. in 100 ml. of water.)
3. Potassium mercuric iodide for Nessler's solution: (a) Using a 1-liter Erlenmeyer flask, 22.5 Gm. of iodine are dissolved in 20 ml. of water containing 30 Gm. of potassium iodide. (b) After the solution is complete, 30 Gm. (about 2.5 ml.) of mercury are added and the mixture is shaken vigorously in order to break the mercury into globules, cooling it from time to time by immersing the flask in cold water. The shaking is continued until the supernatant fluid has lost all color due to iodine. (c) The supernatant is decanted from the excess mercury and tested for free iodine by adding a drop or two of the solution to 1 ml. of a 1-percent starch solution. If the result of the starch test for iodine is negative, a few drops of an iodine solution of the same concentration as described in (a) are added until a faint excess of iodine can be detected by the starch test. (d) The double iodide solution is diluted to 200 ml. with distilled water and mixed thoroughly.
4. Nessler's reagent. (By titration a 10-percent sodium hydroxide solution is accurately prepared from a saturated solution of sodium hydroxide that has been allowed to stand until all carbonates have settled. To 975 ml. of this solution is added the entire solution (200 ml.) of potassium mercuric iodide prepared as described, after which it is mixed thoroughly and allowed to settle.)
5. Ammonium sulfate standard solution. (Prepared by dissolving 4.716 Gm. of pure, dry ammonium sulfate in 0.2 N sulfuric acid and making up to a volume of 1,000 ml. with the 0.2 N sulfuric acid (1 ml. = 1 mg. of nitrogen).)
6. Dilute nitrogen standard solution. (Five ml. of stock standard solution is diluted to 100 ml. with 0.2 N sulfuric acid (3 ml. = 0.15 mg. nitrogen).)

Procedure

To 2.5 ml. of protein-free tungstic acid plasma filtrate in an ignition tube graduated at 35 ml. is added 1 ml. of 50-percent sulfuric acid solution, together with a glass bead to prevent bumping, and it is boiled vigorously until it becomes brown and dense white fumes appear. A funnel is then placed in the tube and the solution is digested for about one minute, when the flame and funnel are removed, 5 drops of potassium persulfate are added, and the mix-

[4] In Hawk, P. B., and Bergeim, O. Practical Physiological Chemistry. 10th ed. Philadelphia, Blakiston, 1931, p. 415.

ture is boiled gently for several minutes. If a brown color persists, another 5 drops of potassium persulfate are added and the mixture is again boiled gently. (A greenish-yellow color at this point indicates an excess of tungstic acid. This color will clear up after the addition of the Nessler's reagent.) It is cooled, diluted to the 35-ml. mark with water, and mixed by inversion.

Into an identical ignition tube are placed 3 ml. of working standard and 1 ml. of 50-percent sulfuric acid solution; this is made up to the 35-ml. mark with water and mixed by inversion. Into a third ignition tube is placed 1 ml. of the sulfuric acid solution, water is added to the 35-ml. mark, and it is mixed by inversion. This is the blank. Next, 3.5 ml. each of the sample, the standard, and the blank are transferred to a small cuvette (12 by 75 mm.), 1.5 ml. of Nessler's reagent is added, the contents are mixed by inversion, and read in the Coleman Junior Spectrophotometer at 440 mμ on the optical density scale, blanking out with the blank solution.

If the nonprotein nitrogen value is high, 2 ml. of the solution and 1.5 ml. of the blank are nesslerized. In this case the final value is multiplied by seven-fourths. Other appropriate dilutions that bring the color intensity into the standard range can be used.

Calculation

The working nitrogen standard is equivalent to 60 mg. of nitrogen per 100 ml. of plasma. (Rs = OD of the standard. Ru = OD of the sample.)

$$\frac{60}{Rs} = \frac{x}{Ru}$$

$$\frac{60 \times Ru}{Rs} = \text{mg./100 ml. nitrogen in plasma sample.}$$

Comment

The method as modified has the following advantages: (1) Nessler's solution is used sparingly; less than 10 percent of the quantity used in the standard procedure is necessary. (2) The procedure is expedited by the digestion of half the quantity of filtrate ordinarily used. (3) An objective reading of the nesslerized solutions increases the accuracy of reading the yellow color. (4) In the event the nonprotein nitrogen level is extremely high, a further dilution of the initial digestion can be made, rather than repeating the entire analysis. (5) The use of saturated potassium persulfate in the oxidation provides a substance which is nitrogen-free, stable, and unlike superoxol, is non-injurious.

Creatinine in Plasma—Modified from Folin and Wu[5]

Reagent.—Alkaline picrate solution. (Five volumes of saturated picric acid are mixed with 1 volume of 10-percent sodium hydroxide solution. This is freshly prepared before each series of analyses.) A reference curve is prepared from standard creatinine solutions read on the spectrophotometer at 500 mμ after following the conditions of the test.

Procedure.—Five ml. of tungstic acid plasma filtrate are placed in one cuvette, and 5 ml. of water in another. To each of the samples and the water blank are added 2.5 ml. of alkaline picrate solution and they are allowed to stand for 10 minutes. The blank is set at 100-percent transmission and the percentage transmission of each sample is read at 500 millimicrons.

Calculation.—Reference of the observed percentage transmission to the standard curve gives the milligrams of creatinine per 100 ml. of plasma. If very high creatinine values are anticipated, appropriate dilutions of the tungstic acid filtrate are made with water before addition of the alkaline picrate.

Uric Acid in Plasma—Modified from Folin[6]

Reagents

1. Standard solution of uric acid. (Exactly 1 Gm. of uric acid is transferred to a 1-liter volumetric flask. To 0.5 Gm. of lithium carbonate in a beaker, 150 ml. of water are added and this solution is heated to 60° C. until all the carbonate has dissolved. All of the hot carbonate solution is then added to the uric acid in the volumetric flask. As soon as a clear solution is obtained, it is cooled, diluted to about five hundred ml. with water, and 25 ml. of formaldehyde are added. This is well mixed and 3 ml. of glacial acetic acid are added. The mixture is shaken to remove most of the carbon dioxide, diluted to 1 liter, mixed, and stored in brown bottles.)

2. Working standard. (Immediately before each series of analyses, 0.4 ml. of the standard solution is diluted to 100 ml. with water.)

3. Five-percent sodium cyanide solution.

4. Uric acid reagent. (To 100 Gm. of sodium tungstate (molybdate-free) in a 500-ml. Florence flask is added dilute phosphoric acid, made by dissolving 33 ml. of 85-percent phosphoric acid in 150 ml. of water, and the solution is mixed. Several glass beads are added to the flask and the mixture is boiled gently for 1 hour, using a funnel containing a flask of cold water as a condenser. It is decolorized with a little bromine water, the excess bromine is boiled off, and the mixture is cooled and diluted to a volume of 500 ml.)

[5] In HAWK, P. B., and BERGEIM, O. Practical Physiological Chemistry. 10th ed. Philadelphia, Blakiston, 1931, p. 421–423.

[6] In SIMMONS, J. S., and GENTZKOW, C. J. Laboratory Methods of the United States Army. Philadelphia, Lea & Febiger, 1944, p. 207.

Procedure

To 1 ml. of tungstic acid filtrate in a cuvette are added 3 ml. of water. Into another cuvette is pipeted 1 ml. of dilute standard, and 3 ml. of water are added. This is the standard solution corresponding to 4 mg. of uric acid per 100 ml. of plasma. Four ml. of water in a third cuvette constitutes the blank tube. To each of the samples, the uric acid standard, and the blank tube, 4 ml. of sodium cyanide are added, using an automatic pipet, and the solutions are mixed, after which 2 ml. of the uric acid reagent are added to each tube, and the solutions are again mixed and are allowed to stand for 30 minutes. The blank is set at 100-percent transmission on the spectrophotometer and the optical density of the standard and each of the samples at 650 mμ is noted.

Calculation

The calculation of milligrams per 100 milliliters of plasma is obtained by setting up a proportion comparing the optical density of the standard of known strength with the observed reading of the sample.

Example: OD of sample 0.150
OD of standard . . . 0.200
Standard = 4 mg./100 ml.
Sample (calculated) = 3 mg. of uric acid per 100 ml. of plasma.

Comment

The advantages of the method as modified are that it (1) yields a nonclouding color development when sodium cyanide and phosphotungstic acid are used, (2) avoids the danger of color development varying with the temperature by the preparation of standard and blank at the same time and by reading the color on the optical density scale of the spectrophotometer, and (3) insures against decomposition of the working standard by preparation of a fresh standard before each series of analyses.

Urea Nitrogen in Plasma—Modified from Karr[7]

Reagents

1. Urease solution. (A mixture of 0.3 Gm. of double-strength urease in 2.5 ml. of water and 7.5 ml. of glycerin is centrifuged and decanted. The supernatant solution is the urease extract and lasts for at least 3 months.)

[7] In HAWK, P. B., and BERGEIM, O. Practical Physiological Chemistry. 10th ed. Philadelphia, Blakiston, 1931, p. 418.

2. Acetate buffer solution. (To 15 Gm. of sodium acetate dissolved in 50 ml. of water is added 1 ml. of glacial acetic acid, and the mixture is diluted to 100 ml. with water.)
3. Dilute standard nitrogen solution. (Same as for nonprotein nitrogen.)
4. Potassium mercuric iodide. (Same as for nonprotein nitrogen.)
5. Urea Nessler's reagent. (Thirty ml. of potassium mercuric iodide are mixed with 30 ml. of water and 140 ml. of 5-percent sodium hydroxide solution are added.)
6. 2/3 N sulfuric acid.
7. Sodium tungstate, 10-percent solution.

Procedure

To 1 ml. of plasma in a tube are added 6.7 ml. of water, 2 drops of urease solution, and 4 drops of acetate buffer, and the tube is incubated at 40° to 50° C. for 15 minutes. One ml. each of the sulfuric acid and the sodium tungstate solution are added, the solution is mixed, allowed to stand for several minutes, and filtered. Into another tube are placed 2 ml. of filtrate and 7 ml. of water. Into a tube graduated at 22.5 ml. are placed 1.5 ml. of the working nitrogen standard, the solution is diluted to the mark, mixed, and 9 ml. of this dilute standard is placed in a tube. To each of the samples and the dilute standard solution is added 1 ml. of urea Nessler's reagent, they are mixed and read in the colorimeter.

Calculation

The unknown is set at 15 mm. and the reading of the standard will be the milligrams of urea nitrogen per 100 ml. of plasma. In the event that a high urea nitrogen is expected, aliquots of the 2-ml. sample of filtrate are taken and the contents of the tube made up to 9 ml. with water. The observed level is then multiplied by the proper factor.

Example: 0.5 ml. taken instead of 2.0 ml.; multiply answer by 4 for mg. of urea nitrogen per 100 ml. of plasma.

A urease blank should be determined about every 3 days. The urease blank usually averaged between 2 and 3 mg. expressed as urea nitrogen per 100 ml. of plasma and was subtracted from the observed values.

Comment

The method as modified has the following advantages: (1) It yields a nonturbid, stable solution upon direct nesslerization; (2) the reagents are stable at room temperature and are used sparingly, and (3) if the urea nitrogen level is extremely high, a further dilution of the initial filtrate of the incubation mixture can be made, rather than repeating the entire analysis.

Acid-Base Analyses

Blood pH (from Hawkins, Hastings, and Sendroy[8])

Preparation of the bicolor standards was taken from Peters and Van Slyke's *Quantitative Clinical Chemistry* (cited below) p. 797, Table 65. The preparation of the reagents (p. 796) and Hawkins' modification (p. 801) for using a sample of whole blood were also followed.

Procedure

The phenol red tube and the saline tube are prepared immediately before the analysis, using tubes similar to those for the preparation of standards. (*Phenol red tube:* After placing 5 ml. of freshly adjusted saline solution (which contains 11 ml. of 0.0075-percent phenol red solution per 100 ml.) in a tube, about one-quarter inch of liquid petrolatum is stratified above this solution. *Saline tube:* Five ml. of freshly prepared saline are put into a similar tube.)

Drawing blood samples: A glass bead is placed in the barrel of a 2-ml. syringe with needle attached, about 0.5 ml. of sterile liquid petrolatum and a small drop of saturated potassium oxalate are added, and the plunger is inserted in the syringe. The syringe is inverted so that the needle is pointing upward, the droplet of potassium oxalate is allowed to fall to the bottom of the solution, and all the air and excess petrolatum are slowly expressed until the movement of the plunger is arrested by the glass bead. The excess petrolatum is wiped off the needle, a blood sample of about 1.5 to 2 milliliters is taken, and the syringe is inverted several times to insure mixing with the oxalate. After waiting a moment for the petrolatum to stratify to the top of the syringe, the needle is placed under the petrolatum layer of the phenol red tube and exactly 0.5 ml. of blood is expressed into the tube. In a similar manner 0.5 ml. of blood is placed in the saline tube. The petrolatum is siphoned off from the phenol red tube, which is then sealed with 1/4 inch of paraffin, and the contents of both tubes are mixed by inversion and centrifuged.

[8] In Peters, J. P., and Van Slyke, D. D. Quantitative Clinical Chemistry. vol. II: Methods. Baltimore, Williams & Wilkins, 1932, p. 796–801.

Color comparison is made by arrangement of the tubes in the comparator as illustrated in Fig. 87 of Peters and Van Slyke's *Quantitative Clinical Chemistry*. Readings are made between 18° and 20° C., noting the temperature in the saline tube.

Correction of Observed pH to pH at 38° C.

Since the standards were prepared to read pH at 38° C., it is necessary only to subtract the observed temperature from 38° C., multiply this difference by 0.005 and subtract this product from the observed pH to obtain blood pH at 38° Centigrade.

Example:

1. Observed pH 7.48 at 20° C.
2. 38 — 20 = 18
3. 18 x 0.005 = 0.09
4. 7.48 — 0.09 = pH 7.39 at 38° C.

Normal controls are run with each series of analyses.

Serum Sodium—Modified from Weinbach's Modification of Butler and Tuthill's Method[9]

Reagents

1. Trichloracetic acid, 20-percent solution.
2. Sodium reagent (uranyl zinc acetate). ((a) Uranium acetate, 38.5 Gm., and glacial acetic acid, 14 ml., are dissolved in 150 ml. of distilled water with the aid of heat. (b) Zinc oxide, 37.5 Gm., and glacial acetic acid, 63 ml., are dissolved in 150 ml. of distilled water with the aid of heat. (c) The two solutions are combined, mixed, cooled, and made up to 500 ml. with distilled water. (d) This solution is transferred to a reagent bottle, about 0.5 Gm. of the salt sodium uranyl zinc acetate is introduced, and this mixture is shaken to effect saturation with the sodium uranyl zinc acetate.)
3. Standard sodium solution, 330 mg. of sodium per 100 milliliters. (Sodium chloride, 0.840 Gm., is diluted to 100 ml. with water and stored in a paraffin-lined bottle.)
4. 95-percent ethyl alcohol.
5. Acetone wash. (Sodium uranyl zinc acetate, 0.5 Gm., is introduced into a bottle containing about one liter of acetone, the bottle is well shaken and allowed to stand at least overnight before using.)
6. A 0.0348 N solution of sodium hydroxide.

[9] In Hawk, P. B., and Bergeim, O. Practical Physiological Chemistry. 11th ed. Philadelphia, Blakiston, 1937, p. 472–473.

7. Sodium uranyl zinc acetate. (One ml. of a 5-percent solution of sodium chloride is added to 15 ml. of the sodium reagent in a 50-ml. Erlenmeyer flask, and 1 ml. of 95-percent ethyl alcohol is added at 5-minute intervals until 5 ml. have been added. The mixture is filtered, using suction, and the precipitate of sodium uranyl zinc acetate is washed three times with alcohol and three times with ether, sucking dry after each washing.)

Preparation of Glassware.—Two clean graduated centrifuge tubes for each determination and two for the standard are prepared by rinsing them four times with distilled water and drying in an oven.

Procedure

One volume of serum, 3 volumes of water, and 1 volume of 20-percent trichloracetic acid are mixed in a tube by inversion, and the process is repeated, using 1 volume of the standard sodium solution instead of serum. Into each of two of the specially prepared centrifuge tubes are placed 0.5 ml. of the serum filtrate, and into each of the two other specially prepared centrifuge tubes 0.5 ml. of the dilute standard. Five ml. of filtered sodium reagent are then added to each tube, followed by 0.3 ml. of 95-percent ethyl alcohol at 5-minute intervals until 2.1 ml. have been added to each, when the supernatant fluid is centrifuged and decanted, allowing the tubes to drain and taking care not to dislodge the residue. Five ml. of filtered acetone wash are blown into the residue, the tubes are centrifuged, and the supernatant is decanted and drained. This process is repeated two more times, making three washings in all. Using 25 ml. of distilled water, the residue is dissolved and transferred quantitatively to a 125-ml. Erlenmeyer flask and titrated with 0.0348 N sodium hydroxide using phenolphthalein as the indicator.

Calculation

1 ml. of 0.0348 N sodium hydroxide = 100 mg. of sodium per 100 ml. of serum.

Example:

Titration of Sample I		*Sample II*	*Average*
Serum	3.43	3.45	3.44 or 344 mg./100 ml.
Standard	3.38	3.36	3.37 or 337 mg./100 ml.

Actual strength of standard: 330 mg./100 ml.
Determined strength of standard: 337 mg./100 ml.
Difference (blank): 7 mg./100 ml.
Therefore, 344 — 7 = 337 mg. of sodium per 100 ml. of serum.
Mg./100 ml. sodium x 10/23 = milliequivalents of sodium.

Comment

The modified method used was further modified (1) by changing the strength of the sodium hydroxide used, thus simplifying the calculation, (2) by using a standard of known sodium concentration to ascertain the reagent blank, and (3) by an additional acetone washing.

Serum Potassium (Kramer and Tisdall[10]*)*

The standard procedure was followed, with duplicate analyses of each sample and potassium standards for every analysis.

Serum Calcium (Clark-Collip Modification of Kramer and Tisdall Method[11]*)*

The standard procedure was followed.

Magnesium in Plasma—Modified from Herschfelder and Serles[12]

Reagents

1. Titan yellow, 0.05-percent solution. (This keeps for about two weeks.)
2. Sodium hydroxide, 10-percent solution.
3. Trichloracetic acid, 10-percent solution.
4. Stock magnesium standard solution. (One Gm. of magnesium sulfate heptahydrate is dissolved with a little water and then made up to a 100-ml. solution.)
5. Working magnesium standard solution. (1.45 ml. of stock standard diluted to 100 ml. with water. (7 milliliters = 0.1 mg. magnesium.) A standard reference curve is prepared, using this solution according to conditions of the test. The color is read at 535 mμ in the spectrophotometer.)

Procedure

To 2 ml. of plasma are added 4 ml. of water and 4 ml. of 10-percent trichloracetic acid. The solution is mixed, allowed to stand for several minutes,

[10] In Todd, J. C., and Sanford, A. H. Clinical Diagnosis by Laboratory Methods. 10th ed. Philadelphia, W. B. Saunders, 1943, p. 420–421.

[11] In Hawk, P. B., and Bergeim, O. Practical Physiological Chemistry. 10th ed. Philadelphia, Blakiston, 1931, p. 460–461.

[12] Herschfelder, A. D., and Serles, E. R.: A simple adaptation of Kolthoff's colorimetric method for the determination of magnesium in biological fluids. J. Biol. Chem. **104**: 635, March 1934.

centrifuged, and filtered. To 5 ml. of plasma filtrate in a cuvette, 1.6 ml. of water is added, and 7 ml. of water in another cuvette serves as the blank. One ml. of titan yellow is then added to each of the samples and to the blank. Two ml. of the sodium hydroxide solution are added to the blank tube, the contents are mixed, and the tube is set to read at 100-percent transmission on the spectrophotometer at 535 millimicrons. Similarly, 2.4 ml. of the sodium hydroxide solution are added to each of the samples, and the solution is mixed and read immediately on the spectrophotometer at 535 millimicrons.

Calculation

Milligrams of magnesium per 100 ml. of plasma are determined by reference of the observed percentage transmission to the standard curve.

Comment

This method is a simple, rapid procedure. Recoveries of added magnesium and comparisons of normal range of plasma magnesium with that of other methods (1.5-2.0 mg. per 100 ml.) indicate its accuracy.

Phosphorus in Plasma—Modified from Bodansky[13]

The method was modified by making up the standard in trichloracetic acid. This permitted of more exact color comparison and eliminated the need for the two molybdate solutions which the original method demands.

Carbon-Dioxide Combining Power of Plasma (Van Slyke and Cullen[14]*)*

Chlorides in Plasma (Schales and Schales[15]*)*

Plasma chlorides were determined by the method of Schales and Schales.

[13] In TODD, J. C., and SANFORD, A. H. Clinical Diagnosis by Laboratory Methods. 10th ed. Philadelphia, W. B. Saunders, 1943, p. 404–411.

[14] The procedure was followed as described in *Methods for Laboratory Technicians,* War Department Technical Manual 8–227, October 1946, p. 123–129.

[15] In SIMMONS, J. S., and GENTZKOW, C. J. Laboratory Methods of the United States Army. Philadelphia, Lea & Febiger, 1944, p. 209.

Lactic Acid in Plasma—Modified from Mendel and Goldschieder[16]

Reagents

1. Metaphosphoric acid, 5-percent solution, prepared daily.
2. Copper sulfate, 15 percent by weight of pentahydrate.
3. Blank-free concentrated sulfuric acid. (The quality of the sulfuric acid should be such that no yellow color develops on the addition of 0.1 ml. of 0.125-percent veratrole to 3 ml. of acid. A good reagent grade of sulfuric acid is satisfactory.)
4. Lactic acid, 100 mg. per 100 ml., prepared from lithium lactate.
5. Sodium fluoride, 0.1-percent solution.
6. Veratrole, 0.125 percent in absolute alcohol.

Procedure

To 1 ml. of plasma separated from freshly drawn blood are added 5 ml. of water, 1 ml. of sodium fluoride, and 1 ml. of metaphosphoric acid. The whole is shaken vigorously, allowed to stand for several minutes, and filtered. To 4 ml. of the protein-free filtrate in a centrifuge tube are added 1 ml. of copper sulfate solution and 1 Gm. of calcium hydroxide, the mixture is allowed to stand about 30 minutes, shaking several times, and is then centrifuged. The pellicle of copper hydroxide is broken with a glass rod and the supernatant is decanted into another tube and centrifuged again, resulting in a clear, sugar-free filtrate. The standard lactic acid solution is diluted 1:10, corresponding to 100 mg. of lactic acid per 100 ml. of plasma, according to the conditions of the test. Weaker dilutions corresponding to 75, 50, 25, and 12.5 mg. of lactic acid per 100 ml. of plasma are also prepared.

To 0.5 ml. of the clear sugar-free filtrate (obtained by centrifugation only), to 0.5 ml. of each standard, and to 0.5 ml. of water in a carefully cleaned test tube, 3 ml. of concentrated sulfuric acid are slowly added while the tubes are cooled in cold water. The tubes are then placed in a boiling water bath for exactly 4 minutes, removed and immersed in cold water for 5 minutes. To each tube 0.1 ml. of the veratrole solution is added, and the solution is mixed and allowed to stand for 20 minutes, after which it is decanted into small cuvettes (12 by 75 mm.) and read in the spectrophotometer at 545 mμ, blanking out with the water reagent blank and reading the optical density scale.

[16] In PETERS, J. P., and VAN SLYKE, D. D. Quantitative Clinical Chemistry. vol. II: Methods. Baltimore, Williams & Wilkins, 1932, p. 618–620.

Note: In the process of color development, a brown color may form in addition to the pink of the test color. This is due to unclean glassware and contaminated filtrate. In these instances the analysis is repeated.

Calculation

A proportion is set up comparing the reading of the sample with that of the nearest standard.

Comment

The test was set up on the spectrophotometer, and readings were made on the optical density scale, using a series of standards with each run, since color development is not reproducible from day to day as required for using a permanent chart. The color development does not satisfactorily follow Beer's law, and the optical density reading of the closest standard was used in calculating the value of the sample.

The use of 1 ml. of sodium fluoride in the dilution of the plasma permits preservation of the lactic acid level until a series of samples has accumulated.

Glucose in Plasma

The standard procedure of Folin and Wu[17] was followed for the determination of glucose in plasma.

Sulfonamides in Whole Blood

The method of Bratton and Marshall[18] was followed.

Determination of Methemoglobin

The method of Paul and Kemp[19] was followed.

[17] In Simmons, J. S., and Gentzkow, C. J. Laboratory Methods of the United States Army. Philadelphia, Lea & Febiger, 1944, p. 207–208.

[18] In Simmons, J. S., and Gentzkow, C. J. Laboratory Methods of the United States Army. Philadelphia, Lea & Febiger, 1944, p. 219–220.

[19] Paul, W. D., and Kemp, C. R.: Methemoglobin; a normal constituent of blood. Proc. Soc. Exp. Biol. & Med. 56: 55–56, 1944.

Plasma Bilirubin (van den Bergh)

The method of Evelyn and Malloy[20] was followed.

Hemoglobin, Hematocrit, and Plasma Protein

The method of Phillips et al.[21] for the calculation of hemoglobin, hematocrit value, and plasma proteins by means of copper sulfate was followed with the exception that, since a chemical balance was available, all the solutions were checked and standardized so that they were correct to within ±2 units in the fourth decimal place, using a 25-ml. pyknometer and water at the same temperature as the standard solution. Each bottle was prepared in 1-liter quantity and replacements were made from this stock. Bottles were prepared for each unit difference in the third decimal place.

Plasma Hemoglobin Determination

Plasma Hemoglobin—Modified from Bing and Baker[22]

Reagents

1. Benzidine reagent. (Five Gm. of a good quality of benzidine are dissolved in 50 milliliters of glacial acetic acid, warming gently to effect solution. The mixture is cooled, diluted to 250 ml. with distilled water, about 2 Gm. of decolorizing charcoal are added, and the solution is thoroughly mixed, allowed to stand for approximately 10 minutes, and filtered into a brown bottle.)
2. Hydrogen peroxide, 3-percent solution.
3. Hemoglobin standard solution. (A 20-mg. per 100 ml. solution of hemoglobin is prepared in 1-percent boric acid by diluting blood of known hemoglobin content.)
4. Acetic acid, 20-percent solution.

Procedure

To 0.2 ml. of each sample and of the standard in separate tubes are added

[20] In Simmons, J. S., and Gentzkow, C. J. Laboratory Methods of the United States Army. Philadelphia, Lea & Febiger, 1944, p. 214–215.

[21] Phillips, R. A.; Van Slyke, D. D.; Dole, V. P.; Emerson, K., Jr.; Hamilton, P. B., and Archibald, R. M.: Copper sulfate method for measuring specific gravities of whole blood and plasma. BUMED News Letter, U. S. Navy, June 25, 1943, p. 1-16.

[22] Bing, F. C., and Baker, R. W.: The determination of hemoglobin in minute amounts of blood by Wu's method. J. Biol. Chem. 92: 589–600, August 1931.

2 ml. of the benzidine reagent, and each is thoroughly mixed. One ml. of the 3-percent hydrogen peroxide is then added to each tube and they are allowed to stand for 30 minutes, at the end of which time the mixtures are diluted with 6.8 ml. of the acetic acid and allowed to stand until all the tubes have developed the red color (about 30 minutes), when they are compared in the colorimeter.

Calculation

The sample is set on 20 millimeters. The reading of the standard equals milligrams of benzidine-reacting substance per 100 ml. of plasma. As has been explained in Chapter VIII of the text, this entire benzidine-reacting substance was termed "plasma hemoglobin" because a means for its further breakdown was not available to us.

Liver Function Test

Bromsulfalein Test—Modified from Rosenthal[23]

Reagents

Bromsulfalein, 5-percent solution, in sterilized, sealed ampules.
Sodium hydroxide, 10-percent solution.
3. Sodium chloride, 0.9-percent solution.

Procedure

The patient's weight is recorded in kilograms and the amount of dye to be injected is calculated on the basis of 5 mg. per Kg. of body weight. A simple procedure is to divide the body weight in kilograms by 10 to yield the exact amount in milliliters of bromsulfalein to be used for injection. The required amount of dye is drawn into a 10-ml. syringe and slowly injected into a vein in the patient's arm, the exact time of injection being recorded. Forty-five minutes after injection, a sample of blood from the opposite arm is collected in the standard lithium oxalate bottle, the blood specimen is centrifuged, and the plasma is collected.

[23] In TODD, J. C., and SANFORD, A. H. Clinical Diagnosis by Laboratory Methods. 10th ed. Philadelphia, W. B. Saunders, 1943, p. 428–429.

To 1 ml. of plasma placed in a cuvette 5 ml. of a 0.9-percent solution of sodium chloride are added. The contents are well mixed and the spectrophotometer is set to read 100-percent transmission at 575 millimicrons with this solution. Three drops of a 10-percent solution of sodium hydroxide are then added to the same tube and it is inverted and read on the spectrophotometer. The transmission percentage is noted and the percentage of dye retention is obtained from the curve plotted from a standard bromsulfalein solution, following the conditions of the test wherein 10 mg. per 100 ml. is considered 100-percent retention.

Comment

The standard procedure for the determination of dye retention using the Hynson, Westcott & Dunning Comparator Block was abandoned because various degrees of hemolysis in the samples would result in readings that indicated as much as 5-percent retention when no bromsulfalein was present. Low retention figures, therefore, could not be expressed with any degree of certainty, as results were often not reproducible to within ±5-percent retention. Furthermore the method was time-consuming.

The test was set up on the Coleman Junior Spectrophotometer Model No. 6, using a 1:6 dilution of plasma and reading the color of the alkalinized bromsulfalein at 575 millimicrons.

Renal Function Tests

Determination of Mannitol—Modified from Smith, H.[24]

MEASUREMENT OF GLOMERULAR FILTRATION RATE

Reagents

1. A 20-percent yeast suspension. (Bakers' yeast, 25 Gm., is placed in about 100 ml. of water, allowed to incubate overnight, and then washed by repeated centrifugation until a clear supernatant is obtained (about 6 washings are necessary). The resulting suspension is diluted to contain 20 percent by volume of yeast. This is washed several times each day

[24] In GOLDRING, W., and CHASSIS, H. Hypertension and Hypertensive Disease. New York, The Commonwealth Fund, 1944. Appendix D.

before using and readjusted to the 20-percent volume.)

2. 1.1 N sodium hydroxide.

3. Zinc sulfate solution. (A solution of zinc sulfate is prepared and adjusted so that 6 ml. of zinc sulfate are equivalent to 2.2 ml. of 1.1 N sodium hydroxide.)

4. 0.005 N sodium thiosulfate. (The normality is determined by using 10 ml. of 0.010 N potassium iodate. The factor for 0.005 N thiosulfate is: 1 ml. = 4.6 mg. of mannitol. The factor for the determined normality is calculated daily rather than adjusting the strength of the thiosulfate.)

5. Potassium periodate, 0.1-percent solution. (Prepared with the aid of heat.)

6. Sulfuric acid, 5 percent by volume.

7. Acid potassium periodate. (A solution of three parts of 0.1-percent potassium periodate and two parts of 5-percent sulfuric acid is prepared daily.)

8. Potassium iodide, 50-percent solution. (Prepared just before the analysis is made.)

9. Starch, 1-percent solution. (Prepared just before the analysis is made.)

Procedure

Six ml. of the 20-percent yeast suspension are placed in each of as many tubes as there are specimens and in a blank tube.

For plasma analyses, 1 ml. of water is first added to each of the yeast tubes and then 1 ml. of each mannitol-containing plasma specimen is added. Similarly, to another yeast tube are added 1 ml. of water and 1 ml. of blank (mannitol-free) plasma.

For urine analyses, the urine samples are diluted to contain from 100 to 150 mg. of mannitol per 100 ml. of urine. Two ml. from each such diluted sample are added to 6 ml. of yeast. Another tube containing 2 ml. of water and 6 ml. of yeast serves as the urine blank.

The yeasted tubes are shaken at intervals, and allowed to stand for 20 minutes, then centrifuged, and the supernatant fluid is decanted. Four ml. of each supernatant are measured into 6 ml. of zinc sulfate solution, mixed, and 2 ml. of 1.1 N sodium hydroxide are added. The tubes are shaken vigorously, and allowed to stand for 10 minutes, centrifuged, and filtered. Two ml. of each filtrate are placed in a 50-ml. Erlenmeyer flask, and exactly 5 ml. of acid potassium periodate are added with scrupulous care with an Ostwald pipet. A glass bead is placed in the flask and a glass stopper is placed in the mouth of the flask to effect condensation. The contents are boiled gently for 5 minutes and when cooled 1 ml. of 50-percent potassium iodide is added. The liberated iodine is titrated with sodium thiosulfate, adding 0.5 ml. of starch just before the end-point and titrating until the blue color disappears.

956507 O—52——27

Calculation

Plasma

ml. of thiosulfate used for plasma blank — ml. of thiosulfate for sample = ml. of thiosulfate for mannitol in plasma.

mg. of mannitol per 100 ml. of plasma = ml. of thiosulfate used x 4.6 (thiosulfate factor) x 24 (dilution factor).

Urine

ml. of thiosulfate for water blank — ml. of thiosulfate used for urine sample = ml. of thiosulfate for mannitol in urine.

mg. of mannitol per 100 ml. of urine = ml. of thiosulfate used x 4.6 x D x W x 12 (dilution factor).

Where:

4.6 = thiosulfate factor
D = urine dilution
W = washout dilution factor
12 = dilution factor for analysis

Mannitol Clearance (rate of glomerular filtration):

$$\text{Cm (in ml./minute} = \frac{\text{V x Um}}{\text{Pm}}$$

Where:

Cm = mannitol clearance
V = urine volume in ml. per minute
Um = mg. mannitol in 1 ml. of urine
Pm = mg. mannitol in 1 ml. of plasma

Para-Amino Hippuric Acid

MEASUREMENT OF EFFECTIVE RENAL PLASMA FLOW AND MAXIMUM TUBULAR EXCRETORY CAPACITY

The method of Homer Smith[25] was followed.

Phenolsulfonphthalein Test—Modified—Analytical Procedure[26]

Reagents

1. Sodium hydroxide, 2-percent solution.

[25] Ibid.

[26] In Todd, J. C., and Sanford, A. H.: Clinical Diagnosis by Laboratory Methods. 10th ed. Philadelphia, W. B. Saunders, 1943, p. 163–167.

2. Acetic acid, 10-percent solution.

A standard curve is prepared from the phenolsulfonphthalein standard solution according to conditions of the test, blanking out with the acid color of the indicator at 540 millimicrons.

Procedure

The volumes of four urine specimens (timed) are measured and aliquots representing one-hundredth of the volume of each specimen are each pipeted into two cuvettes, one being designated as the acid tube and one the alkaline tube for the individual specimens. All the samples are diluted to 9.75 ml. with water, and to the alkaline tubes 0.25 ml. of the sodium hydroxide solution is added, and 0.25 ml. of the acetic acid to the acid tubes. Unless the solutions are absolutely clear, they are filtered. The alkaline tube is read in the spectrophotometer at 540 mμ, blanking out with the corresponding acid tube. The percentage transmission is noted for each alkaline tube and the milligrams of phenolsulfonphthalein content are recorded from the chart. In the event that excretion is markedly diminished, the procedure is repeated, using one-tenth aliquots of each specimen and dividing the chart readings by ten.

Comment

This method is much more accurate than methods depending on the usual comparator block because color due to urinary pigments is entirely blanked out.

Urinalyses

Routine Urinalysis

Specific Gravity.—Specific gravity is measured with a urinometer. If the specimen is not sufficient, the specific gravity is determined by weighing.

Appearance.—The color and appearance of the urine are noted.

Albumin.—Approximately 8 ml. of the specimen are placed in a test tube, the upper part of which is heated gently to the boiling point, any change in turbidity being carefully observed. Three drops of acetic acid in 20-percent solution are added and the upper portion is again heated to boiling. The heated portion is compared with the portion in the bottom of the tube, and depending upon the density of the precipitate, is read as negative, trace, 1-plus, 2-plus, 3-plus, or 4-plus.

pH.—Indicators used: Phenol red, bromcresol purple, and methyl red.

Procedure for determining hydrogen ion concentration: Three tubes of the same size as the indicator tubes are used, each of two of them containing 1 ml. of urine and 4 ml. of water, and the third containing 5 ml. of water only. To one of the tubes containing urine 0.25 ml. of bromcresol purple is added. The color resulting is compared with the standard solutions,[27] arranging the tubes so the diluted urine to which the indicator has been added is backed by distilled water and the standard tube is backed by the other diluted urine tube. If the pH is above 7.0, phenol red is used in a similar manner. If the pH is below 5.8, methyl red is used. Methyl red ranges from red to yellow between pH of 4.4 and 6.0.

The Benzidine Test.—Reagents: (1) Benzidine solution. (Five Gm. of a reagent grade of benzidine are dissolved in 50 ml. of glacial acetic acid with the aid of gentle heat, cooled, and diluted to 250 ml. with distilled water, 1 Gm. of animal charcoal is added, and the mixture is shaken and filtered into a brown bottle. It should be kept cool.) (2) Hydrogen peroxide, 3-percent solution. (3) Hemoglobin standard, 20 mg. of hemoglobin per 100 ml. in boric acid, 1-percent solution. (Lasts a week or 10 days.)

Procedure for performing the benzidine test: To 2 ml. of benzidine reagent in a clean tube are added 0.2 ml. of urine and 1 ml. of hydrogen peroxide. This is allowed to stand for from 30 to 60 minutes, the shorter time being for higher temperatures, and is then diluted to 10 ml. with 20-percent acetic acid solution. The red color may turn blue at this point, in which case the solution is allowed to stand in a warm place until the red color again develops. The standard is prepared exactly as if it were a sample. The solutions are filtered and compared in the colorimeter, with the unknown set on 20 millimeters. The reading of the standard yields the milligrams of hemoglobin per 100 ml. of urine.

Bile (Rosenbach's Modification of Gmelin's Test[28]*).*—A portion of the urine is filtered and a drop of fuming nitric acid is introduced into the cone of the filter paper. A succession of colors—green, blue, violet, and red in a ring pattern —is interpreted as a positive result.

The following urinalyses were performed by the standard methods indi-

[27] Preparation of the Clark and Lubs standard buffer mixture is described on p. 24 of HAWK, P. B., and BERGEIM, O. Practical Physiological Chemistry. 10th ed. Philadelphia, Blakiston, 1931.

[28] Ibid. Page 762.

cated: Ammonia (Folin and Bell[29]); urea nitrogen (Folin and Youngburg[30]); titratable acidity (Henderson and Palmer[31]); chlorides (Schales and Schales[32]).

Organic Acids in Urine—Modified from Van Slyke and Palmer[33]

Reagents

1. Calcium hydroxide.
2. Thymol blue indicator solution. (0.1 Gm. of thymol blue and 2.1 ml. of 0.1 N sodium hydroxide are made up to 100 milliliters.)
3. 0.50 N hydrochloric acid.
4. Phenolphthalein. (1 percent in 50-percent alcohol.)

Procedure

The urine is tested for albumin. If the albumin is 1-plus or higher, a noted volume of urine (greater than 100 ml.) is acidified with 0.5 ml. of concentrated hydrochloric acid, boiled for several minutes to coagulate the protein, cooled, made up to the initial volume, and filtered. If the urine is protein-free, it is used directly. Next, 0.5 ml. of phenolphthalein is added to 100 ml. of urine (or the protein-free urine filtrate) and powdered calcium hydroxide is added until the body of the solution turns pink (about 2 to 4 Gm. are required). The mixture is allowed to stand for 1 hour. It is then filtered and 50 ml. of the filtrate are measured into a 125-ml. Erlenmeyer flask, decanting the remaining filtrate into an identical flask. To discharge the phenolphthalein color in both flasks 0.5 N HCl is added.

Two ml. of thymol blue are added to the 50-ml. sample of the urine, and 2 ml. of thymol blue and 0.3 ml. of 0.5 N hydrochloric acid to 50 ml. of distilled water, and the flasks are arranged for titration. (The 50-ml. urine flask is placed in front of a flask of distilled water, and the flask containing the dilute

[29] In Hawk, P. B., and Bergeim, O. Practical Physiological Chemistry. 10th ed. Philadelphia, Blakiston, 1931, p. 829.

[30] Ibid. Page 825.

[31] In Peters, J. P., and Van Slyke, D. D. Quantitative Clinical Chemistry. vol. II: Methods. Baltimore, Williams & Wilkins, 1932, p. 827.

[32] In Simmons, J. S., and Gentzkow, C. J. Laboratory Methods of the United States Army. Philadelphia, Lea & Febiger, 1944, p. 209.

[33] In Peters, J. P., and Van Slyke, D. D. Quantitative Clinical Chemistry. vol. II: Methods. Baltimore, Williams & Wilkins, 1932, p. 647–651.

hydrochloric acid and thymol blue is placed in front of the urine flask that does not contain thymol blue.) The 50-ml. urine specimen is titrated until its color matches the other set of flasks.

Calculation

$$\left[(\text{ml required} - 0.3 \times \frac{\text{24-hr. urine volume}}{100}\right] - \left[\frac{\text{Gm. creatinine in 24-hr. urine}}{100}\right]$$

= ml. of 1 N acid

Comment

The original method was modified by the use of thymol blue as the indicator instead of tropeolin 00, which was not available for the study, and by introducing into the comparator-block system a sample of the phosphate-free urine to compensate for urinary pigments in the titration flask.

Creatinine and Creatine in Urine—Modified from Folin and from Folin-Benedict and Myers[34]

Reagents

1. Saturated picric acid.
2. Sodium hydroxide, 10-percent solution.
3. 1 N hydrochloric acid.
4. 0.25 N sodium hydroxide.
5. Alkaline picrate. (Made by combining 5 volumes of saturated picric acid with 1 volume of 10-percent sodium hydroxide solution. It is freshly prepared before each series of analyses.)

Procedure for Determination of Creatinine

One-thousandth of the volume of a 24-hour urine specimen is made up to 10 milliliters. This is designated as the first tube. One milliliter of the contents of this tube is then diluted to 10 ml. with water, and designated as the second tube. Three ml. of the contents of the second tube are diluted to 10 milliliters, forming the third tube. Five ml. of the contents of this third tube are placed in a cuvette, and 2.5 ml. of alkaline picrate are added. The color is allowed to

[34] In Hawk, P. B., and Bergeim, O. Practical Physiological Chemistry. 10th ed. Philadelphia, Blakiston, 1931, p. 835–837.

develop for 10 minutes and is then read in the spectrophotometer at 500 mμ, blanking out with a solution containing 5 ml. of water and 2.5 ml. of alkaline picrate solution prepared at the same time as the sample. Grams of creatinine per 24-hour urine specimen are calculated by reference to the chart used for plasma creatinine and dividing by three.

Procedure for Determination of Creatine

To 2.5 ml. of the first creatinine tube, placed in a 25-ml. volumetric flask, is added 1 ml. of 1 N hydrochloric acid and the flask is placed in an autoclave at 120°C. for 15 minutes, cooled, and made up to volume with water. A portion of the contents of the flask is titrated with 0.25 N sodium hydroxide, using phenolphthalein as an indicator to determine the amount required to neutralize 3 milliliters. A 3-ml. aliquot is neutralized and made up with water to 10 ml., 5.0 ml. are transferred to a cuvette, 2.5 ml. of alkaline picrate are added, and the color is read as for creatinine.

The turbidity correction factor is determined and subtracted in this manner: The autoclaved solution in the volumetric flask is placed in a cuvette, blanked out with the contents of the second creatinine tube, and its value in terms of optical density is determined. The value is muliplied by 0.3, changed to the transmission percentage at the creatine reading, and added to that reading.

Example: Creatinine plus creatine reading: 50-percent T. (transmission)
OD of flask contents: 0.003
0.003 x 0.3 = 0.0009 = 0.001
OD of 0.001 corresponds to 1.5% T. at 50% T., making the corrected creatine reading 51.5-percent transmission.

The corrected creatine plus creatinine reading is converted to grams per 24-hour urine specimen by reference to the chart and then dividing by three.

The creatine content is determined by subtracting creatinine from the combined creatinine and creatine.

Comment

The method as modified had these advantages: (1) The analysis was set up on the spectrophotometer, which yielded more accurate colorimeter readings, and equipment and reagents were used sparingly, and (2) a turbidity correction factor was introduced into the creatine analysis which compensates for turbidity formed during the autoclaving process.

Determination of Myoglobin

Myoglobin, the red coloring matter of muscle, is a conjugated protein consisting of a protein part called globin and the iron pyrol compound known as hematin; it has a molecular weight of 17,000.

As stated in Chapter VIII, a spectroscope sufficiently sensitive to distinguish between hemoglobin and myoglobin was not available to us, and it did not prove possible to separate the two pigments in the plasma. The measurement of myoglobin in tissue and urine involved the following considerations: (1) It was necessary to find some property of myoglobin which would permit its quantitative separation from hemoglobin; (2) a convenient procedure for measuring the ultimately separated myoglobin, one that would be sufficiently sensitive to measure the small quantities anticipated in urine, was required, and (3) a rapid urine test was deemed essential since identification of myoglobin in the urine might influence the treatment of the patient.

Quantitative determination by means of the benzidine reagent was determined as the most satisfactory method. This test, however, was not satisfactory in media containing large amounts of phosphates and sulfates which caused gross precipitation of the benzidine reagent. These ions were present when it was attempted to separate myoglobin from hemoglobin by fractional crystallization procedures as described by Morgan[35] and Rossi-Fanelli,[36] using lead acetate in 3 M phosphate buffer solutions or in concentrated ammonium sulfate. An efficient means of dialysis was not available at the time of the study and this method of separation was not pursued.

The myoglobin for further experimentation was extracted from perfused normal human skeletal muscle. A saline extract was made of finely minced muscle, eluting with constant shaking for 1 hour, using 2 ml. of saline for each gram of muscle tissue and allowing it to stand overnight in a refrigerator. The suspension was centrifuged to eliminate any red cells and then filtered (the muscle was completely bleached).

The concentration of myoglobin in this extract was determined by the benzidine test. The benzidine test measures the hematin part of the hemo-

[35] Morgan, V. E.: The solubility of myoglobin in concentrated ammonium sulfate solutions. J. Biol. Chem. **112**: 557–563, January 1936.

[36] Rossi-Fanelli, A.: Crystalline human myoglobin; some physicochemical properties and chemical composition. Science **108**: 15–16, July 2, 1948.

globin, or myoglobin molecule, and since the relationship of myoglobin (one hematin molecule, molecular weight 17,000) to hemoglobin (four hematin molecules, molecular weight 68,000) indicates the same proportion of benzidine-positive substance per unit weight of protein, reference can be made to standard hemoglobin solutions for quantitative measurement of myoglobin.

A portion of the stock myoglobin solution obtained as described above was diluted with normal urine to yield a level of 50 mg. per 100 ml., and a control solution containing 50 mg. of hemoglobin in 100 ml. of urine was prepared. On the addition of 0.5 ml. of 2.5 N sodium hydroxide to 10-ml. of each sample, a striking difference in the behavior of the two solutions was noted. The solution containing the myoglobin retained its reddish tint, while that containing the hemoglobin turned brown with the formation of alkali hematin. When acid, in equivalent amount to that of the alkali previously added, was added to each of the samples, the one containing myoglobin precipitated as a brownish-red protein, while in the hemoglobin tube the precipitation yielded a white protein material and the supernatant fluid remained brown due to the hematin. The contents of the tubes were then centrifuged.

The following chemical pattern indicates the different properties of the two proteins:

Myoglobin $\xrightarrow{\text{alkali}}$ myoglobin $\xrightarrow{\text{acidify and centrifuge}}$
myoglobin (precipitate) + hematin-free supernatant
[benzidine-positive] [benzidine-negative]

Hemoglobin $\xrightarrow{\text{alkali}}$ alkali hematin + globin $\xrightarrow{\text{acidify and centrifuge}}$
globin (precipitate) + hematin supernatant
[benzidine-negative] [benzidine-positive]

The supernatant fluid of the hemoglobin tube reflects the original concentration of the hemoglobin as hematin. The precipitate in the myoglobin tube was the myoglobin present. This dissolved readily in a little weak alkali and was made up to the 10-ml. volume. Quantitative estimation of myoglobin could then be made by the benzidine test.

Determinations made with hemoglobin solutions in urine indicated that on the average 90 percent of the hemoglobin could be recovered as hematin in the supernatant fluid while the precipitate would contain 10 percent of benzidine-positive material in the form of undecomposed hemoglobin. Determinations with myoglobin solutions in urine indicated that from 65 to 85 percent could be recovered in the precipitate (the myoglobin fraction of the reaction) and that the remainder had been decomposed by the alkali to alkali hematin, yielding different proportions (15 to 35 percent) of myoglobin which would be measured as hemoglobin in the supernatant.

Recoveries from mixtures of myoglobin and hemoglobin indicated that separation could be effected between the two proteins, and that quantitative estimation of myoglobin in urine as well as in tissue was feasible. The following standards were established for interpretation of the findings:

1. A urine sample reflecting an analysis as 90 percent of the total benzidine-positive substance as hemoglobin and the remainder as myoglobin was considered to be all hemoglobin, while an analysis reflecting between 80 and 90 percent as hemoglobin was considered doubtful for myoglobin, and was also recorded as myoglobin-negative. A sample of urine yielding a level of less than 4 mg. of myoglobin per 100 ml., with a higher level in the hemoglobin fraction, was considered doubtful for myoglobin and recorded as negative.

2. A sample was considered to contain myoglobin beyond a doubt if it turned red or retained its reddish tint on addition of alkali and if, after separation of the protein, the precipitate was 20 percent or more of the total benzidine-positive substance. Recoveries in the myoglobin tube were considered as 70 percent; the value found was divided by 0.7 and the result reported in terms of the recovery factor.

For the first month of the survey each day's run of benzidine-positive urines was accompanied by control recovery tubes of hemoglobin and myoglobin. Solutions of methemoglobin or hematin failed to show the analytical pattern described.

DETERMINATION OF MYOGLOBIN IN URINE

Following are the details of performing the test on urine.

Reagents

1. Benzidine solution. (As for plasma hemoglobin.)
2. Hydrogen peroxide, 3-percent solution. (As for plasma hemoglobin.)
3. Hemoglobin standard solution, 20 mg. per 100 cc. (As for plasma hemoglobin.)
4. Sodium hydroxide, 10-percent solution.
5. 2.5 N hydrochloric acid.
6. 0.1 N sodium hydroxide.

Procedure

To 10 ml. of urine in a test tube is added 0.5 ml. of the 10-percent sodium hydroxide solution. (Reddening of the urine at this time serves as a qualitative test for the presence of myoglobin.) The solution is allowed to stand for 5 minutes, 0.5 ml. of the 2.5 N hydrochloric acid is added dropwise, mixing between each drop, and the solution is allowed to stand for 10 minutes, after which the tube is centrifuged for 10 minutes and the supernatant carefully decanted into another tube to be called the hemoglobin tube. To the residue in the first tube are added 9 ml. of water and 1 ml. of the 0.1 N sodium hydroxide, and this is mixed to effect complete solution of the protein precipitate. This is called the myoglobin tube. The "plasma hemoglobin" test is then made on the contents of both the hemoglobin and myoglobin tubes, using 0.2 ml. of each.

Calculation

mg. of hemoglobin per 100 ml. found in the hemoglobin tube x 11/10 = mg. of hemoglobin in 100 ml. of urine.

mg. of myoglobin per 100 ml. in the myoglobin tube divided by 0.7 = mg. of myoglobin per 100 ml. of urine.

If the urine contains over 100 mg. of benzidine-positive pigments per 100 ml., it is diluted to contain no more than from 50 to 75 mg.; the dilution is accounted for before making the final calculation. If the concentration in the myoglobin tube is low, instead of making the contents of this tube up to 10 ml., the precipitate is dissolved and made up to 2.5 ml. and the resulting calculation is divided by four.

DETERMINATION OF MYOGLOBIN IN TISSUE

The procedure followed for the determination of myoglobin in tissue is essentially the same as that for the determination of myoglobin in urine. The wet tissues are minced, finely ground, and weighed. Two ml. of saline are added for each gram of wet tissue and the mixture is shaken for 30 minutes and allowed to stand overnight. The contents of the tube are then centrifuged and filtered. Two ml. of the filtrate (corresponding to 1 Gm. of tissue) are placed in a tube, 8 ml. of water are added, and from this point the sample is handled as a urine sample.

Calculation

$$\frac{\text{mg. of myoglobin per 100 ml. of diluted extract}}{0.7 \times 10} = \text{Gm. of myoglobin per Kg. of wet tissue.}$$

APPENDIX D

Survey of Case Records

COMPOSITION OF GROUP

The 186 patients studied, the majority of them American infantrymen, were largely battle casualties classified under U. S. Army policy as "wounded in action" (WIA). Wounds were inflicted by gunshot, bullet, shell fragmentation, grenade, mine explosion, and collapse of buildings. In addition, there were two patients seriously injured in truck accidents, one in a plane crash, one in a tent fire, and three who had been accidentally shot or stabbed. Two medical cases were included for comparison of renal lesions. Six patients were civilians wounded during combat, and 13 were wounded German prisoners of war. The term "severely wounded" (nontransportable wounded or injured patients) has been used to designate the entire group because the distinctions between those wounded by direct enemy action, by other agent, or injured accidentally are military ones, and because the causative agent was not a significant factor in any phase of this report.

DEATH RATES

Of the 186 patients studied, 65 died, a case fatality rate of 35 percent. With few exceptions, these deaths all occurred in the forward hospitals. It was impossible in most instances for the Board to follow a case once the patient had left the forward area, so the death rate applies only to the evacuation or field hospital level (field hospital as it operated in the Mediterranean Theater of Operations). The death rate of these seriously wounded was approximately double that of the field hospital average death rate, which included *all* wounded, at the time this study was being made.

Fifty, or nearly 70 percent, of the 73 patients with high azotemia included in the study died, and of these 73 patients, uremia appeared to be the major cause of death in thirty-five. The importance of uremia as a cause of death in the severely wounded is evident when the number dying of this complication is compared with the total number of severely wounded. Of the 35 patients dying of uremia, 32 were battle casualties. Since it was estimated that there were, during the period of this study, between 201 and 252 severely wounded men among the 10,073 battle casualties admitted to forward hospitals in the area where the study was conducted, it is apparent that at least 14 to 17 percent of the severely wounded were dying of uremia.

CLASSIFICATION OF CASE RECORDS

A table in which the cases have been classified so that they may be readily located according to various aspects of the study follows. Cases 10, 46, 59, and 94 were discarded because data were inadequate; hence the omission of these numbers between Cases 1 and 150.

The "A" series (A-1 through A-40) represent a group in which attention was focused primarily on blood-volume data. For these data to have significance, a large number of determinations was needed. Therefore a temporary branch of the Board's activities was established in a field hospital during a period of heavy combat activity in the vicinity. All pertinent data possible were obtained on these patients at the time of their entry to this forward hospital but, with the exception of a few cases and of outcome, no follow-up studies were made by us, and no intake-output records were kept on these cases. Therefore the A series records are, for the most part, very brief. Two patients of this group died.

Résumés of the case records on which the study is based are on file in the Treadwell Library, Massachusetts General Hospital, Boston, Massachusetts.

TABLE 121.—TOTAL CASES CLASSIFIED ACCORDING TO SHOCK ON ADMISSION, MAJOR WOUNDS OR INJURIES, AND OUTCOME

Case No.	Age	Shock on Admission	Major Wound or Injury	Patient's Outcome
1	21	Moderate (*B*)	Soft part with fracture	Lived.
2	22	Moderate (*B*)	Soft part with fracture	Lived.
3	29	None (*B*)	Soft part without fracture	Lived.
4	23	Severe (*B*)	Intra-abdominal; bladder; soft part with fracture.	Died.
5	27	Slight	Soft part without fracture.	Lived.
6	31	Slight (*B*)	Thoracic	Lived.
7	20	None	Soft part without fracture.	Lived.
8	24	Severe	Intra-abdominal; bladder.	Died.
9	25	None	Thoracic (transfusion reaction).	Died.
11	19	Moderate (*B*)	Soft part with fracture	Lived.
12	26	Severe	Intra-abdominal; kidney (nephrectomy done)	Died.
13	19	Moderate (*B*)	Soft part with fractures; intra-abdominal; liver	Lived.
14	22	Severe	Thoraco-abdominal; kidney (nephrectomy done).	Lived.
15	22	Slight (*B*)	Soft part without fracture.	Lived.
16	?	Moderate (*B*)	Soft part with fractures.	Lived.
17	20	None	Soft part with fracture.	Lived.
18	22	Slight	Soft part without fracture.	Lived.
19	?	Moderate	Traumatic amputation of extremity	Died.
20	20	None	Soft part with fracture	Lived.
21	25	None	Ureteral obstruction (disease).	Lived.
22	19	None	Soft part with fractures.	Died.
23	28	None (*B*)	Soft part with fracture	Lived.
24	28	Moderate	Intra-abdominal; liver	Died.
25	19	Severe	Intra-abdominal; liver; kidney (nephrectomy done).	Died.
26	20	Unclassified	Thoraco-abdominal; liver; kidney.	Died.
27	25	Moderate	Thoracic	Lived. (recovery diuresis)
28	21	Moderate	Spinal cord; soft part with fractures.	Lived.

(*B*): Cases that were classified by the Board and that had admission laboratory data.

TABLE 121.—TOTAL CASES CLASSIFIED ACCORDING TO SHOCK ON ADMISSION, MAJOR WOUNDS OR INJURIES, AND OUTCOME—*Continued*

Case No.	Age	Shock on Admission	Major Wound or Injury	Patient's Outcome
29	18	Moderate	Intra-abdominal	Lived.
30	19	Moderate	Intra-abdominal	Lived. (recovery diuresis)
31	?	Moderate	Thoraco-abdominal; spinal cord; liver; kidney (nephrectomy done).	Died.
32	?	Severe	Thoraco-abdominal; intra-abdominal; liver	Died.
33	25	Slight (*B*)	Soft part with fractures	Lived.
34	30	Severe (*B*)	Soft part with fractures	Died.
35	18	Moderate (*B*)	Soft part with fracture	Lived.
36	?	Severe (*B*)	Soft part with fracture	Lived.
37	?	Moderate	Thoracic; liver	Lived.
38	22	Severe	Intra-abdominal (volvulus)	Lived.
39	19	Moderate (*B*)	Soft part with fracture	Lived.
40	40	Severe (*B*)	Traumatic amputation of extremity	Lived.
41	33	Slight	Thoracic	Died.
42	28	Severe	Soft part with fractures	Lived.
43	25	Slight	Intra-abdominal	Lived. (recovery diuresis)
44	19	Moderate	Thoracic	Lived. (recovery diuresis)
45	20	Severe	Intra-abdominal	Died.
47	23	Slight	Soft part with fracture	Died.
48	22	Moderate (*B*)	Soft part without fracture	Died.
49	32	Severe	Intra-abdominal; transection, ureter	Died.
50	23	Moderate (*B*)	Soft part with fracture	Lived.
51	20	Severe	Intra-abdominal	Died.
52	31	Severe	Intra-abdominal	Died.
53	26	Moderate (*B*)	Thoracic	Lived.
54	27	Moderate	Soft part with fractures	Lived.
55	29	Severe	Intra-abdominal; kidney (nephrectomy done)	Died.

TABLE 121.—TOTAL CASES CLASSIFIED ACCORDING TO SHOCK ON ADMISSION, MAJOR WOUNDS OR INJURIES, AND OUTCOME—*Continued*

Case No.	Age	Shock on Admission	Major Wound or Injury	Patient's Outcome
56	25	None (*B*)	Crush	Lived.
57	29	Slight	Soft part with fracture	Lived.
58	28	Moderate (*B*)	Spinal cord	Lived.
60	26	Severe (*B*)	Soft part with fracture	Lived. (recovery diuresis)
61	22	Slight	Thoracic	Lived.
62	20	Slight (*B*)	Intra-abdominal	Lived.
63	26	Moderate	Intra-abdominal	Lived.
64	20	Moderate (*B*)	Intra-abdominal; bladder; soft part with fracture.	Lived.
65	23	Severe	Thoraco-abdominal; liver	Died.
66	20	Severe	Intra-abdominal	Died.
67	26	Severe	Intra-abdominal; urinary tract	Died.
68	36	None	Kidney (disease)	Lived.
69	21	None (*B*)	Crush	Died.
70	25	None	Crush	Died.
71	23	Moderate	Intra-abdominal	Lived.
72	16	Severe (*B*)	Intra-abdominal; kidney	Lived.
73	34	None	Crush	Lived.
74	25	Slight	Burn	Died.
75	?	Slight	Thoracic	Lived.
76	25	Moderate (*B*)	Soft part with fracture	Lived.
77	27	Severe	Thoraco-abdominal; liver	Died.
78	19	Slight (*B*)	Crush	Died.
79	27	Slight (*B*)	Soft part with fractures	Lived.
80	19	Severe	Thoracic; liver	Died.
81	25	Severe (*B*)	Thoracic	Lived.
82	21	Severe	Thoraco-abdominal; liver; kidney (nephrectomy done).	Died.
83	28	Slight (*B*)	Thoraco-abdominal; liver	Lived.
84	30	Slight (*B*)	Soft part with fractures	Lived.

956507 O—52——28

TABLE 121.—TOTAL CASES CLASSIFIED ACCORDING TO SHOCK ON ADMISSION, MAJOR WOUNDS OR INJURIES, AND OUTCOME—*Continued*

Case No.	Age	Shock on Admission	Major Wound or Injury	Patient's Outcome
85	38	Severe	Thoracic	Died.
86	29	Severe	Soft part with fractures	Died.
87	?	Severe (*B*)	Soft part with fractures	Lived.
88	25	Severe	Intra-abdominal; kidney (nephrectomy done)	Died.
89	24	Severe (*B*)	Traumatic amputation of extremity	Lived.
90	34	Moderate (*B*)	Thoraco-abdominal; liver; kidney (nephrectomy done).	Lived.
91	27	None (*B*)	Soft part with fracture	Lived.
92	29	Slight	Soft part with fracture	Died.
93	32	Severe (*B*)	Crush	Died.
95	28	Severe	Intra-abdominal	Died.
96	27	None	Soft part with fracture	Lived.
97	27	Severe	Intra-abdominal	Died.
98	20	Moderate	Intra-abdominal; bladder	Died.
99	23	None (*B*)	Crush	Lived.
100	24	Severe (*B*)	Soft part with fractures	Died.
101	20	Moderate	Intra-abdominal	Lived.
102	32	None (*B*)	Intra-abdominal	Died.
103	35	Unclassified	Soft part with fractures	Lived.
104	32	Moderate	Intra-abdominal; bladder	Lived. (recovery diuresis)
105	34	Severe	Intra-abdominal	Died.
106	21	None (*B*)	Soft part without fracture	Lived.
107	?	Moderate (*B*)	Intra-abdominal	Died.
108	27	Severe (*B*)	Soft part with fracture	Died.
109	29	None (*B*)	Intra-abdominal; liver	Lived.
110	35	Severe (*B*)	Soft part with fracture	Lived.
111	35	Slight (*B*)	Intra-abdominal	Lived.
112	21	Severe (*B*)	Traumatic amputation of extremity	Lived.

Table 121.—Total Cases Classified according to Shock on Admission, Major Wounds or Injuries, and Outcome—*Continued*

Case No.	Age	Shock on Admission	Major Wound or Injury	Patient's Outcome
113	23	Slight (*B*)	Thoracic	Lived.
114	35	Moderate	Traumatic amputation of extremity	Died.
115	24	Moderate	Intra-abdominal; liver	Died.
116	20	Moderate	Thoraco-abdominal; kidney	Died.
117	25	Moderate	Intra-abdominal; liver	Died.
118	18	Severe	Thoracic	Died.
119	31	Severe	Thoraco-abdominal.	Died.
120	23	None	Soft part without fracture	Died.
121	20	Severe	Thoraco-abdominal; liver	Died.
122	22	Severe (*B*)	Thoraco-abdominal; kidney (nephrectomy done)	Died.
123	19	Severe	Traumatic amputation of extremity; thoracic.	Died.
124	23	None (*B*)	Crush.	Lived.
125	34	Severe (*B*)	Soft part with fractures; thoracic.	Lived. (recovery diuresis)
126	23	Moderate (*B*)	Thoraco-abdominal; liver; kidney.	Died.
127	32	Slight (*B*)	Soft part with fractures	Lived.
128	21	Slight (*B*)	Soft part without fracture	Lived.
129	20	Moderate (*B*)	Soft part with fractures; kidney	Died.
130	27	Severe (*B*)	Soft part with fractures	Lived.
131	27	Severe (*B*)	Intra-abdominal; thoracic	Died.
132	22	None	Crush.	Died.
133	26	Severe	Intra-abdominal	Lived. (recovery diuresis)
134	33	None (*B*)	Intra-abdominal	Lived.
135	21	Severe	Intra-abdominal; liver	Died.
136	22	Moderate	Thoraco-abdominal; kidney	Died.
137	22	None	Soft part without fracture	Lived.
138	32	None	Thoracic	Lived. (recovery diuresis)
139	26	Severe (*B*)	Thoracic; soft part with fractures	Lived.

TABLE 121.—TOTAL CASES CLASSIFIED ACCORDING TO SHOCK ON ADMISSION, MAJOR WOUNDS OR INJURIES, AND OUTCOME—*Continued*

Case No.	Age	Shock on Admission	Major Wound or Injury	Patient's Outcome
140	23	Slight (*B*)	Intra-abdominal	Lived.
141	19	Slight (*B*)	Thoraco-abdominal; liver	Lived.
142	24	Moderate (*B*)	Thoracic	Lived.
143	28	Moderate (*B*)	Thoraco-abdominal; liver	Died.
144	32	Slight (*B*)	Soft part with fractures	Lived.
145	41	Slight (*B*)	Soft part with fractures; thoracic.	Lived.
146	39	Severe	Thoraco-abdominal; liver; kidney (nephrectomy done).	Died.
147	23	Severe (*B*)	Intra-abdominal	Died.
148	25	Moderate (*B*)	Traumatic amputation, both extremities.	Lived.
149	26	Severe (*B*)	Intra-abdominal; bladder	Died.
150	27	Moderate	Thoraco-abdominal	Lived. (recovery diuresis)
A–1	23	Slight (*B*)	Thoracic	Lived.
A–2	21	Slight (*B*)	Intra-abdominal	Lived.
A–3	25	Moderate (*B*)	Intra-abdominal; kidney (nephrectomy done)	Lived.
A–4	37	None (*B*)	Soft part without fracture	Lived.
A–5	17	Slight (*B*)	Traumatic amputation of extremity	Lived.
A–6	22	Moderate (*B*)	Intra-abdominal; liver	Lived.
A–7	30	Unclassified (*B*)	Head injury	Lived.
A–8	31	Slight (*B*)	Soft part without fracture	Lived.
A–9	18	Moderate (*B*)	Thoracic	Lived.
A–10	24	Slight (*B*)	Soft part without fracture	Lived.

TABLE 121.—TOTAL CASES CLASSIFIED ACCORDING TO SHOCK ON ADMISSION, MAJOR WOUNDS OR INJURIES, AND OUTCOME—*Continued*

Case No.	Age	Shock on Admission	Major Wound or Injury	Patient's Outcome
A-11	?	Slight (*B*)	Thoracic	Lived.
A-12	22	Moderate (*B*)	Thoracic	Lived.
A-13	21	None (*B*)	Traumatic amputation of extremity	Lived.
A-14	22	Moderate (*B*)	Thoracic	Lived.
A-15	21	Moderate (*B*)	Soft part with fracture	Lived.
A-16	23	None (*B*)	Thoraco-abdominal; liver; kidney	Lived.
A-17	21	Slight (*B*)	Traumatic amputation, extremity; intra-abdominal.	Lived.
A-18	35	Moderate (*B*)	Traumatic amputation of extremity; soft part with fracture.	Lived.
A-19	26	None (*B*)	Soft part with fracture	Lived.
A-20	29	Slight (*B*)	Traumatic amputation of extremity	Lived.
A-21	21	Severe (*B*)	Soft part with fractures	Lived.
A-22	21	None (*B*)	Intra-abdominal; liver; kidney	Lived.
A-23	18	None (*B*)	Soft part without fracture	Lived.
A-24	19	None (*B*)	Intra-abdominal	Lived.
A-25	23	Slight (*B*)	Soft part with fracture	Lived.
A-26	32	Slight (*B*)	Thoracic	Lived.
A-27	25	None (*B*)	Intra-abdominal	Lived.
A-28	20	Severe (*B*)	Soft part with fractures	Lived.
A-29	20	Severe (*B*)	Soft part without fracture	Lived.
A-30	24	Moderate (*B*)	Soft part with fracture	Died.
A-31	20	Moderate (*B*)	Thoracic	Lived.
A-32	19	Moderate (*B*)	Thoracic	Lived.

TABLE 121.—TOTAL CASES CLASSIFIED ACCORDING TO SHOCK ON ADMISSION, MAJOR WOUNDS OR INJURIES, AND OUTCOME—*Continued*

Case No.	Age	Shock on Admission	Major Wound or Injury	Patient's Outcome
A-33	19	Moderate (*B*)	Traumatic amputation of extremity	Lived.
A-34	31	Severe (*B*)	Soft part with fractures	Lived.
A-35	25	Moderate (*B*)	Soft part with fractures	Lived.
A-36	21	Moderate (*B*)	Soft part without fracture	Died.
A-37	19	Moderate (*B*)	Soft part with fracture	Lived.
A-38	19	Severe (*B*)	Soft part with fracture	Lived.
A-39	19	None (*B*)	Thoracic	Lived.
A-40	25	Slight (*B*)	Thoraco-abdominal; kidney	Lived.

Index

U. S. GOVERNMENT PRINTING OFFICE: 1952—956507